MEDICAL TRANSITIONS IN TWENTIETH-CENTURY CHINA

MEDICAL TRANSITIONS
IN TWENTIETH-CENTURY CHINA

Edited by Bridie Andrews
and Mary Brown Bullock

Indiana University Press

Bloomington & Indianapolis

This book is a publication of

Indiana University Press
Office of Scholarly Publishing
Herman B Wells Library 350
1320 East 10th Street
Bloomington, Indiana 47405 USA

iupress.indiana.edu

Telephone orders   800-842-6796
Fax orders   812-855-7931

Library of Congress Cataloging-in-Publication Data

Medical transitions in twentieth-century China / edited
by Bridie Andrews and Mary Brown Bullock.
   p. ; cm.
   Includes bibliographical references and index.
   ISBN 978-0-253-01485-6 (cloth : alk. paper) — ISBN 978-0-253-
01490-0 (pbk. : alk. paper) — ISBN 978-0-253-01494-8 (ebook)
   I. Andrews, Bridie, editor. II. Bullock, Mary Brown, editor.
   [DNLM: 1. History of Medicine—China. 2. History,
20th Century—China. 3. Public Health—history—China.
4. Public Health—trends—China. WZ 70 JC6]
   R601
   610.951—dc23

                                                2014 011883

1 2 3 4 5   19 18 17 16 15 14

Contents

Preface

THIS VOLUME IS one of several projects which celebrate the centenary of the China Medical Board (CMB). Our aim is to provide a broad overview of the history of medicine in China rather than a narrow institutional history of the CMB, but readers may find it helpful to have a summary of the mission and history of the CMB here.

The CMB's work began in 1914 when it was created by the Rockefeller Foundation to manage philanthropic funding for the Peking Union Medical College (PUMC), "the cradle of modern medicine in China." In the first half of the twentieth century, most of the CMB's resources went toward the construction and development of PUMC, which was the largest investment project in Rockefeller Foundation history. In 1928, the CMB was endowed as an independent American foundation for the continuing support of PUMC. Through war and chaos, PUMC not only endured but flourished. Its faculty and graduates founded many key clinical specialties in China and developed innovations such as a three-tiered rural health system. The CMB continued to work in China after the establishment of the People's Republic of China in 1949, but two years later, in 1951, the Chinese government nationalized PUMC, ending the decades-long relationship.

Starting in the 1950s, the CMB expanded its capacity-building work into other Asian countries: Japan, Korea, Hong Kong, the Philippines, Thailand, Indonesia, Malaysia, Singapore, and Taiwan. Today, the CMB remains active in mainland Southeast Asia, supporting universities to strengthen education and research in medicine, nursing, and public health.

In 1980, the CMB accepted an invitation to return to China and has since expanded its support of medical education and research to more than a dozen medical universities. From 1980 to 2008, the CMB invested strategically in medical research and education. In medical education, it developed the Global Minimum Essential Requirements (GMER), seeded innovations, and established four centers at Central South University, China Medical University, Sichuan University, and PUMC.

In 2008, the CMB launched a fresh initiative to strengthen scientific excellence in "critical capacities" among Chinese and Asian institutions in order to promote equitable access to primary and preventive health services. This initiative refocused the CMB's efforts on advancing the field of health policy and systems sciences (HPSS), building capacity in health professional education, and directing resources to rural health.

Conventions

For consistency, all our authors are listed by given name followed by family name. Chinese names within the chapters have been given in the Chinese style, family name first, using pinyin romanization. For the Republican era (1912–1949), it has been necessary to make some exceptions to this rule. Before the pinyin system was designed in the 1950s, many Chinese published in English using other romanizations (for example, Jin Baoshan, who published as P. Z. King; and Wu Liande, who published as Wu Lien-teh). In these cases, we have attempted to provide all versions (Chinese, modern pinyin, and the author's preferred romanization) on first usage. When citing publications written in Chinese, we have indexed names according to pinyin. When citing publications written in English, we have used the authors' preferred rendering of their names and supplied the pinyin versions in parentheses following those names in the Chinese-language section of the bibliography. For institutions and publications during the Republican era, we have rendered Chinese using traditional (unsimplified) characters; for the People's Republic of China we have used simplified characters.

Acknowledgments

THIS VOLUME HAS been a couple of years in the making, with input and assistance from many quarters, which we are happy to acknowledge here.

Lincoln Chen first conceived of a series of history volumes to mark the 2014 centenary of the China Medical Board, of which he is president, and provided the resources and enthusiasm that have made it possible. We owe the existence of the volume and the wonderful intellectual exchanges it has generated to his vision. Emma Rothschild helped shape the project and brought the leadership and editorial personnel together over some wonderful dinners, and William Summers, Paul Cohen, and Charles Rosenberg provided essential scholarly orientation during the planning phase.

Our papers got their first readings at a conference held at MIT's Endicott House with the help of Camilla Harris and Betty DaSilva. Logistical and translation assistance was provided by Bentley University graduate students Angie Mengxi Luo, Wei Wang, Lily Guan, and Ying Zheng, and the complexities of U.S. visa and tax requirements were ably handled by Maria Bergmann, James Fuerst, Donna DeIulio, and Donna McKnight at Bentley. We were saddened that illness prevented one of our attendees, Professor Hu Cheng of Nanjing University, from continuing with the project but would nonetheless like to express our appreciation for his contribution here.

In Beijing, CMB staff Echo Zong, Mariel Reed, Roman Xu, and Linda Zhou were gracious hosts, as were Peking Union Medical College staff members Yuhong Jiang and Zhang Xia. Susan Gatewood made sure that everyone arrived safely.

During the editing process, we were fortunate to have the translating expertise of Sabine Wilms and the English editing of Michelle Renshaw. The process of romanizing Russian names correctly was made easy with the kind assistance of Leonid Trofimov, historian of Russia at Bentley. The difficult task of creating a uniform style and bibliography was achieved with great skill and good humor by Rebecca Scofield and Mary Augusta Brazelton. At the CMB Cambridge office, Jennifer Ryan's editorial professionalism and encouragement was essential to the management of our multiple agendas and deadlines. She was ably assisted by Joshua Bocher. CMB staff Shenique Bennett, Sally Paquet, and Sarah Wood provided essential administrative support.

At Indiana University Press, our project editor Michelle Sybert and copyeditor Eric Levy were expert and conscientious guides through the publishing process, providing consistency and attention to detail that are rare and precious in today's publishing world. Thank you.

MEDICAL TRANSITIONS IN TWENTIETH-CENTURY CHINA

Introduction

Mary Brown Bullock and Bridie Andrews

THE MODERN HISTORY of medicine and public health in China is dramatic and complex. Transnational forces propelled medical ideas and practice both within and between East and West. Health concerns moved from an intimate, relatively private personal realm to a concern of the state which imposed often draconian regulations but also introduced state responsibility for health care. The efficacy of newly discovered vaccinations, sulfa drugs, and antibiotics contributed to the epidemiologic transition from infectious to chronic diseases as the main threats to health, while simultaneously transforming Chinese perceptions of Western medicine. The technological discoveries that advanced an understanding of disease causation and sometimes cure led, as the century progressed, to costly technological innovations that greatly escalated the costs of medical care. The emerging new medical institutions and professions were challenged by domestic political and economic forces, including several wars and revolutions. Having weathered those challenges today, China's health care system, like many worldwide, faces challenges of quality, costs, and unequal care across populations.

Nonetheless, China is no longer "the sick man of Asia." A hybrid system of modern medicine which includes traditional Chinese medicine and the most advanced Western medicine is well established. Chinese life expectancy rates doubled in the twentieth century, and today approaches those of the most advanced economies. Infectious diseases, often associated with poverty and poor living conditions, have declined dramatically even as some persist, often in virulent forms. Chinese medicine is one of China's most successful cultural exports and China is a significant provider of health assistance to Africa.

The work collected here is published on the occasion of the centennial of the China Medical Board, which was established by the Rockefeller Foundation in 1914 to create and manage the Peking Union Medical College (PUMC), which in turn quickly became the preeminent medical education and research institution in China. When PUMC was closed in 1951 the China Medical Board extended its work to medical schools in other parts of East and Southeast Asia. Since 1980, the CMB has returned to China, supporting thirteen medical schools and initiating programs in health policy and rural health. Although several of the chapters refer to the activities of the CMB, this volume is not intended as an encomium to Rockefeller medical philanthropy. Indeed, our authors were charged with *not* paying special attention to the activities of the China Medical Board. As Lincoln Chen—current president of the CMB—and Ling Chen argue in their chapter, the greatest improvements in population health and longevity occurred during the Maoist era, after U.S. agencies were expelled by the Chinese Communist Party in 1952. Nonetheless, our study of a century of medical history in China, focusing on the activities of medical professionals (doctors, nurses, midwives, health advisors) and on disease management, reveals that many of the CMB-trained professionals were key to the construction of the health care system both before and after the establishment of the People's Republic of China. Indeed there is much evidence in this volume that the medical institutions, research, and health care programs of the Republican period, many of which were funded by the Rockefeller Foundation and the China Medical Board, were key to the later advances made by the People's Republic of China. As Chinese society has opened up to market economics since the 1980s, and the "iron rice bowl" of government welfare has disappeared, problems of refractory infectious diseases and unequal access to health care have reemerged. It is striking to note how similar today's proposed solutions are to those proposed in the 1930s by delegates from the League of Nations Health Organization and the CMB.

The voices of patients are never far from the surface, and they are often critical of the schemes of government. For example, in Daqing Zhang's chapter we hear of vaccination programs with low acceptance rates. We also observe in Xinzhong Yu's chapter that because of Communist Party authoritarianism in the past, today's Chinese citizens are no longer willing to cooperate with government-led mass movements in health. We see this confirmed in Miriam Gross and Kawai Fan's chapter on schistosomiasis: patients were happy to accept the Praziquantel drug treatments when they became available, but were reluctant to engage in (largely futile) snail eradication efforts. The mistrust the public now has for mass health movements may be what is driving the enthusiasm for U.S.-style health insurance schemes today, with their health savings accounts which, while inadequate for dealing with major individual health crises, do have the virtue of remaining in the control of individual patients.

Western medical missionaries, key to any understanding of how modern medicine was transmitted to China, deserve a volume of their own. They feature here as instigators of many modern health initiatives: they brought a model of health care that was firmly rooted in the specialist institution of the hospital, as we see in Michelle Renshaw's chapter; and they attempted to medicalize the treatment of the mentally ill, starting with John Kerr's Refuge for the Insane in late nineteenth-century Canton, described here by Veronica Pearson. Sonya Grypma and Cheng Zhen describe how missionaries set up nursing education programs and Tina Phillips Johnson and Yi-Li Wu describe missionary-run medical schools for women, both of which created new roles for Chinese women in public life. Missionaries translated the first Western medical texts for use by Chinese students, and we should not forget that in rural areas, many farmers' only experience of Western medicine before 1949 came from mission clinics, as missionaries would go to practice in impoverished areas when the newly qualified Chinese medical elites would not.

The economics of health care feature in several of our chapters, most notably in Xiaoping Fang's chapter on the barefoot doctor movement, Xi Gao's account of the reasons China adapted different foreign models of health care, and Volker Scheid and Sean Hsiang-lin Lei's account of the institutionalization of Chinese medicine. In recent years the rising cost of health care and increasing income disparities between urban and rural areas have recreated a crisis in access to health care in China. The government is attempting to ameliorate these disparities through a series of reforms that health economists, health policy advocates, and scholars of medical history are watching closely. The very great economic as well as technical challenges involved in extending medical provision are demonstrated in almost all of our chapters, perhaps in none more than Veronica Pearson's overview of the development of mental health services.

No single volume can possibly provide a comprehensive record of these developments. The history of medicine and health has become an important endeavor of scholars worldwide, precisely because it operates at this nexus of governmental power and local and individual agency, with important things to say about culture and ideology as well as access to economic resources. With its long historic records and complex evolution this is especially the case with medicine and health in China. Drawing on scholarship from China, Australia, Taiwan, Germany, Canada, and the United States, this book presents, for the first time, an overview of medical transitions in the twentieth century. Drawing on scholarship from Australia, Canada, China, Hong Kong, Singapore, Taiwan, the United Kingdom, and the United States, this book presents, for the first time, an overview of medical transitions in the twentieth century. Of particular note are chapters by four scholars—Daqing Zhang, Xinzhong Yu, Xi Gao, and Cheng Zhen—who usually write for a Chinese audience. Several chapters notably include the roles of both Chinese medicine and traditional-style doctors. Our study also highlights how new drugs and vaccinations depended on both individual and state-led efforts for their therapeutic successes.

The factors influencing medicine are many, and include social, political, and economic conditions as well as new understandings of hygiene and science. Geographical proximity to medical care, most often differentiated by urban or rural location, is also of the utmost importance. All of these were in flux in twentieth-century China. Likewise, changes in the delivery of health care from the home to the hospital, from laypersons to specialists, brought marked changes to the ways in which illness is treated and health maintained. In this book these medical transitions are discussed in four sections: health transitions, disease transitions, adaptations and innovations, and professional transitions.

Health Transitions

Historians and political scientists have tended to view China's twentieth century as segmented between the late Qing, the Republican, and the People's Republic eras. In different ways the chapters in this section demonstrate how transitions in health care occur continuously across the century, sometimes, but not always, marked by political change. Other factors, notably scientific advances in medical therapies and changes in economic and social systems, contribute to dramatic health changes. Beginning with an overview of China's mortality and demographic changes, we turn to three specific examples of these macro-level changes across the century: the health transitions in the city of Beijing, in the maternal and child health sector, and in tobacco and smoking usage.

Lincoln Chen and Ling Chen's chapter, "China's Exceptional Health Transitions," sets the theoretical stage for this section, and the statistical stage for the entire book, as it explores the major causes of mortality and demographic change across twentieth-century China. The transitions examined are the epidemiologic, demographic, and health transitions. The *epidemiologic transition* occurs as populations progress from higher to lower mortality levels associated with rising incomes and improving health systems. Whereas poverty-linked diseases such as childhood infections, malnutrition, and maternity-linked burdens characterize low-income societies, the noncommunicable chronic diseases like cancer and heart disease dominate in higher-income countries. *Demographic transition* theory captures changes of fertility and mortality from high to low levels. The time gap between an earlier reduction of mortality and the later decline of fertility generates a gap between birth and death rates that accelerates population growth. In addition to rates of growth, demographic change may also affect the spatial distribution, age structure, and other parameters of human populations. These two theories of transition are brought together in the theory of the *health transition*, which integrates not only epidemiologic and demographic parameters but also changes in sociocultural perceptions, health-seeking behavior, and the structure and operations of health systems. This chapter uses health transition theory as an interdisciplinary framework to outline the multiple dimensions of changes related to the health of the population of twentieth-century China.

From this macro-overview we turn to health transitions in a specific place, the city of Beijing, analyzed by Daqing Zhang. This longitudinal study discusses how the social and political environment in modern China has undergone dramatic changes from periods of continuous warfare to political chaos to peace. From the foundation of the Republic of China in 1912 to the mid-1930s, the new national medical administration system had to be restructured several times in accordance with the changing political environment. Despite these changes, the causes of disease mortality transitioned from infectious diseases to chronic and degenerative conditions.

Another way to examine health transitions is through the status of maternal and child health, a universal indicator of a nation's health. Certainly the welfare of childbearing women and children has been a prominent concern in Chinese culture from ancient times to the present. Many older, indigenous practices are still relevant in maternal and child care practices today. At the same time, the social context and intellectual content of medicine in China has changed significantly as a result of the Chinese pursuit of modernization beginning in the late nineteenth century. Tina Phillips Johnson and Yi-Li Wu trace this evolution in their chapter on maternal and child health, observing that whereas maternal and child health was a family-directed, household-centered issue during the Qing, under both the Republican and Communist regimes it became a crucial ideological component of state building, modernization, and economic growth. As a result of both individual and state initiatives, the past century has witnessed dramatic drops in maternal and child mortality. Economic reforms since 1978 have also vastly increased the resources potentially available for maternal and child health. But as China attempts to achieve a standard of health care consistent with its level of economic development, it will also have to negotiate systemic problems engendered by the very policies that have driven its breathtaking economic growth. These include particularly the policies that removed state subsidies from hospitals and made them profit centers.

The final chapter in this section is Carol Benedict's "Tobacco Smoking and Health." This chapter traces changing ideas about tobacco and health in China across the twentieth century, beginning with new medical discourses about tobacco that were constructed early in the century in dialogue with the transnational anti-cigarette movement centered in Great Britain and the United States. It explores popular views of tobacco's harms in the 1930s "literature of leisure" and advice columns of women's magazines. The chapter also describes changing patterns of tobacco consumption across the twentieth century that had implications for health and concludes with a brief history of recent tobacco control efforts in the People's Republic of China.

Disease Transitions

Changes in global disease patterns during the twentieth century were dramatic, in part due to scientific discoveries which brought more effective prevention and treatment as well as economic improvements in many people's lives. While the diseases discussed in this section have been universally prevalent, they are selected here because their trajectory in China has been distinct. Writing from the discipline of history, the authors illustrate how the convergence of political, cultural, ideological, and scientific forces can dramatically influence the course of diseases. Three of the four chapters focus on infectious diseases because these were responsible for the highest mortality rates for the first two-thirds of the century. Today, noncommunicable diseases (cancer, heart disease, and diabetes) claim more lives and they are well-covered in medical journals and most recently in a series of articles in the *Lancet*. Mental health, however, is now considered China's number one medical problem. Here, as in other chapters in this section, Chinese culture and political ideology have dramatically affected the course and treatment of mental health–related diseases.

The first chapter on disease patterns, Xinzhong Yu's "Epidemics and Public Health in Twentieth-Century China: Plague, Smallpox, and AIDS" reminds us that the century began and ended with virulent epidemics, even as vaccinations rendered smallpox obsolete. The twentieth century demonstrated what William McNeill termed a homogenization of disease, facilitated by new forms of more rapid transportation, the imposition of Western institutions with their circulation of personnel and their diseases, and the increasingly hegemonic role of biomedicine in identifying and controlling infectious diseases. Yu argues that although public health measures were developed primarily to control disease, they were also undertaken to reinforce the power and legitimacy of the state under the Qing, the Republican, and the People's Republic of China governments.

Schistosomiasis, a water-borne and snail-transmitted disease, has a storied political history, well illustrating the intersection of politics and medicine in China. Chairman Mao's historic campaign against schistosomiasis is widely considered by the Chinese government and most Chinese people as one of their most successful and well-run health crusades. It became a symbol of the Communist Party's care for the people, brought international attention to the Chinese public health model, and still serves as an important model for current campaigns against SARS, avian and swine flu, and AIDS. Since the construction of the Three Gorges Dam, schistosomiasis has garnered increasing notice as a critical public health issue in contemporary China, and the disease has been growing at epidemic rates since 2001. Miriam Gross and Kawai Fan's chapter on schistosomiasis examines the history of the disease and the Chinese government's campaign to eradicate it against the political background that made treatment of Chinese troops a strategic priority, and encouraged Mao to encourage the anti-schistosomiasis campaign as a model mass movement.

Rachel Core's chapter, "Tuberculosis Control in Shanghai: Bringing Health to the Masses, 1928–Present," turns to one of the most deadly diseases in early twentieth-century China. Throughout the century biomedical discoveries combined with political and socioeconomic forces to modify TB control efforts worldwide; however, given China's massive population, developing a system to bring scientific advances to the wide population presented a special challenge. In Shanghai, the speed of the city's urbanization, and the resulting size and heterogeneity of the population, amplified these challenges. This chapter examines a century of efforts to connect the population to the health and public health system in order to control TB in China's largest city. The chapter is divided chronologically into three sections, each of which coincides with larger socioeconomic developments. The first section examines limited success in bringing primary and tertiary TB prevention to affected individuals during the period 1914–1949. The second section considers widespread efforts to bring the disease under control after the 1949 Communist Revolution. During the height of the Socialist era, 1958–1978, TB control programs became systematized, with district prevention and treatment stations overseeing efforts within individual workplaces. The relationship between district stations and individual workplaces, which provided an effective link ensuring that scientific advances could reach the masses, continued through the 1980s. In the 1990s, China adopted the World Health Organization's Directly Observed Therapy, Short-Course (DOTS) TB control program at the same time that the workplace-based urban health insurance system began to collapse. The final section discusses the ongoing challenges of bringing TB control to the masses in an era of wide-scale in-migration.

Today China views mental health as one of its most significant health issues. Veronica Pearson's chapter reviews the history of attempts to provide humane health care for the mentally ill. She outlines the many obstacles that stand in the way, perhaps most seriously the stigma that is still associated with mental illness. By the 1950s, the study of such "bourgeois" subjects as sociology and psychology had been banned in Chinese universities, precluding any study of the particular sociocultural aspects of mental health in China. Yet, ironically, the centralized education and job assignment system of the Mao years meant that mental hospitals were assigned medical staff, even if the staff members themselves were often reluctant. Now that students may choose their own specialties and apply for their own jobs, it has become even harder to find and train mental health professionals. The chapter ends on a hopeful note, documenting the government's new initiatives to reform mental health care both in the community and in institutional settings.

Adaptations and Innovation

The twentieth century was an era of three revolutions (Nationalist, Communist, and Cultural) and four wars (World War I, the Sino-Japanese War, the Civil War, and the Korean War). Across this turbulent period there were significant adaptations and innovations in China's medical theory, practice, and professions. During the first half of the century foreign spheres of influence included medicine and public health. For much of the second half of the century more indigenous forces adapted foreign models and modified traditional models to shape new China's medical system. The first chapter in this section views adaptation and innovation from the perspective of foreign medical systems. It differentiates among the German, British, American, and Japanese influences in the first half of the century and also includes a critique of Soviet influence during the first decade of the People's Republic of China. The second two chapters cover the less well-known but formative evolution of public health during the Republican period. Both chapters argue that well-trained professionals worked with the Nationalist government and regional provincial governments to improve the health conditions of the Chinese people. Although the health statistics from the 1920s to the 1940s reveal little change (see figure 1.1), the dramatic progress in the 1950s was due in no small measure to the institutions, health models, and professional experience gained in these earlier decades. The most significant adaptation of the twentieth century was surely that of traditional Chinese medicine. New perspectives on the institutions and popular practice of traditional medicine are transforming our knowledge of the extraordinary evolution of this classical medical tradition. The last two chapters in this section, one on the institutionalization of Chinese medicine and the other on barefoot doctors as transmitters of both traditional and Western medicine, illustrate these newer findings and interpretations.

Xi Gao's chapter, "Foreign Models of Medicine in Twentieth-Century China," describes how the adaptation of modern medicine in China drew on several national styles, most notably Anglo-American missionary and secular models, German-Japanese-style state medicine, and the socialist model developed in the Soviet Union. This chapter examines each of these influences and discusses the ways in which elements of each were adapted for use in China. Different models have waxed and waned in influence, and the reasons for this and for regional variations in medical styles are explored. Broadly speaking, during the first half of the twentieth century Anglo-American influence was most strongly felt in the south of China, but Chinese distrust of foreign motives and paternalism led Canton to lead the way in establishing independent medical schools and an urban public health infrastructure based on this model. In northern China and especially Manchuria, German-inspired Japanese-style medicine was more frequently studied and emulated. In the Communist-held areas and in the first few years of the PRC, the Soviet influence was most closely followed, while market reforms and the opening to the West have expanded the medical marketplace in recent years. China (like the United States) has still to settle on a satisfactory health care delivery system that can meet national development goals and provide basic medical care while at the same time fostering excellence and innovation in medicine.

John B. Grant (1890–1962) has been praised as the "spirit of public health" for modern China. Liping Bu's chapter, "John B. Grant: Public Health and State Medicine," focuses on three interrelated aspects of Grant's work that had long-term implications for China's public health profession and health care system. First, the development of the Department of Public Health at PUMC to train public health professionals; second, the creation of health stations in rural and urban settings as experiments of pilot projects to study health conditions and deliver health services; and third, Grant's assisting the Chinese government in establishing a modern national health administration with state medicine. For Grant, the first priority in the establishment of state medicine was to train high-caliber personnel, which he implemented both at PUMC and in the fieldwork settings of his innovative health stations. Second, as Grant wrote, "the most important would be the establishment of a centralized medical authority with power to execute the adopted policy on a nation-wide scale" (1928, 79). Grant's promotion of state medicine set in motion an extensive debate in China. Many Chinese medical leaders supported state medicine but they seemed to understand the concept differently. Some focused on health service to all—rich or poor, rural or urban—while others emphasized the importance of a centralized health administration. This chapter explores these debates and their long-term consequences through Grant's activities in China and the careers of his students.

In their chapter titled "The Influence of War on China's Modern Health Systems," Nicole Barnes and John Watt come to the counterintuitive conclusion that this war, by causing so much human suffering, greatly stimulated the development of public health care in Nationalist China. Public health organizations developed in the war years were stronger in western than in eastern China, dependent on visionary leadership, opposed by conservative leaders particularly in the military, deprived for much of the time of essential resources, and subject to enemy destruction. The chapter's focus on medical institutions in Chongqing vividly demonstrates the progress that was made under wartime conditions. The medical organizations developed new systems of management in both urban and rural settings, and trained thousands of individuals in hygiene, sanitation, and preventive medicine. This body of trained health care leaders and workers was one of Nationalist China's lasting contributions to postwar China.

Volker Scheid and Sean Hsiang-lin Lei's chapter on the institutionalization of Chinese medicine argues that the process that led to the creation of a pluralistic combination of Western and Chinese medicine was neither linear nor the outcome of a well-thought-out master plan. Rather, it was the product of an underdetermined and piecemeal process that owed more to a careful manipulation of Chinese medicine's value as a cultural legacy than to any consideration of its actual therapeutic value. The emergence of plural health care in contemporary China thus might be said to mirror the tortuous, painful, and frequently contradictory path the country itself has taken into the present. It is important to remember that the Communist victory in the Civil War of 1945–1949 and the proclamation of the People's Republic in October 1949 did not augur well for the future of Chinese medicine as an independent medical tradition. Under the slogan "cooperation of Chinese and Western medicine" (*zhongxiyi hezuo*) the Communist Party (CCP) in Yan'an had utilized Chinese medicine to gain the support of the rural population and to meet health care needs in settings where Western drugs and technological resources were scarce. Ideologically, however, the party's leadership was committed to establishing a health care system modeled on the West, in particular Russia, in which there was little room for a medicine considered to be a remnant of feudal society and its irrational superstitions. In Nationalist-controlled areas, meanwhile, the Chinese medical infrastructure created during the 1920s and '30s was all but dismantled. And yet, less than ten years later a large-scale effort was underway to rebuild Chinese medicine as a modern tradition that would make a unique contribution to the health care of China and even the world. Another quarter of a century later, in 1982, the principle of "paying equal attention to Chinese and Western medicine" was enshrined in the Constitution. Ever since, the country has enjoyed the fruits and problems of an officially plural health care system.

Xiaoping Fang's "Barefoot Doctors and the Provision of Rural Health Care" makes the unexpected claim that barefoot doctors played a pivotal role in introducing Western medicine and displacing Chinese medicine in rural China. The barefoot doctor program was one of a series of landmark events in the long-term historical development of rural health and medicine in China since the early twentieth century, alongside the initiation of the experimental rural health programs in the 1930s, the founding of the Communist regime in 1949, the popularization of the barefoot doctor program in 1968, the disintegration of the barefoot doctor group around 1983, and the recent rural medical reforms. The essence of this developmental trend remained the same: the introduction of Western medicine (i.e., modern medicine) in terms of its institutionalization, the development of new professional roles, and the promotion of science. The barefoot doctor program, which lasted from 1968 to 1983, was a pivotal stage in the displacement of Chinese medicine by Western medicine in rural China. During this process, the state played a significant role by mobilizing private medical practitioners into establishing union clinics, implementing the barefoot doctor program, mandating large reductions in pharmaceutical prices, creating a new hierarchical and coordinated medical system, and redefining medical legitimacy. Within this context, Western medicine was introduced into Chinese villages under socialism within just three decades. The significance of the barefoot doctors lies in their role in the contest between Chinese and Western medicine in the village arena, the evolution of the three-tier medical system, and the formation of a new professional group. Entering the twenty-first century, the state still plays the leading role in the transformation of rural medicine through the recent medical reforms.

Professional Transitions

The relationships between doctors, patients, and the state went through several dramatic changes in the course of the twentieth century. Until the Nanjing decade, there was almost no licensing of physicians: anyone could practice as a doctor. To distinguish themselves from traditional doctors and self-taught or only partially trained practitioners of modern medicine, Chinese doctors with biomedical degrees organized themselves into professional organizations starting in 1915. During the 1930s, these associations merged in order to be able to negotiate with one voice with the Nationalist Government. The profession fought hard to gain and protect its privileges as the only legitimate representative of modern medical practitioners, but it was always in competition with less qualified practitioners who were never effectively banned. In 1949, the Ministry of Health regulated medical practice, including the work of medical doctors (MDs), middle- and lower-level health workers, and Chinese medical practitioners. The modern nursing profession was dramatically downgraded. Although biomedicine was never able to achieve a monopoly on medical practice, the presence of many highly educated doctors in powerful positions in the Ministry of Health provided a buffer between medicine and some of the worst political excesses of the 1950s and 1960s. The prestige of doctors was highest during the 1980s, but decollectivization has required hospitals to become economically self-supporting, leading to a fee-for-service environment in which many patients suspect that they are being charged for unnecessary but expensive tests, drugs, and interventions. In China today, the profession is in a crisis brought on by these fiscal changes and the concomitant loss of patient trust.

The chapters in this section review three aspects of the changing status and role of medical professionals and institutions, which shed light on the medical professional crisis today: the early formation of American-trained medical and public health personnel, the evolution of the nursing profession, and the primacy of hospitals in China's health care systems. Elite physicians and the Flexnerian educational model, the nursing profession, and the modern hospital are all aspects of the Western medical system that was introduced to China. In each case, however, the particular professional model was either incomplete or limited in its appropriateness for a heavily populated, developing country such as China. Today's medical reforms are attempting to address these challenges.

Transnational flows of medical personnel were an important aspect of the internationalization of medicine in the twentieth century. For most of the century Chinese medical personnel traveled to and from Japan, Europe, and the United States. Mary Brown Bullock's "A Case Study of Transnational Flows of

Chinese Medical Professionals" examines this intellectual migration through an analysis of the medical fellowship programs of the China Medical Board and the Rockefeller Foundation, primarily during the period 1914–1951. Utilizing fellowship files for 350 physicians, nurses, and public health specialists it identifies the primary Chinese home institutions and American training institutions as well as sheds light on the subsequent professional careers of those trained abroad. The data reveals that Harvard and Johns Hopkins Universities became critical nodes in this trans-Pacific program, especially for those in the field of public health. It also reveals that China's Republican-era National Health Administration was a primary beneficiary of the program: nearly one hundred of its key leaders were trained in the United States. The overall significance of this program includes the fact that almost all returned to progressively important positions in China's health system and that the American Flexnerian model of medical education had an extensive influence in China. After the renewal of diplomatic relations in 1979, the trans-Pacific flow of medical personnel resumed—reuniting many of the same institutions but on a much larger scale.

Sonya Grypma and Cheng Zhen's chapter on nursing begins with the intersecting nursing careers of Nie Yuchan and Zhou Meiyu, who illustrate the interrelatedness of key people and organizations in the first half of the twentieth century. As students at PUMC and Rockefeller Fellows, both perceived nursing as a way to provide patriotic service to China, were offered leadership roles in PUMC and Nurses Association of China (NAC), and made career decisions in response to wartime needs. Yet they had differing ideas about the best form of education for nurses. Whereas Nie followed the American model of (baccalaureate) nursing education established at PUMC and recreated at the West China Union University, Zhou responded to urgent army needs by creating a modified version of the Ministry of Education nursing curriculum, along with a series of shorter courses for emergency technical personnel (X-ray technician, sanitary engineering, laboratory technician). While PUMC, Rockefeller Fellowships, and the NAC provided the educational and other preparation and advancement opportunities for a small number of highly capable nurses—a Chinese nursing elite—it was wartime that helped shape Chinese nursing from a form of Christian and professional service administered by foreigners, into a patriotic, nationalized service administered by highly qualified Chinese nurses. Under the PRC, nursing training was abolished until the late 1970s, and since then nursing activists have been negotiating to reestablish professional training and expanded fields of activity for Chinese nurses.

The hospital is so dominant an institution in the Chinese health care system that 90 percent of all in- and outpatient services in the country occur in one—a remarkable feat for an introduced institution with no indigenous counterpart. In her chapter "The Evolution of the Hospital in Twentieth-Century China," Michelle Renshaw describes the introduction of the hospital and dispensary as sites for the distribution of medicine and evangelism by Christian missionaries, the establishment of government hospitals as sites of modernization and control in the early twentieth century, the Republican government's experiments with state medicine centered on hospitals, and the continued centrality of the hospital under CCP rule. Noting that patients still decide for themselves which clinics and specialties to attend, the chapter ends by describing health care reforms that aim to allocate a supervising general practitioner to every patient, following a modern Russian model, while implementing the new universal health care insurance system.

By concluding with the professional and institutional challenges of health care in China today this volume demonstrates that China's twentieth-century health transitions are continuing. In the early twenty-first century the People's Republic of China embarked on massive health reforms only briefly touched on in these chapters. The vibrant history of health transitions depicted herein provides a benchmark for understanding the future trajectory of health and medicine in China.

PART I
HEALTH TRANSITIONS

1 China's Exceptional Health Transitions

Overcoming the Four Horsemen of the Apocalypse

Lincoln Chen and Ling Chen

Introduction

Many of the world's countries experienced major health transitions over the course of the twentieth century. China is no exception, but its passage has been distinctive in many ways. China's achievement in life expectancy has been truly spectacular, with average longevity more than doubling over the course of the century. Perhaps unique to China, however, have been major health catastrophes, human calamities that call forth the death theme of "the four horsemen of the apocalypse." In overcoming these dramatic setbacks, China's health transitions have been marked by distinctive phases, where health conditions have been shaped by its health care systems as well as powerful social determinants of health. These phases have exhibited both distinctiveness among countries and continuity across time.

This chapter reviews the unique and exceptional transitions of health in China over the course of the twentieth century. It should be noted that this paper's term "health transition" has different connotations than the title of this volume's reference to "medical transitions." Medical transitions imply changes in the field of medicine—science, perceptions, practice, and institutions. Health transition is a broader concept dealing with the health of populations, not individuals.

By using the term "health transition," this chapter brings together several major transition theories. The theory of the "epidemiologic transition" describes the changing pattern of disease and cause of death as populations progress from higher to lower mortality levels associated with rising incomes and improving health systems (Omran 1971). Whereas poverty-linked diseases such as childhood infections, malnutrition, and maternity-linked burdens characterize low-income societies, noncommunicable chronic diseases like cancer and heart disease dominate in higher-income countries. "Demographic transition" theory, similarly, captures changes in fertility and mortality from high to low levels (Caldwell 1976; Davis 1963; Frederiksen 1969). The time gap between an earlier reduction in mortality to the later decline in fertility generates a gap between birth and death rates that accelerates population growth. In addition to rates of growth, demographic change may also affect the spatial distribution, age structure, and other parameters of human populations. These two theories of transitions are brought together in the theory of the health transition, which integrates not only epidemiologic and demographic parameters but also changes in sociocultural perceptions, health-seeking behavior, and the structure and operations of health systems (Caldwell 1990; Frenk et al. 1989; Frenk et al. 1994; Mosley and Chen 1984). As such, health transition theory is comprehensive, holistic, and interdisciplinary in describing the multiple dimensions of simultaneous changes related to the health of populations.

Using the framework of health transitions, this paper opens with an assessment of changing health conditions in China over the course of the twentieth century. Though they started with health backwardness in the beginning of the century, China's current health conditions rival those of more economically advanced countries. Perhaps uniquely in the world, China demonstrates these remarkable health achievements by overcoming unprecedented health catastrophes. The chapter then probes the nature of these health changes by examining patterns in the cause of death, again showing China's shift from poverty-linked to affluent lifestyle patterns in the burden of disease. Assessment of China's epidemiologic transition is followed by a review of China's demographic transition. The chapter concludes by looking to the future through an analysis of the reform of China's health system, a recurring theme throughout the century.

Two caveats are indicated. First, the data sources for China's health conditions, causes of death, and population size and distribution are variable; there is better availability of data in recent decades with increasing lacunae as one moves back in history. Especially difficult are estimations of health conditions during times of political crisis, when data collection systems are disturbed or misrepresented. There is also insufficient transparency and openness of access to data for academic study. We recognize these imperfections, but we believe that our estimations are sufficiently robust to substantiate the basic conclusions. Second, we recognize that China is a vast country with great internal diversity. This chapter focuses only on the national level. The variability within China is recognized; indeed, many estimations of the national pattern are derived from microstudies

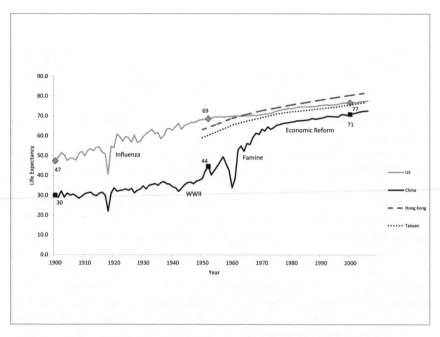

Figure 1.1. Life expectancy, China (with Hong Kong and Taiwan) and United States, 1900–2000. *Sources:* For United States, data from Arias (2010). For China, 1950–2000, data from Peng (1987); Sen (1990); United Nations (2011). For China, 1900–1950, data from Campell (1997); Ni (1986); Rao and Chen (1995); Seifert (1935); You, Quan, and Xu (1991); Zhao (1990). For Hong Kong, data from United Nations (2011). For Taiwan, data from Ministry of the Interior (2011).

in China's different regions. But focusing on the national level better captures the pattern and velocity of change over the course of a century.

Health Transitions

Figure 1.1 charts China's remarkable achievements in health across the twentieth century. With an estimated average life expectancy of only thirty years in 1900, it is no wonder that China was denigrated as the "sick man of Asia." By the end of the century in 2000, however, China's life expectancy had more than doubled, to an estimated seventy-one years.

The trend line for the United States is shown to highlight the nature of China's achievements. Whereas China was seventeen years behind America's life expectancy in 1900, that gap had narrowed to only six years by 2000. Noteworthy is that the gap had widened to twenty-five years at mid-century—China at forty-four years and the United States at sixty-nine years—underscoring China's stagnated health gains in the first half of the century followed by markedly accelerating improvements in the second half of the century.

For comparative purposes, available data on Taiwan and Hong Kong since 1950 is superimposed on the time trends. Relatively unencumbered by the effects of war, Taiwan and Hong Kong began with a higher life expectancy around 1950 and also performed well in the second half of the twentieth century, even surpassing the United States in longevity (United Nations 2011; Ministry of the Interior 2011).

The weak progress in mainland China in the first half of the century, 1900–1950, was undoubtedly related to political chaos, war, and weak health care infrastructure associated with the collapse of the Qing dynasty, the emergence of the Guomindang, the Japanese invasion, World War II, and the postwar civil conflict. The marked acceleration of improvements characterizing the second half of the century, 1950–2000, was achieved due to political stability followed by strong government commitment to equitable health interventions.

The two phases of retarded and accelerated health achievements match well with the theory of the twin engines of health development: direct health action and social determinants of health. The revolution in health sciences, modern knowledge, its derived technologies, and their application has undoubtedly had an important impact on health conditions. While not dismissing the usefulness of traditional medicine as well as modern, there is strong evidence of the life expectancy impact of the application of modern science through health institutions of hospitals and field-based health systems operated by well-trained modern health professionals. These direct health actions parallel the influence of powerful social determinants. Political stability can enable populations to reduce their risk and vulnerability to disease and provide the institutional foundation for direct health interventions. Economic growth brings not only food, clothing, housing, and other material provisions but the physical infrastructure of health care systems. Perhaps most important among social determinants are universal literacy and education, including gender equality. Literate populations are able to understand and act on theories of disease caution, utilize health services, and adapt their behavior to enhance disease prevention and the use of earlier and more effective treatment.

Four Horsemen of the Apocalypse

Figure 1.1 also shows that, more than any major world country, China has experienced some of the greatest health catastrophes in human history. "The four horsemen of the apocalypse" describes the major life-threatening crises due to war, famine, disease, and death (Cunningham and Grell 2000). Unfortunately for the Chinese people, the country experienced all four horsemen. We discuss in turn China's experiences of invasion, war, famine, and epidemics.

Invasion, war, and conflict characterize China's turmoil over the decade and a half of 1937–1949. In 1937 Japan launched a massive invasion of China called the Second Sino-Japanese War (the first war occurred in 1894–1895). After the Japanese attack on Pearl Harbor in 1941, the invasion became part of the greater conflict of World War II as a major front of what is broadly known as the Pacific War. The conflict did not cease with the surrender of Japan in 1945, as the Guomindang and the Communists fought a protracted civil war in 1945–1949. The official government statistics for Chinese military and civilian casualties in the Second Sino-Japanese War from 1937 to 1945 are twenty million dead and fifteen million wounded (Guo 2005). Other estimates suggest that the total population of about 500 million suffered ten to twenty million deaths, or 2–4 percent of the population (Clodfelter 2001).

Famine, unfortunately, killed more Chinese than epidemics or war in the twentieth century! Indeed the worst famine in recorded history hit China during the Great Leap Forward in 1959–1962. The causes and toll of the famine have received extensive and intensive academic attention (Ashton et al. 1984; Lin and Yang 1998), and excess famine deaths have been estimated at twenty to forty-five million (Peng 1987; Sen 1987). Grain production dropped by 15 percent in one year and then to about 25 percent below its previous level for two further consecutive years. Birth rates dropped by 50 percent and the number of births during 1958–1962 was about thirty-three million fewer than expected. Population annual growth rate dropped from 2 percent in 1958 to negative in 1961 (Ashton et al. 1984). Long term effects were also significant, as fetal and early childhood malnutrition carried adverse consequences for adult health as well as a range of socioeconomic outcomes, including literacy, labor market status, wealth, and marriage markets. An estimated fifteen to twenty years of loss in life expectancy was caused by the famine (Banister 1984; Sen 1990).

The causes of the famine were officially claimed to be natural disasters, including drought and flooding, which had periodically affected China. The bad weather contributed to the significant drop in output (Ashton et al. 1984), but as Amartya Sen points out in his entitlement theory, some of the worst famines have occurred without a significant decline in food availability (Sen 1990). What is important is that affected individuals ceased to have the ability to command food. It is widely accepted that a set of misguided policies in China's Great Leap Forward played a critical role in the massive food shortage. Especially detrimental were misreports of local food production to demonstrate political correctness imposed by top-down policies irrespective of conditions on the ground—policies for which millions suffered and lost their lives.

The total human toll of all of these health catastrophes over the century will never be known with certainty. What appears well documented is that China's twentieth century witnessed at least between 45 to 74 million excess deaths due to these disasters.

Disease epidemics have hit China throughout the century, such as the Manchurian plague early in the century, the worldwide influenza epidemic, and SARS early in the twenty-first century. Mortality data on the Manchurian plague of 1910–1911 is limited. The mortality toll of the SARS epidemic of 2003 was miniscule in comparison to its impact on public fears and the paralysis of international trade and commerce. The 1918–1919 influenza epidemic was likely the most deadly infectious crisis in China in the course of the century.

Deemed one of the most devastating epidemics in human history, three extensive pandemic waves of influenza spread globally in 1918–1919, killing worldwide an estimated 20 to 50 million people. The case fatality rate was over 2.5 percent (Luk, Gross, and Thompson 2001; Taubenberger and Morens 2006), with the highest mortality impact concentrated in young adults. In the United States, about a third of the total population of about one hundred million was infected and at least 675,000 people were killed. The impact was so profound that average life expectancy declined by ten to twelve years, from fifty-one years in 1917 to thirty-nine years in 1919 (Cheng and Leung 2007; Crosby 2003). Estimates for the mortality toll in another country, India, was 12 to 20 million deaths (Patterson and Pyle 1991).

Records for the influenza pandemic of 1918 in China are very sparse, but there is evidence that influenza did hit the country, whose population was then 450 to 475 million (Patterson and Pyle 1991). The overall estimated flu death rate in China was 1 to 2 percent, suggesting five to nine million deaths. The virus spread from the south (Shanghai, Guangzhou) to the north as far as Harbin, and even to remote regions like Yunnan Province (Cheng and Leung 2007). Regions like Peking and Manchuria reported "serious epidemic with a high percentage of death" (Patterson and Pyle 1991). In many other places in southern China, including Hong Kong and Shanghai, influenza mortality was relatively lower (Cheng and Leung 2007).

Were the impact of all epidemics, violence, and famine to be totaled—including violence and dislocation imposed during internal political upheavals—the human toll would surely exceed one hundred million people!

Epidemiologic Transition

China's patterns of disease and causes of death changed over the course of the twentieth century. Times of crisis inherently affect some people more than others, and the causes of death may vary considerably. Epidemics impact on age-sex groups differentially, with young adults suffering the highest mortality risk due to the influenza epidemic. The toll of war is usually borne by innocent civilians rather than combatants, and children and women are particularly vulnerable to health crises (Dower 1993). The impact of famine, too, is absorbed disproportion-

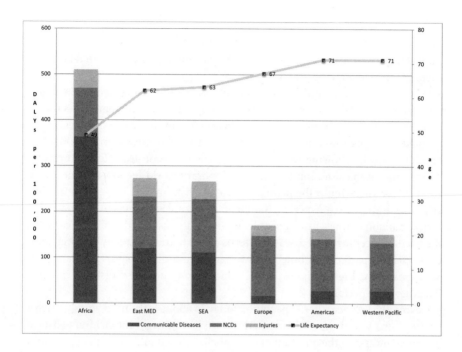

Figure 1.2. Burden of disease (DALYs, or disability-adjusted life years) in world regions (2004) (Low- and middle-income countries grouped by WHO region, 2004). *Source:* Mathers et al. (2008).

ately by children and women, and in the case of China, political background and affiliation may have affected vulnerability (Ashton et al. 1984).

But what has been the pattern of causes of death during non-crisis time periods? These causes ultimately result in more suffering and death and challenge the people, government, and health care system. Fortunately, causes of death may be estimated for China based on indirect techniques derived from contemporary data from different world regions.

China has few comprehensive assessments of major diseases, although special isolated studies of specific diseases may be found in the literature. The current epidemiologic profile in China, however, is well established. Recent analyses confirm that noncommunicable diseases account for more than 80 percent of all deaths. In addition to cardiovascular disease, stroke, cancer, and diabetes, chronic diseases also include mental illness, which is now considered the disease imposing the greatest health burden (WHO Department of Mental Health and Substance Abuse 2005). Communicable diseases and injury have not been entirely eliminated, of course, and new threats are emerging on the horizon, including new infectious pathogens like SARS, environmental pollution, and sociobehavioral pathologies including alcoholism, drug abuse, and sexually transmitted diseases. The huge burden of noncommunicable diseases underscores the critical importance of controlling such risk factors as smoking, diets rich in fats, lack of exercise, and car-driving practices.

In contrast with China's exceptionality in the four horsemen of the apocalypse, its causes of death conform to the theory of the epidemiologic transition, in which societies shift from communicable to noncommunicable diseases. Figure 1.2 offers insights into how the pattern of causes of death in China is likely to have changed by showing the three major categories of death (communicable, noncommunicable, and injury) for contemporary world regions (Mathers et al. 2008). Overwhelmingly, the primary cause of death in China today, as in Western Europe and North America, is noncommunicable disease. Due to sparse historical data on China's health profile, we can only assume that China earlier in the twentieth century had disease patterns closer to those of today's poorer countries. Disease patterns in other world regions like sub-Saharan Africa suggest analogies to the higher disease burden due to communicable diseases in China in earlier time periods.

Note that Africa's life expectancy today is about forty-nine years, which is where China was at the mid-twentieth century. An insight into China's past can be gained by asking the question of how much China at mid-century experienced a pattern of death that resembles that of Africa today. While recognizing that there are distinctive epidemiologic patterns between China and Africa, insights on contemporary societies are one approach to historical situations in other societies. One could extrapolate back further and assume that at the beginning of the twentieth century, the communicable and poverty-linked diseases—such as common childhood infections and tuberculosis—would have been even more dominant in China, along with malnutrition and maternity-linked risks.

Though it shares similarities with other countries, it is important to recognize that Africa, of course, has unique crises with such diseases as HIV/AIDS, malaria, and other tropical threats, while China has some unique pathologies not common to other countries, such as nasopharyngeal and esophageal cancer, schistosomiasis, and other afflictions. Some specific Chinese health issues and diseases like leprosy, plague, HIV/AIDS, tuberculosis, and sexually transmitted diseases have received individual attention.

Demographic Transition

Changing fertility and mortality has shaped China's population size and age structure. Despite the huge loss of human life, China is the most populous country in the world at about 1.3 billion people in 2000. China tripled its population size in a century, representing a gain of 870 million people from a base of 430 million estimated in 1900. Like most modernizing societies, China underwent

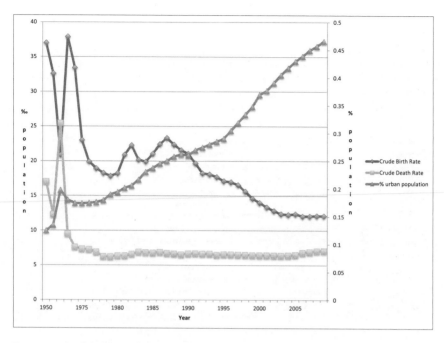

Figure 1.3. Crude birth rate (‰), crude death rate (‰), and percent urban population of China. *Source:* Zhonghua renmin gongheguo weishengbu (2010).

an especially marked demographic transition in the second half of the twentieth century.

Figure 1.3 shows the trend of birth and death rates in 1950–2010. Annual birth rates of over thirty per thousand at mid-century have declined to about fifteen per thousand today, and death rates have similarly declined from twenty-plus to seven per thousand. The dramatic disjunctions in the trend line were due to the famine of 1959–1962, when births temporarily plummeted and mortality sharply rose, both demonstrating fluctuations in their return to long-term equilibrium.

The People's Republic of China since its inception has set startling precedents in managing its great and burgeoning population (Ding and Hesketh 2006). It is the first country to try to popularize the ideal of a one-child family. The PRC's one-child policy has sparked much controversy. The government claims that the policy has prevented 250 to 300 million births, facilitating China's economic development and environmental sustainability. The total fertility rate decreased from 2.9 to 1.7 children per couple between 1979 and 2004, creating a distinctive demographic pattern of urban families with predominantly one child and rural families with predominantly two children. The small family norm

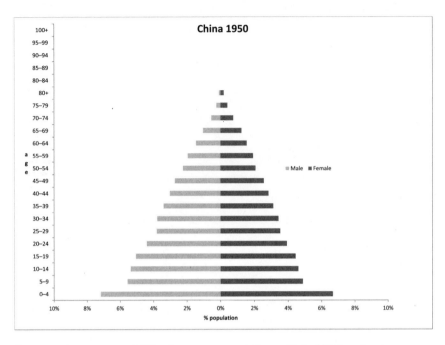

Figure 1.4. Age structure of China (1950, 2000, 2050). *Source:* United Nations (2011).

appears to have taken root in China, with 35 percent of couples preferring one child, 57 percent expressing preference for two children, and only 5.8 percent wanting more than two children (Hesketh, Li, and Zhu 2005).

The fertility impact of the one-child policy is, however, debatable. The more dramatic decrease in China's fertility actually occurred before the policy was imposed. Between 1970 and 1979, the largely voluntary "later, longer, fewer" policy, which called for later childbearing, greater spacing between children, and fewer children, had already been accompanied by the halving of the total fertility rate, from 5.9 to 2.9. In addition, the introduction of universal basic education, improved child survival, and greater gender equality were among key development measures that would have themselves powerfully dampened the desire for large families (Lapham and Mauldin 1984; Poston and Gu 1987). Other Asian countries without compulsory one-child family policies have experienced substantial declines in fertility during the same time period, with China's East Asian neighbors having some of the lowest fertility rates in the world.

Equally marked have been changes in China's gender and age structures as well as the population's spatial distribution. China is among a handful of countries with a severe deficit of female births due to sex-selective abortions. There has been a steady increase in the reported sex ratio of male to female births, from 1.06

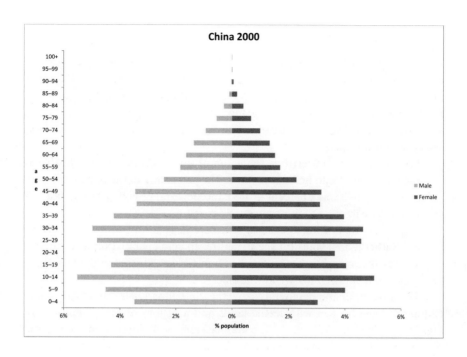

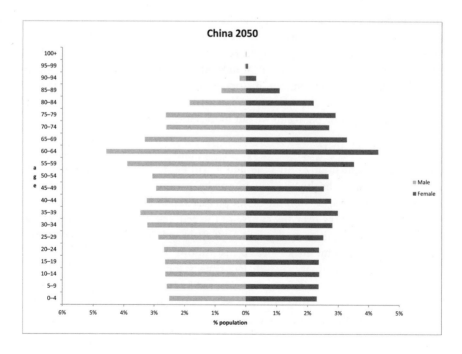

in 1979, to 1.11 in 1988, to 1.17 in 2001. This implies that 17 percent of males do not have demographically matched females. The Chinese government has acknowledged the potentially disastrous social consequences of this sex imbalance. The shortage of women may increase mental health distress and socially disruptive behavior, leaving many men unable to marry and rear children. The scarcity of females has also sparked kidnapping and the trafficking of women for marriage, and has also fueled the commercial sex work industry, with a consequent rise in sexually transmitted diseases.

With the decline in fertility, the aging of the population is inescapable as fewer children enter into new age cohorts. The percentage of the population over the age of sixty-five was 5 percent in 1982 and now stands at 7.5 percent, but it is expected to rise to more than 15 percent by 2025.

Figure 1.4 shows China's age-sex structure in 1950, in 2000, and projected to 2050. Rather than a youthful age structure, an aging population will generate greater pressures on costly health care and home-based care in households which have only a few children to care for the elderly.

The most dramatic demographic change in China relates to urbanization. China has been blessed with fertile lands and a history of many centuries of highly organized government. This combination favored population growth and resulted in extremely dense settlements in arable land by the middle of the nineteenth century. Therefore, the PRC upon its founding inherited a huge population densely packed in agricultural areas. With rapid economic and social transition, more people have migrated to urban areas. Figure 1.3 shows that whereas only 12 percent of China's population was urban in 1950, the urbanization level has now reached 50 percent. The wholesale movement of rural people to urban settings involving a total urban population of more than six-hundred million people is entirely unprecedented in human history, and has generated huge challenges in terms of jobs, education, health care, urban infrastructure, and the decay of rural communities as young people move out to the cities.

Looking to the Future

China's health transition is ongoing and it will be determined by its socioeconomic development, health challenges, and health system performance. China's health transitions mirror well the major phases of political and economic development of the country over the course of the century. The early decades of the collapse of the Qing dynasty brought with them political chaos and economic difficulties. While some major health institutions were established during the Republican period, there was insufficient time, stability, and cohesion to sustain major advances that were severely interrupted by the Japanese invasion, World War II, and the civil war. The Communist victory, with its political stability and a national ideology of universal access to health, irrespective of economic conditions, undoubtedly contributed to the significant acceleration of health in the second half of the century. In 1968, the program of barefoot doctors was introduced as a national policy focused on quickly training paramedics to meet rural needs. Most barefoot doctors, who graduated from secondary school education, practiced after training at the county or community hospital for three to six months. Hence medical coverage in the countryside expanded rapidly (Zhang and Unschuld 2008). But the commune-based health care system collapsed after the Cultural Revolution, and health gains have been moderate during the early decades of economic liberalization.

The rapid, continuing decline of the cooperative medical system affected many important elements in health care. The number of barefoot doctors diminished greatly as many of them left for full-time work. There was also a serious impact on the continuing education of barefoot doctors when its costs were no longer being covered by the cooperative medical system. The financial burden of illnesses borne by the peasants increased, which also affected hospitals' financial situations (Hsiao 1984). The problems of people left uncovered by insurance, rising health care costs, drug-company kickbacks to providers, and fragmented health services made it imperative for the Chinese government to reform its health care system. Starting in the early 1990s, several rounds of health reforms have been implemented. The latest round, begun in 2009, focused on "securing essential health care services, strengthening primary health care and building up institutions and mechanisms." The overall goal is to establish a basic health system and achieve primary health for all by 2020.

The reforms have five pillars of action: universal health insurance, primary health care, essential drugs, disease prevention, and reform of public hospitals. For the implementation of these five reform priorities, an additional 850 billion RMB (around $134 billion) from governments at various levels are allocated, of which 331.8 billion RMB is from the central government.

Health insurance coverage has expanded quite rapidly since the early 2000s, with China now achieving nearly universal coverage. 1.27 billion Chinese people, or 95 percent of the total population, are covered by some kind of health insurance, up from 15 percent in 2000. The central government has invested 41.2 billion RMB to improve the hardware of grassroots-level health facilities, and to develop a partnership between large urban hospitals and grassroots health institutions, recruit licensed medical practitioners, train general practitioners, and take other measure to enhance health services at local levels. The total number of outpatient visits to the grassroots-level clinics reached 3.61 billion in 2011, a 22 percent increase compared to 2008. By the end of June 2011, the essential drug system was implemented in 98 percent of government-run community health institutions and township hospitals. The government has provided ten kinds of national basic public health programs, covering such necessities as disease prevention, and health education. Provinces all over the country launched pilot public hospital reform, and seventeen cities were chosen as national pilot areas. A series of measures which facilitate seeking medical care have been taken, including appointment and registration systems, 24/7 outpatient care, quality nursing care, and clinical pathways. Meanwhile, explorations have been made in reforming systems and mechanisms, such as management systems, operation mechanisms, compensation mechanisms, and pricing mechanisms.

Whatever progress these reforms will achieve in the coming decade, the basic contours of health challenges to China are already etched in its earlier health transition. China's population will stabilize in size, but its structure will be dramatically changed into more elderly, urbanized, and smaller nuclear family households. The noncommunicable diseases will impose great challenges to China's health prevention programs as well as huge burdens on its health care system. In addition to these chronic diseases will be new threats ushered in by the risk of pollution, sociobehavioral pathologies, and new infectious epidemics.

There are still some problems pending in the health care system, including insufficient health care resources, the ever-increasing medical costs that have become a heavy burden to residents, the inadequate coverage of health insurance, and large gaps in basic medical service between rural and urban areas among different regions and between different populations. Apart from those issues, the allocation efficiency of the health system and the microefficiency of medical facilities is low, and the safety and quality of health care services need to be improved.

China has established a three-tiered organization for the delivery of health care. First-tier hospitals generally serve communities with basic services and treatment of common diseases. A wider range of medical services and treatment of more diverse diseases is offered by second-tier hospitals to patients across a municipality. Third-tier hospitals are not only providing superior services, but are also usually connected to a medical university and therefore are involved in medical research and the education of medical students. But China's incremental reform of health care delivery has failed to produce an efficient system. There is a mismatch of services and needs, with more than 80 percent of health care delivered in urban areas even though 50 percent of the population resides in rural areas. Third-tier hospitals operate at full capacity, while community hospitals and township health centers have bed occupancy rates below 50 percent. Doctors at some hospitals see over seventy patients daily, while doctors at other hospitals see far fewer patients, ranging from 4.5 to 6.9 outpatient visits per day in some studies and from 5.8 to 15.3 in Ministry of Health statistics. China's health care system reform will depend centrally on whether its three-tier health system is able to reestablish primary services at the lower level to ensure affordable, high-quality services (see chapter 13). China currently faces a disequilibrium, where patients bypass the primary and secondary level of services due to lack of qualified providers and perceptions of poor quality, and flock instead to tertiary facilities, which are incentivized to draw such income streams into for-profit tertiary public hospitals.

By 2003, there were 1.4 physicians and 1.0 nursing and midwifery personnel per thousand people in China, which is slightly below the threshold of 2.5 health care professionals (counting only physicians, nurses, and midwives) per thousand people necessary to achieve adequate coverage rates for selected primary health care interventions. A more notable fact is the lack of qualified health care professionals. In 2003, less than 1 percent of all health care professionals had either a master's degree or a doctorate, and only 13 percent had a four-year college degree. Fewer than 30 percent of doctors have four years or more of university education. Furthermore, rural communities depend on care from former barefoot doctors, who were never well-trained and who now earn their keep mostly by selling drugs and providing intravenous infusions, a popular form of therapy for all kinds of problems in China. In particular, it has been estimated that one-third of drugs dispensed in rural areas are counterfeit, enabling their vendors to earn huge markups (Hsiao 2004).

Successful reform will ultimately depend upon the capacity of the system to develop primary- and secondary-level services that are affordable and of high quality, overcoming patient perceptions. This will critically depend upon training professional doctors and nurses to staff such facilities, which will require a revamping of the health professional education system in China, which will in turn depend upon institutional reforms in both the health and the educational sectors (Yip et al. 2012). Ultimately, China's health transitions will be determined by the harmonization of its health and educational systems' generating a universal, high-quality, affordable health care system balanced by equitable development of the social determinants of health for all of its citizens.

2 Changing Patterns of Diseases and Longevity

The Evolution of Health in Twentieth-Century Beijing

Daqing Zhang

WHILE BEIJING, THE capital of China, cannot be said to be typical of the country as a whole, the relatively ample documentation of the health of its citizens will be used in this chapter to provide a window into the process of health modernization in China over the twentieth century.

Hygienic Modernization: From Agency to Action

The process of health modernization in Beijing began during the late Qing reforms, or "New Policies" era (1901–1911). In 1905 the Board of Police, set up under the new Ministry of Police, had three departments, one of which was the Department of Health Services (*weisheng shu*). The department was divided into four sections:

1. Street Cleaning: cleaning streets, public toilets, garbage disposal, and controlling sewage and litter.
2. Disease Prevention: preventing epidemics by vaccination and surveillance of hospitals, slaughterhouses, and food shops.
3. Medicine: administering medical schools and hospitals, certifying doctors, publishing medical books, and keeping statistics of births and deaths.
4. Health Services: treating diseases, inspecting sanitary conditions in factories, and manufacturing pharmaceuticals.

The Department of Health Services also established a laboratory for bacteriological and drug testing. At the same time, it issued a series of sanitary regulations and public health laws, including rules for preventing epidemics and managing vaccination, and charters for the government-run Inner- and Outer City hospitals. The establishment of a health system was a landmark of Late Qing modernization. Although it is difficult to evaluate the system's effectiveness in improving health and controlling disease, a number of the practical actions taken had lasting value: the founding of smallpox vaccination stations, street cleaning, management of wells, and the establishment of tap water supplies and water treatment plants.

When the Republican government was established in 1911, the sanitation work in cities, including Beijing, remained entirely in the hands of the police. The Health Services Section of the Board of Health continued to issue rules and regulations, but persistent political instability meant they were not able to be put comprehensively into effect. For instance, during the epidemic of scarlet fever in 1915, the Northern Warlord government established the Capital Hospital for Infectious Disease at the tenth Hu-tong of Dongsi Pailou (东四牌楼十条胡同) with a capacity of only ten beds. It was obvious that the hospital was only minimally effective when confronted with a rapidly spreading infectious disease.

In 1928, a Bureau of Health was established within the municipality of Peiping—as the city was called under the new Nationalist (*Guomindang*) government—and Dr. Huang Tse-fang (Huang Zifang), who was studying at the Harvard School of Public Health, was invited to become its first commissioner. The Bureau of Health, now administratively independent from the police, was better able to act and could initiate the development of a public health system. The bureau rearranged the organization's administrative and advisory structures, formulated health plans, issued a series of laws and regulations, and initiated regular sanitary campaigns to gradually improve health conditions in Beijing. Specifically, the bureau promulgated a series of regulations for the registration of medical practitioners, street cleaning, the management of hospitals, and the examination of prostitutes. In the meantime a Health Council, with membership drawn from the social elite and medical specialists, was established to advise on health policy and to supervise medical services (BSWJ 1928a). As the Health Policy Guidelines, formulated in 1928, stated,

> Public health, as a matter of population health, can relieve the suffering of people and enhance the capacity for social service, and also prolong life and preserve the nation. All modern states attach high importance to this issue, recruiting excellent specialists and allocating a great deal of financial resources. . . . The situation is different in every country, hence sanitary measures should be tailored with consideration to the particular conditions. Based on Beijing's peculiar customs and local conditions, the health issues that the government should pay special attention to are listed as follows: 1. Administration 2. General sanitation 3. Health statistics 4. Health education 5. Prevention of com-

municable diseases 6. Inspection of clinics and pharmacies 7. Development of public health stations in demonstration districts 8. Treatment of venereal diseases and tuberculosis 9. Maternal and child health care 10. School health 11. Public health nursing and 12. Plant/factory health. (BSWJ 1928b)

The priority given to each of the twelve obligations was to depend on the financial situation of the local government, but sixteen public health tasks were given high priority; these included vaccinating against smallpox, establishing a midwifery school to train old-fashioned birth attendants as modern midwives, street cleaning, providing clean drinking water, upgrading toilets, managing and regulating hospitals, certifying doctors, and setting up a registry of births and deaths.

Financial deficiency was one of the greatest obstacles to public health implementation in the Republican era. In 1928, the funding for the administration of the Beijing Bureau of Health was no more than Mex$40,000 and for street cleaning and garbage disposal was only Mex$120,000 (Wu 1929). The Nanking government, founded in 1928, slightly increased the health budget, but it was still tight. Dr. Huang Tse-fang, the director of the Bureau of Health, appealed to the municipal government for financial support four times. According to the administrative plans and temporary standards formulated by the authority, the annual health expenditure per hundred thousand urban residents should be no less than Mex$148,000, that is, 1.5 yuan of health funding per capita. In fact, the total health expenditure of Beijing in 1931, for approximately one million residents, was only Mex$263,000. Although this amount was increased to Mex$570,000 in 1936 (ZGDE n.d.b), between 30 and 50 percent was spent on street cleaning and garbage disposal. The expenditure on medical facilities was about 50 percent and the expenditure on disease prevention, school health, maternal and child health, health education, and life statistics combined was less than 5 percent.

Another obstacle was insufficient human resources in the health field. According to a survey in 1929, compared with European and North American countries there was a huge shortage in the number of physicians in China. The ratios of doctors to population in the United States, the United Kingdom, Japan, and China were, respectively, 1:800; 1:1,500; 1:1,000; and 1:400,000. In the same year, a survey carried out by the Beijing Public Health Station in the second district of the Inner City found that 34.9 percent of people died having received no medical diagnosis and treatment, 44.3 percent had been diagnosed and treated by traditional Chinese medical practitioners, and 16.3 percent had been treated by Western medical practitioners (Chen 1929b). As the statistical data reveals, in 1935 there were 230 certified Western medical practitioners and 886 certified traditional Chinese medical practitioners in Beijing, serving a population of about 1,550,000. Thus, on average, there were 0.15 Western medical practitioners and 0.57 traditional Chinese medical practitioners per 1,000 people: that is, 0.72 physicians of any sort per 1,000 people (Ono 1935, 406). The situation did not change until 1949, by which time there was approximately 1 physician per 1,000 people (BWZBW 2001, 840, 860).

The People's Republic of China (PRC) was founded in 1949, with Beijing as the capital city, which restored its status as the political, economic, and cultural center of the country. Thereafter, the health situation in Beijing significantly and rapidly improved in various aspects. First there was the improvement in environmental health, in particular a hygienic water supply and efficient disposal of garbage and night soil. In the 1920s, about 80 percent of the water supply for Beijing residents had come from wells and 20 percent from tap water. A tap water supply system had been basically completed in the central urban area by 1952 and the well water supply in suburban areas had been improved, ensuring the safety of drinking water. The street cleaning and garbage disposal problems were eventually resolved, essentially giving the lie to the sarcastic slang, "Three feet of soil on a clear day; all streets of mud on a rainy day." The story of how the drainage ditches and the environment around them were changed so that the lower-class people living there moved from a miserable situation to a happy life was vividly told in the play *Dragon's Beard Ditch*, written in 1951 by one of China's most notable novelists, Lao She.

Second was the effective control of infectious diseases: when the PRC was founded, the government implemented active preventive and curative measures against fulminating infectious diseases, including smallpox, cholera, and plague, which can devastate people's health. Through large-scale smallpox vaccination programs, including compulsory vaccination for newborns (initiated in 1950), epidemic prevention and quarantine institutions, health education and promotion, and improvements in the environment, these three infectious diseases had been basically controlled in the Beijing area by the end of 1950. By the end of the 1950s, several other infectious diseases had also been severely curtailed: the incidence of diphtheria had been reduced to 1.39 per hundred thousand in 1959 from 15.5 per hundred thousand in 1950; the incidence of typhus had dropped to 0.1 per hundred thousand in 1958 from 1.18 per hundred thousand in 1950; and relapsing fever and kala-azar were also under control. Infectious disease dropped from the top cause of death to the second cause of death in 1956, and the fifth in 1964, and had disappeared from the top eight causes of death in Beijing by 1979. With social and economic development and improvements in living standards, the general health of Beijing residents had been greatly improved. A series of health regulations and laws issued by the government ensured the effective fulfillment of city health, disease prevention and control, and delivery of residents' medical services. Life expectancy increased to 70.86 years in 1990, from 35 years in 1936. According to data provided by the *Statistical Bulletin of Beijing Health Enterprise 2011*, the life expectancy of Beijing-registered residents had reached 81.12 years in

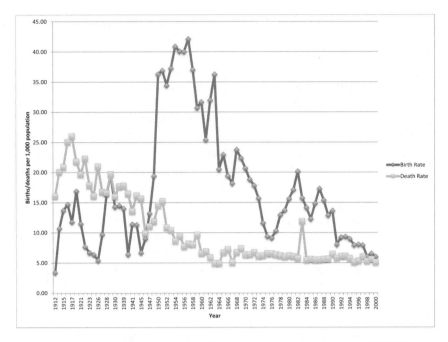

Figure 2.1. The demographic transition: Beijing, 1912–1999. *Sources:* Data from BWZBW (2001); BWNW (1992–1999).

2011, 8 years more than the national average and equal to the advanced countries worldwide.

However, with an aging population, changes in lifestyle, the emotional pressure of fierce competition, lack of physical activity and exercise, and changes in dietary habits, the disease spectrum has been altered. The residents of Beijing are facing new challenges. As shown by the relevant data, the top three causes of death in Beijing are chronic noncommunicable diseases: heart disease, cerebrovascular disease, and malignant tumors. Cancer has become, and remains, the top cause of death among Beijing residents. The Beijing municipal government has already initiated the Sunshine Great Wall Program 2012 for healthy Beijing citizens, that is, the prevention and control of heart and brain diseases, cancer, and oral diseases.

The Demographic/Epidemiological Transition

As outlined above, the health situation of residents of Beijing has gone through tremendous changes during the past century, and the major disease pattern has changed from infectious diseases and malnutrition to chronic diseases and lifestyle-related diseases. We will use some basic demographic parameters and essential indicators for population health to examine the specific changes.

Birth rates and death rates are the fundamental data for assessing all health work, and the police, who were responsible for health in the early twentieth century, had endeavored to secure the statistics on which these rates are based. After the Peiping Health Board was established in 1933, demographic data became more reliable.

The first phase of the demographic and epidemiological transition (before 1950) was characterized by a universally high level of mortality which fluctuated annually but was slowly declining. The second phase, which corresponds to the conditions in Beijing from 1950 to 1975, was characterized by a universally reduced mortality rate and a high birth rate. Gradually but steadily, the dominance of infectious diseases began to subside. The last phase is still ongoing and is characterized by a historically low level of mortality, dominated by such ailments as cardiovascular disease and cancer (otherwise known as noncommunicable diseases) and injuries, while infectious diseases play a relatively insignificant role in the cause of death.

The Role of Social Factors in Health

Our knowledge of the impact of social factors on health in early twentieth-century Beijing is limited and hampered by the lack of reliable demographic data. While S. D. Gamble, in his *Peking: A Social Survey,* described "the health of Peking" as "on the whole very good" (Gamble 1921, 31), endemic and infectious diseases were hard to avoid for most. Generally, death was democratic; it did not take notice of a person's social and economic standing. It is a difficult task to accurately describe health conditions in Beijing in the early twentieth century, but we can infer the general picture of health conditions from some historical documents.

Changing Health Status of Teenagers

The Medical Director of Tsing Hua College, Richard A. Bolt, introduced the medical inspection of young students at Tsing Hua College, and described the findings in a July 1913 article in the *China Medical Journal* (Bolt 1913). The article gave information on the general health condition of young students.

As shown in figures 2.2 and 2.3, while the young students were judged to be generally in good condition, they were not strong. The medical inspection found many students with lesions (figure 2.4), especially of the eyes and nose and throat. Conjunctivitis of varying degrees was found in about 36 percent of students, and about 71 percent had hypertrophied tonsils and/or pharyngitis. It is notable that most cases are related to everyday health customs and behavior.

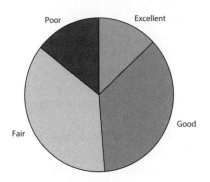

Figure 2.2. General health of students entering Tsing Hua College in 1913.
Source: Bolt (1913).

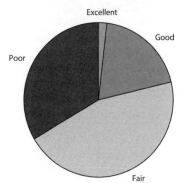

Figure 2.3. Muscular development of students entering Tsing Hua College in 1913.
Source: Bolt (1913).

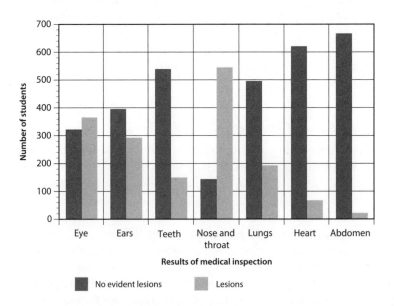

Figure 2.4. Locations of lesions detected in students entering Tsing Hua College in 1913.
Source: Bolt (1913).

**Table 2.1. Incidence of trachoma among the students in
selected schools in Beijing**

Schools	Prevalence of trachoma %
Police School	22.1
Zhao Yang University	26.0
Zhi Cheng Middle School	20.8
Women Professional Training School	41.5
Hot Spring Middle School	34.3
No. 4 Middle School	32.3
Comte School	24.3
No. 21 Elementary School	20.2
Sino-French University	17.0
Primary School Attached to Normal College	7.9
Tsinghua University	19.5

Source: Data from Lu (1930).

Some twenty years later, according to the 1934 annual report of the second health district of Beijing, it was found that the major disorders among students were trachoma (26.4 percent), tooth impairment (12.6 percent), ear diseases (12.4 percent), nose diseases (11.1 percent), and lymph gland enlargement (5.7 percent) (BSWC 1934, 53). Trachoma was the most severe of the diseases that affected adolescents and teenagers in China, especially young students, and foreign governments imposed restrictions on Chinese students entering their countries if they were suffering from it. According to the report in the *China Yearbook* (1924–1925), trachoma was excessively prevalent, affecting almost 30 percent of the total population. Children had higher morbidity rates: in one orphan asylum in Beijing, 68.4 percent of the children suffered from trachoma. In 1930, Lu Yong-chun carried out a survey of the incidence and prevalence of trachoma among the students in several selected schools in Beijing. The results are reproduced in table 2.1 above.

As the prevention of trachoma in Beijing was paid more attention in the 1950s, its prevalence gradually decreased. A middle school in the rural exurban Daxing district is a good example: trachoma prevalence was reduced from its peak of 60 percent in 1950 to 56 percent in 1961, 28 percent in 1971, and 22 percent by 1979. Similarly, the prevalence of trachoma in an urban middle school was reduced from 20 percent in 1964 to 11 percent in 1979 (BWZBW 2001, 511).

Malnutrition was another significant factor that endangered the health of adolescents. Poverty played a role but the cause of nutrition-related diseases was almost entirely ignorance and consequent errors in feeding. Not only did people fail to adapt an infant's food to the stage of development of the digestive organs, but too great attention was paid to the age of the child and too little to its individual stage of development. Although nutritive diseases caused many deaths in the first two years of life, their danger lay chiefly in making the individual vulnerable to other diseases, which, according to their virulence, could lead to irreparable crippling and even death.

With improvement in living standards, the nutritive status of adolescents has been changed greatly. There are three main health issues facing teenagers today. The first is their being overweight or obese. A study of Beijing students aged seven to eighteen reveals that the prevalence of overweight and obesity increased quickly from 1995 to 2005 and shows the tendency of obesity to spread from urban to rural areas (Song et al. 2008). The second is myopia, the incidence of which among Chinese primary and middle school students ranks fourth in the world according to statistics published in 1998; and the third is mental and psychological illness (Ji n.d.).

Maternal and Child Health

Maternal and infant mortality rates are regarded as fundamental indicators of population health: they stand for the strength of a nation and the success or failure of public health. In the 1920s, medical personnel in China were aware of this, and wanted to improve the situation. As Marian Yang (1891–1983), the instructor of the Department of Public Health in the Peking Union Medical College and director of the Health Care Department in the First Special Health Station, stated,

> The high death rate of China is caused by nothing but the birth attendants' lack of obstetric knowledge. First, their inability to tell the difference between physiological and pathological conditions in the field of obstetrics means that few survive a difficult labor. Second, they have no knowledge of disinfection and sterilization methods: puerperal fever or infantile tetanus result in many deaths. Third, lack of knowledge of dietary hygiene causes maternal malnutrition during and after pregnancy and inappropriate breastfeeding of infants, which leads to gastrointestinal or respiratory disorders. It is known that millions of deaths are the consequences of these conditions. (Yang 1928b)

Based on such advocacies, maternal and child health care began to attract more attention. In 1928, the Health Bureau issued regulations on reforming childbirth. The National First Midwifery School was established in November 1929, with Marian Yang appointed as its first principal. There were three kinds of training provided: midwife education consisting of two years for graduates of senior middle school, which aimed to train professionals; six-month midwifery training for nurses who had work experience; and a six-month midwife training course for graduates of senior or junior middle school. It was estimated that in

Table 2.2. Rate of new- and old- method delivery in the First Health Demonstration District in Beijing, 1926–1935

	1926–27	1930–31	1934–35
Western medical practitioners or new-method midwives	17.1%	30.0%	43.3%
Old-fashioned birth attendants	54.3	40.9	38.5
Others	25.8	29.1	18.2
Unknown	2.8	0	0
Total	100.0	100.0	100.0
Total births	1,277	1,842	2,836
Population	51,189	106,547	120,680

Source: Data from Yung (1936).

the 1930s about 65 percent of infants were delivered by old-fashioned birth attendants, only 20 percent were delivered by trained midwives, and the remaining 15 percent were delivered by family members (Yung 1936). In 1934, the Beijing Preparatory Committee for Obstetrics Education was founded, taking charge of the management of obstetricians and midwives as well as the training of traditional birth attendants. The committee maintained a midwife registry and established training schools for birth attendants, with the ambition of having all newborns delivered by trained doctors or midwives (Zhang 1934). Maternal and infant health status showed some improvement but the training courses did not survive political unrest and were terminated. A handful of courses had been held and no more than three hundred trainees benefited. When the first Health Demonstration Station in the east city of Peking was established in 1925, no more than one in five newborns were delivered by Western-style medical practitioners or midwives, while three times as many were delivered by old-fashioned birth attendants. A decade later the percentage of new-method deliveries had more than doubled (see table 2.2).

In 1948 M. Y. Cheng, a researcher in the Maternal and Child Health Department of the National Institute of Health, reported on infant mortality and its causes in China. He pointed out that the average infant mortality rate in urban areas was 130 per thousand, and in rural areas it was 170 per thousand, yielding a national average of 150 per thousand. This was more than two or three times that of Europe and North America. Cheng also compared infant mortality in Peiping, Nanjing, Chengdu, and Lanzhou and noted that the mortality rate did not vary widely and was as high as 130 per thousand. According to his survey, Cheng found that the sex, age, parity, and months of birth and death seemed to have very little influence on infant mortality. About 70 percent of infant deaths

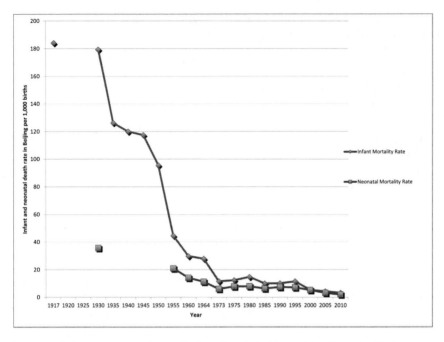

Figure 2.5. Infant and neonatal mortality in Beijing (‰). *Sources:* Data from Gamble (1921, 107); Cheng (1948, 54); BZBZW (2001, 273).

were due to infectious diseases such as tetanus neonatorum, dysentery and diarrhea, measles, pneumonia, congenital syphilis, diphtheria, meningitis, pertussis, scarlet fever, and erysipelas, all of which could be prevented or treated with scientific medicine. Moreover, the 30 percent dying of noninfectious causes such as premature birth, malnutrition, birth injury, malformations, and accidents could also be greatly decreased by modern methods and mass health education (Cheng 1948). Cheng suggested a series of methods to reduce infant mortality. These included establishing and extending public health facilities and agencies, training and educating more maternal and child health personnel, and improving health propaganda through the newspapers, radio, exhibits, lantern slides, and so on. In addition, it was very important to use all ways and means to ameliorate the socioeconomic factors which adversely affect an infant's life and health. These included passing a series of laws on health protection for premarital health examinations, prenatal serological testing for syphilis, special care of employed pregnant mothers, and health education for mother and child.

According to Cheng, the main causes of death of the newborn were premature birth, congenital syphilis, prenatal injury, asphyxia, and deformity. He proposed that the newborn death rate could be lowered through sterile labor delivery, nutrition during pregnancy, appropriate health education to prevent premature labor, and syphilis treatment during pregnancy (Cheng 1948). Congenital syphilis was eliminated in 1961 in Beijing, malnutrition and neonatal tetanus were basically eliminated in 1961 and 1962, respectively, and the death rate fell accordingly. Fewer premature births and cases of neonatal weakness also resulted in fewer deaths (see figure 2.5).

The Epidemiological Transition

As Jin Zizhi, a modern physician in Beijing, described the situation in the early 1920s, "I regret that infectious diseases rage perennial and endless in Beijing; I regret that Beijing's narrow streets and lanes are unbearably filthy and stink; I regret that our nation's tuberculosis sufferers are so numerous, and that we have not taken preventive measures; and I regret that venereal diseases are so widespread, yet we do no inspections of prostitutes" (Jin 1922).[1] Infectious diseases caused the majority of deaths in Beijing, as in other cities in China, in the first half of the twentieth century. Epidemics of smallpox, typhus, and relapsing fever, as well as measles, rubella, and chicken pox came with great frequency, taking thousands of victims. Typhoid claimed its daily victims, and cholera, in the epidemic form, was almost a yearly visitor. Under the Nationalist government, a series of laws and regulations concerning epidemic control and management were issued; infectious disease hospitals and specialized prevention and control institutes targeting tuberculosis and venereal diseases were founded; regular vaccination was carried out; city health campaigns were launched; and mass health education was initiated. As a result, the incidence of communicable diseases was slightly reduced but the overall results were not completely satisfactory.

As discussed earlier, public health promotion and management have been much enhanced since the 1950s, so that several dreadful communicable diseases, including plague, smallpox, and cholera, have almost vanished from Beijing. In addition, some acute infectious diseases such as diphtheria, typhus, relapsing fever, measles, dysentery, and epidemic encephalitis B are also under control.

Accompanying socialist economic development, improvements in public health have resulted in the health of the Chinese improving apace. The incidence of infectious diseases and the death rate have both declined. Average life expectancy has been extended, and marked changes can be seen in the growth and development of young people and children. Some dangerous diseases, such as plague, smallpox, kala-azar, relapsing fever, and typhus have been wiped out. The incidence of acute infectious diseases, such as malaria, poliomyelitis, measles, diphtheria, and whooping cough, has dropped sharply. Since 1970, a comprehensive inoculation program has been carried out in China and significant results have been achieved (see figure 2.6). Average life expectancy rose from thirty-five

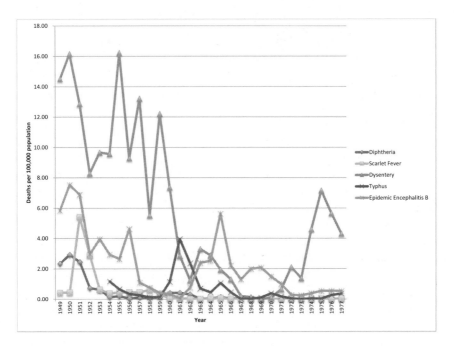

Figure 2.6. Mortality rate of major infectious diseases (unit: per 100,000). *Source:* Wang (2001).

years in 1949 to 72.5 years for males and 75.2 years for female by 1990, close to those in developed counties. According to the statistical bulletin of 2011, the major health indicators for registered residents of Beijing include a life expectancy of 81.12 (exceeding 81 for the first time); a maternal mortality rate of 9.09 per hundred thousand; and an infant death rate which has been reduced to 2.84 per thousand. The top five causes of death, accounting for 87.06 percent of deaths, were cancer, heart disease, cerebrovascular disease, respiratory disease, and injury and poisoning. The report's authors conclude that the health indicators of Beijing residents were on par with those of other international metropolises, such as New York, London, and Paris (BJSWJ 2012).

Social Determinants of Health

As historian of medicine Harold Cook has said, "In considering the health of groups of people, it is generally accepted that many kinds of social interaction have large effects. While individuals may respond positively and negatively to their circumstances, most of the matters that affect health and life expectancy are beyond the control of any single person" (Cook, Battacharya, and Hardy

2009, 1) The history of health changes in Beijing during the twentieth century demonstrate the close and complex interactions between population health and multiple factors, such as society, the economy, culture, and politics. The best evidence for the role of politics is the elimination of smallpox, plague, and cholera in Beijing within about a year of the establishment of the new government in 1949. The technology and methods of preventing and controlling such epidemics had been confirmed much earlier; the holdup was the lack of capacity to scale up these measures. Although preventive vaccination was carried on every year in Beijing during the Republican era, it was difficult to build a complete immunity barrier because of low rates of coverage. After the PRC was founded, the Beijing municipal government proposed an action plan to eliminate smallpox within three years, and a vaccination campaign was carried out throughout the whole city between the fall of 1949 and the spring of 1950. It was estimated that there were 310,000 people vaccinated against smallpox in Beijing in 1949, and a further 400,000 people in 1950; that is, nearly 40 percent of the general population had been vaccinated by 1950. In 1964, a paper in the *Beijing Historical Records of Medicine and Hygiene* declared that no cases of smallpox occurred after May 1950 in Beijing (BYYXBZ 1964, 35).

The prevention and control of venereal disease was another typical case. Prostitutes, who were the largest group vulnerable to sexually transmitted diseases, became the focus of efforts to control the spread of disease. In 1927, the Northern Warlord government created the Screening Institute for Prostitutes, with the responsibility of examining prostitutes and assessing whether they were "qualified" to provide services. In 1928, the newly founded Beijing Bureau of Health expanded the Screening Institute and it began to offer physical examinations free of charge and treatment at discounted rates ("Beijing shi weisheng ju" 1928). In 1948, the government banned brothels and established penitentiaries for prostitutes. Funding problems, however, caused incarceration to be replaced by fines. The new People's Municipal Government of Beijing ordered all the brothels to be closed down on November 12, 1949. On that day 237 brothels were closed, and 1,316 prostitutes were taken into penitentiaries. Examination found that 84.9 percent of them had a venereal disease, and they were given medical treatment. Beijing was one of the earliest cities to achieve control of prostitution and thus control of the major source of venereal diseases. According to the statistics furnished in 1964 by Beijing Medical University, the incidence rate of primary symptomatic syphilis was 24.15 percent in 1949. This was reduced to 2.92 percent in 1951, and was officially at zero after 1953. The incidence rate of primary congenital syphilis, which was 10 percent in 1949, was reduced to 1 percent in 1953, and remained at zero after 1957 ("Beijing shi weisheng ju" 1928, 103).

Tuberculosis, sometimes called the "white plague," is a communicable disease which can severely damage society. Before effective chemotherapy was in-

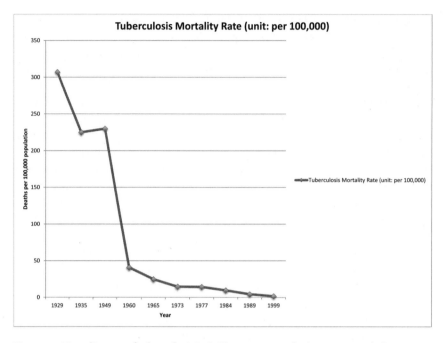

Figure 2.7. Mortality rate of tuberculosis in Beijing, 1929–1999 (unit: per 100,000). *Sources:* Data from Liu et al. (2011b); An (2003); BWZBW (2001, 200).

vented in the 1950s, it was believed to be one of the most common causes of death. According to the statistical data of the Beijing first health district in 1929, the mortality rate of tuberculosis was 307 per hundred thousand, which was twenty times higher than in the United States and ten times higher than in Germany (Lu 1937).

In 1935, Yuan Yijin, G. A. M. Hall, and Qiu Zuyuan founded the Tuberculosis Prevention and Treatment Outpatient Service within Beijing's First Special Health Station, and formulated a package of prevention and treatment measures, including promotion of health education, early detection, early treatment, family follow-up, and local management. They also surveyed the prevalence of tuberculosis among different groups of the population, such as students in elementary and middle schools, colleges, and universities; employees of carpet factories and communal bathing pools; and barbers. The data provided a sound basis to evaluate the epidemiological situation of tuberculosis in Beijing (Wang 2004). In 1946, the Beijing municipal government set up the first government tuberculosis hospital, with a capacity of eighty beds. (Previous tuberculosis hospitals had been operated by missionary societies or by private individuals. See chapter 7 of this volume, on tuberculosis control in Shanghai.) There were eight such hospitals in

Beijing by 1949 but their effectiveness was not as good as was hoped for, with a patient mortality rate remaining as high as 230 per hundred thousand. The municipal government restructured the service and formed the "Beijing sub-committee for BCG vaccination promotion" and "a network of anti-tuberculosis outpatient clinics" in 1950 (BYYXBZ 1964, 84). "Experimental TB prevention and treatment stations" were established in different administrative regions during 1952. Their aim was to popularize BCG vaccination, X-ray examination, and medical treatment. These actions led to greater control of tuberculosis. After 1980, when Beijing introduced "gold therapy" for TB and adopted the World Health Organization's Directly Observed Therapy, Short-Course (DOTS) strategy, the desired effect was achieved and the incidence rate of contagious pulmonary TB was reduced to 16 per hundred thousand in 1990 from 127 per hundred thousand in 2005, or a reduction of 17 percent per year. The incidence of TB in Beijing was one-tenth the average level in China as a whole (An 2003).

According to the World Health Organization there are five necessary components of DOTS: government commitment, including both political will at all levels and a centralized and prioritized system of TB monitoring, recording, and training; case detection by sputum smear microscopy; a standardized treatment regimen directly observed by a health care worker; a regular drug supply; and a standardized recording and reporting system that allows assessment of treatment results (World Health Organization 2013).

Thomas McKeown, a physician and demographic historian from the University of Birmingham, has argued that specific modern medical interventions account for only a small part of the historical fall in the mortality associated with major infectious diseases. For example, economic growth, which made foodstuffs relatively cheap and more widely available throughout the population, led to better resistance to disease and consequently to declining mortality rates (McKeown 1976). But the Beijing TB control story demonstrates that targeted interventions and social change are not dichotomous or opposing choices, but rather complementary to each other. It is essential to integrate technical preventive and curative measures with more broad-based social efforts to improve the health of all people.

The New Culture of Health

In 1938, Hu Shi, in the foreword for Henry S. Sigerist's Chinese edition of *Man and Medicine,* said,

> Because we lack the common sense of modern medicine, we still retain many traditional beliefs and behaviors, which cause us to not take good care of the body, and not focus on individual hygiene. When sick, this can lead us to be thoughtless in selecting doctors and to take random medicines, and even lead us to trust magic cures and witchcraft and not scientific medicine. (Hu 1938)

Hu's critique represented the cultural elite's concern about the public's low level of general health literacy. During the May Fourth period (1919–ca. 1927), a large number of scholars returning from abroad advocated learning from Western science and democracy. Western medicine, as an example of scientific technology, became a powerful weapon with which to criticize traditional culture. This New Culture Movement saw a large number of magazines and journals spring up which spread knowledge of scientific medicine, public health, individual hygiene, and the prevention of epidemic diseases. According to partial statistics, more than ten popular health journals were published between 1912 and 1937 in Beijing. For example, *Health Monthly* was published by the Municipal Health Bureau; *Popular Health* by the First Health Station; *Medical Weekly* by an organization of PUMC alumni, the BinYin Medical Society; and *Popular Medicine Monthly*, renamed *Medicine Monthly* in 1923, was published by the Ai-You Society, an organization of National Medical College alumni. In addition, they published news of health surveys and statistics, health policy and administration, and international medical progress for medical professionals (Wang 1996b, 96).

These efforts of the medical profession and the social elite increased knowledge of scientific medicine and public health, so that concepts of individual hygiene and public health gradually influenced the urban population. The word *weisheng,* which encompasses the notions of health or healthy, sanitary, wholesome, etc., began to be widely used in food advertisements. There was *weisheng* (or "healthy") ice cream, *weisheng* (or "wholesome") plum juice, *weisheng* clean milk, and so on. Many bathhouses, barbershops, and other shops also include *weisheng* in their names (Hou 1939). *Weisheng* became one of the symbols of modernization in modern China.

Since the 1980s, with the changes in the disease spectrum, the biopsychosocial medical model and the concept of holistic health have been increasingly accepted. Today the medical profession has recognized disease as a complex phenomenon which needs a multidimensional, multivariable research approach to develop comprehensive prevention strategies. People's health needs are also increasingly diverse, from improving general health, reducing disease, and extending life, to focusing on the quality and the dignity of life, to selecting the appropriate medical intervention.

Social and Political Mobilization

During the first half of the twentieth century, China's economic development was slow and people's living standards were low. The general public lacked modern medical knowledge. Social mobilization was found to be an effective strategy to popularize knowledge of public health. Peiping's First Clean-Up Campaign, organized by the Health Bureau in 1929, included health exhibitions and vaccinations, as well as the cleaning of streets. To attract the general population the organizers used various means, such as health fairs, plays, movies, free physical examinations, and health counseling. Ahead of time the Health Bureau would issue notices about the campaign, display banners in the streets, and broadcast on the radio in order to attract people to join the campaign (BSDZBW 2000, 105). In 1934, the Clean-Up Campaign Conference changed its name to the Health Campaign Conference and expanded from street cleaning to more comprehensive public health. Wu Jibo, chief editor of *Popular Health*, stated the health campaign's goals as: (1) universal access to health education as quickly as possible so that most people would know about hygiene, and (2) the general public's understanding the importance of public health. In previous years, people had been more concerned with personal hygiene than public health. They had ignored such activities as the pouring of dirty water into the streets and the failure to isolate people suffering infectious diseases. Thus it was an urgent task to improve the public's awareness of public health (Wu 1936). In 1935, 1936, and 1937, the Peiping Health Bureau held public health campaigns, which included exhibitions, dramas, films, physical examinations, and vaccine consultations. The public health campaigns reported good social effects (BSDZBW 2000, 105).

The tradition of public health campaigns continued after 1949 in Beijing under the title of "Patriotic Health Campaigns." During the Korean War, in 1952, in order to deal with the threat of biological warfare, Patriotic Health Campaign Committees were set up at all levels of government, from central to local. These campaigns were a means of both mobilizing the masses to action and educating them in terms of a uniform ideology. They were also a means to lower labor costs and compensate for the lack of health resources. Thus, Patriotic Health Campaigns became regular occurrences. These campaigns have meant that most people now understand the importance of public health, which has paved the way for other public health work.

Conclusion

As we have seen, the history of public health in Beijing can be divided into three phases. The first phase (1900–1949) was characterized by generally higher-level mortality which fluctuated annually but was slowly declining; the second (1950–1975) by a universally reduced mortality rate and a higher birth rate, with the dominance of infectious diseases gradually but steadily beginning to subside; and the third (post-1976) by historically low mortality dominated by cerebrovascular and cardiovascular disease, cancer, and injuries.

We do, however, also find that the extent of the changes has varied at different times, often depending on the political situation, the economy, and cultural traditions, as well as public health measures and medical intervention. For infants and children, before the 1950s Beijing's mortality rates were high in all social groups and were similar to those of other cities such as Nanjing, Chengdu, and Lanzhou. Eighty percent of neonatal deaths were due to preventable causes, such as tetanus neonatorum, premature birth, and congenital syphilis, while about 70 percent of infant deaths were due to infectious diseases which could be prevented or treated with scientific medicine. The sex, age, parity, and months of birth and death seem to have very little influence on infant mortality, but class, or economic level, seems to be more influential. That children were able to access medical services was more important than where they were living.

To understand adult mortality, more factors such as class, income, housing, gender, and access to health care service need to be analyzed. Popularizing the new delivery methods caused maternal mortality to decline rapidly from 7.4 per thousand in 1950 to 0.3 per thousand in 1957. As a developing country with a rapidly growing economy, health resources in China have moved from scarcity to abundance, especially in Beijing, but the challenge of the inequity of distribution remains. For example, according to a survey conducted in 2005, maternal mortality in migrant women is 2.5 times higher than in registered Beijing residents (Shen et al. 2006). Yin Dakui, former vice minister of health, pointed out that 80 percent of government health funding is spent on health insurance for government employees, leading to a grave inequity in health spending (Yan 2006).

Political and social mobilization for public health is a useful strategy to effectively change the living environment and individual hygiene practices in the short term. Beginning in the 1920s, public health advice and motivational campaigns were seen as adequate measures for health promotion, until 2003, when the appearance of SARS in Beijing showed them to be inadequate.

Just as Beijing is the political, cultural, and economic center of China, it is also the center for medical science. Beijing's residents have better and greater access to health care services than those in other parts of the country. But the city is also facing a series of health challenges due to an aging society and changes in the disease spectrum. Beijing today needs to develop new strategies for the prevention and control of chronic diseases, for equity of access to health services, and for wider medical insurance coverage to provide greater access to appropriate health care for its people.

Notes

English-language editing for this chapter was done by Michelle Renshaw.

1. Jin Zizhi (金子直), 1888–?, was born in Dongyang, Zhejiang, graduated from Chiba Medical University, Japan, and was a visiting scholar to the United Kingdom and Germany, researching public health.

3 Maternal and Child Health in Nineteenth- to Twenty-First-Century China

Tina Phillips Johnson and Yi-Li Wu

Introduction

The welfare of childbearing women and children has been a prominent concern in Chinese culture from ancient times to the present. Historically, maternal and child health was a family-directed, household-centered issue. Beginning in the late nineteenth century, however, China's pursuit of modernization significantly changed the context and content of medical practice. For late imperial reformers, as well as the Nationalist and Communist regimes that followed the dynasty's fall, maternal and child health became a crucial component of state building, modernization, and economic growth. While demographic data is spotty or non-existent for the earlier part of this period, modern statistics show that individual and state initiatives have effected dramatic drops in maternal and child mortality over the past few decades. But as China today seeks to attain a standard of health care consistent with its level of economic development, it must also negotiate systemic health problems engendered by the very policies that have driven its breathtaking economic growth.

Maternal and Child Health in the Late Qing Dynasty (1644–1912)

The world of healing in late imperial China was fluid and unregulated, and people selected eclectically from a range of prophylactic and therapeutic methods to promote maternal and child health. The best documented of these is Chinese classical medicine, largely the province of educated men. The ancient, canonical medical texts included discussions of the diseases of women and children, and beginning in the seventh century, these were expanded into systematic, specialized medical writings on gynecological and pediatric ailments (Furth 1999;

Leung 2006; Lee 2008; Wu 2010). Beginning in the eleventh century, "medicine for women" (*fuke*) and "medicine for children" (*erke*) became official departments in the government medical service, with specialized curricula and practitioners. Outside the government, individual practitioners and medical families might also specialize in these areas. Thanks to the growth of medical publishing, especially after the sixteenth century, a plethora of texts on the diseases of women and children were available at a variety of price points, ranging from multivolume heuristic treatises to cheaply printed household handbooks. Many of these texts continue to be standard references for today's practitioners of Chinese medicine (Yang and Liu 1995; Wang and Wang 2000; Wilms 2007).

Typical gynecological topics included promoting fertility and curing menstrual disorders, preventing miscarriage, using drugs to expedite labor or resolve difficulties in childbirth, and protecting a woman's postpartum health. Pediatric topics included how to sever the umbilical cord, how to select a wet nurse, and what kinds of prohibitions women should observe while breastfeeding (Hsiung 1995). People also worried about maternal and infant mortality from illnesses such as "birthing mat wind" and "navel wind," which correspond to tetanus. Pediatric texts also discussed "pox and variola" (*douzhen*), contagious ailments that included measles and smallpox (Wu 2002 [1742]; Hsiung 1999). Throughout, doctors warned that maternal and fetal well-being were intertwined. Such beliefs notably underlay the practice of fetal education (*taijiao*), which taught that a pregnant woman who wished her child to be intelligent, beautiful, and long-lived should regulate her emotions and behavior, engage in salubrious activities, and avoid exposure to inauspicious things.

Midwives and "medicine grannies" also played a central role in caring for women and children (Furth 1999). Childbirth was a female affair, and while male doctors often criticized midwives for inappropriately interfering in labor, they never sought to supplant them as birthing attendants. Instead, learned male practitioners constructed their authority over childbirth in ideological terms. A woman whose body and mind were properly regulated, they taught, would give birth easily, thus making the midwife superfluous. Human ingenuity had its limits, however, and people thus employed religious and ritual practices to promote successful childbearing and protect mother and child. For example, numerous popular deities specialized in curing diseases or promoting fertility, safe childbirth, and infant health. While both men and women made offerings to such deities, women were the main devotees. Such practices overlapped with ritual techniques designed to shield parturient women from evil spirits and to neutralize dangerous cosmic alignments. Families should orient the birthing room in a certain way and affix protective charms to its walls. Similarly, the child's placenta had to be buried in a carefully selected spot. Such practices assumed that childbirth created a form of pollution that had to be carefully managed lest one offend the gods or attract malign forces.

There also was a broad cultural consensus that women should take certain precautions by "doing the month" (*zuoyue*) after childbirth. They were to rest secluded at home, nourishing themselves with warming foods and drugs, and avoiding all drafts and cold water. Bathing and hair washing were proscribed. Such beliefs defined childbirth as a depleting process that left the woman cold, weak, and vulnerable to pathogens. Failure to observe proper precautions would engender dangerous postpartum illnesses as well as later chronic ailments. The practice of doing the month is so deeply rooted in Chinese culture that it continues to shape the postpartum expectations of Chinese women today.

Western Medicine in Late Qing China

In the mid-nineteenth century, European and American Protestant missionaries began to use medicine as a vehicle for Christian evangelization (Tiedemann 2010). Subsequently, missionary dispensaries and hospitals became the most important source of Western medicine in China. These included the hospitals for women and children that were established starting in the 1870s. "Western medicine" was in a state of flux at this time, gradually moving away from a humoral paradigm of disease toward one based on germ theory. Nevertheless, certain features distinguished Western medicine from Chinese: it pursued bodily knowledge via dissection, its practitioners sought authority via educational and professional institutions, its vanguard sought to ally therapeutics to laboratory science, and surgery was an important arena of research and practice. Missionary doctors hoped to impress the Chinese with their skills and thereby make them more receptive to Christianity.

Initially, the medical missionaries were all male. However, Chinese norms of gender segregation meant that female missionaries could interact freely with Chinese women in a way that men could not. After the 1860s, therefore, mission boards actively recruited single women to serve in China, attracting many who felt that the foreign mission field offered professional opportunities not available at home. By century's end, there were more women missionaries (single and married) than men missionaries in China (Hunter 1984; Grypma 2008). These women included physicians and nurses who made possible the growth of a medical ministry aimed specifically at Chinese women and children. This ministry was also driven by missionary perceptions that indigenous health care for Chinese women and children—including that provided by midwives—was appalling (Shemo 2011). Providing Western medical care to women and children would thus produce great returns on the medical and evangelical fronts.

The first female medical missionary in China was the physician Lucinda Combs (1849–1919) of the Methodist Episcopal Church, who arrived in Beijing in 1873. A few years later, she opened a dispensary and a hospital for women and children (Wong and Wu 1936; Tiedemann 2010). She and later female medical missionaries treated their patients for a wide variety of ailments and oversaw obstetrical cases. Missionaries also gave medical instruction to Chinese pupils, who then helped them manage missionary dispensaries and hospitals. Such courses gradually evolved into formal medical schools, typically attached to existing hospitals. In 1879, the medical school of the Canton Missionary Hospital became the first to admit female students (Wong and Wu 1936). In addition to training programs for female doctors and nurses, missionary institutions also started to offer midwifery training starting in the 1890s (Wong and Wu 1936; Johnson 2011).

Western missionaries assumed that their Chinese medical colleagues would play a subordinate role. This assumption was challenged by the Chinese female physicians Shi Meiyu (Mary Stone) and Kang Cheng (Ida Kahn). Both had grown up and been educated in the bosom of the missionary community in Jiujiang (Jiangxi Province), and the Methodist Church's Woman's Foreign Missionary Society later sponsored their medical studies at the University of Michigan. After graduating in 1896, they returned to China as medical missionaries. Shi and Kang saw their medical missions as proof that Chinese women could accomplish just as much as Westerners, and they insisted on being in charge of their own institutions (Shemo 2011). In addition to opening their own hospitals for women and children, these lifelong friends aimed to create a corps of Chinese female medical experts who would use Western medicine to improve the health of Chinese women and children.

This vision, however, did not fit the goals of the Rockefeller Foundation's China Medical Board, whose priorities shaped the contours of medicine in early twentieth-century China. The CMB promoted the ideal of scientific medical training and practice epitomized by Johns Hopkins University, then the premier medical school in the United States. At a time when Shi Meiyu and Kang Cheng were laboring to build independent hospitals for women, the CMB argued that sex-segregated hospitals in China were an inefficient use of limited resources. While Shi and Kang advocated an independent role for Chinese female nurses, the scientific Western hospital model called for female nurses to work under the supervision of male doctors. Ultimately, Shi Meiyu was able to find points of common interest with the CMB, and she received some Rockefeller funding for nurse training. By contrast, Kang Cheng was unable to do so, and she continually struggled to secure adequate resources for her women's hospital in Nanchang (Shemo 2011).

Prior to the 1910s, the direct influence of Western medicine on maternal and infant health in China was geographically and institutionally circumscribed. The vast majority of practitioners of Western medicine worked in missionary institutions, with some also employed by Chinese-founded medical schools in major cities. These practitioners included foreign nationals, Chinese trained by missionaries in China, and Chinese who had studied medicine abroad (China Medical Commission 1914). In 1907, the China Centenary Missionary Conference estimated that "we have now in China 300 fully qualified foreign physicians and 5,000 native assistants, 250 mission hospitals and dispensaries" treating some two million patients a year (China Centenary Missionary Conference 1907, 267). In relative terms, such numbers were miniscule given China's vast territory and huge population. When the Rockefeller Foundation's China Medical Commission visited China in 1914, it estimated that there were at most about forty-five to fifty-five Chinese doctors of Western medicine trained in Europe or the United States, plus a few more trained in Japan (China Medical Commission 1914). Despite these small numbers, medical missionaries and other practitioners of Western medicine were crucial conduits through which this knowledge was promoted and disseminated in China, providing important resources for Chinese modernization and reform movements.

Beginning in the late nineteenth century, maternal and infant health acquired symbolic importance in Chinese modernizing rhetoric. Spurred by ideas of modernism and its associated theories of social Darwinism and eugenics, and inspired by public health movements in the United States, Japan, and Europe, many Chinese intellectuals argued that improvements to public health were essential for China's modernization. Reformers such as Kang Youwei (1858–1927) and Liang Qichao (1873–1929) worried about the ability of the Chinese race to survive the international struggle between nations, and they saw the fate of the Chinese body politic as dependent on the health of maternal and infant bodies. In a similar vein, fiction writers such as Lao She (1899–1966) used tragic images of maternal and infant death as metaphors for the precarious state of the health and well-being of China and the Chinese people (Lao 2005). Other modernizers like Chen Duxiu (1879–1942), Lu Xun (1881–1936), and Hu Shi (1891–1962) heralded science as the savior of China and envisioned a linear progression toward modernity and its attendant prosperity and health for all (Kwok 1965; Lee 2000). By the 1920s, reformers had established journals dedicated to improving public health, while books and magazines like *Funü zazhi* (Ladies' journal) popularized traditional notions of fetal education by cloaking them in the language of modern science (Huang 1931; Li 1935; Song 1936). Such writings imbued modern childbirth with the authority of indisputable scientific discoveries and advancements that would improve lives and save thousands. In this context, motherhood, pregnancy, childbearing, and infant care were no longer private family concerns. Instead, they were now issues that were vital to the future of the country, and thus appropriate targets of public policy (Dikötter 1998; Johnson 2011).

The China Medical Board and the Nationalist Era[1]

Reform and modernization movements in China drew on concepts of global health initiated in the United States and Europe, based on the promises of health and hygiene and rooted in scientific discoveries and theories of eugenics (Bashford and Levine 2010). Science and commercial interests also began to augment religion as an ideological motivation for medical modernization in China. Government and philanthropic organizations like the League of Nations Health Organization and the Rockefeller Foundation's China Medical Board devoted funds and personnel to China, focusing on disease prevention through improved nutrition and hygiene. The most prominent of the China Medical Board's initiatives is the Peking Union Medical College (PUMC), founded in 1921 and modeled on Johns Hopkins University. This school was the locus in China in the 1920s and 1930s for much of the maternal and child health work that had become one of the main concentrations of the global health movement.

The development of modern midwifery was inextricably tied to the modernization process in Republican China. High rates of maternal and infant mortality led Chinese reformers to regulate pregnancy and reform birthing practices. Before the Republican period, and in areas without modern medical resources, infant mortality was estimated at 250–300 per one thousand births, and maternal mortality at 15 per one thousand births (Yang 1928a). Many blamed these deaths on traditional Chinese midwives, whom they accused of employing inadequate and unsanitary methods. Reformers thus promoted aseptic techniques like sterilizing instruments and washing hands to minimize risks to mother and child. As childbirth became linked with scientific medicine and defined as an essential element in the development of a strong and modern nation, local and national governments began to create municipal public health programs and regulate midwives as early as 1913 (Guangdong sheng zhengfu 1913). The so-called "sick man of Asia" (*dongya bingfu*) could become healthy again with good prenatal care and aseptic childbirth.

The period of Guomindang control (1927–1937) saw a significant increase in maternal and child health work in many areas nationwide. Most midwifery reform planning in this period came from the central government in Nanjing. The political weakness of the regime, however, meant that the state lacked the personnel, resources, and commitment to follow through on most of its plans. The Guomindang was trying to build a new, modern state while simultaneously countering political and military threats from regional warlords, the Chinese Communists, and, after 1931, the Japanese. Furthermore, factional infighting within the Nationalist regime prevented consistent policymaking and follow-through in public health, as in other realms (Tien 1972). Despite these impediments, as part of the Nationalist government's mandate to emphasize public health, government officials undertook a concentrated effort to develop maternal and child health programs. In 1929, the Ministry of Health's first Five-Year Plan aimed to provide preventive and clinical maternal and child health care in cities and rural areas. It included strategies to train old-style and modern midwives and public health nurses, as well as to provide a nationwide maternal and child health care network within ten years. Also in 1929, the Ministry of Health and the Ministry of Education jointly established the National Midwifery Board (*Zhuchan jiaoyu weiyuanhui*) to oversee training and regulation of midwives. The First National Midwifery School was the showpiece of the National Midwifery Board and was intended to serve as a "higher normal" school, a training center for midwives who would in turn instruct others around the country. The school was affiliated with PUMC and funded largely by the Rockefeller Foundation's China Medical Board, with additional support from the Nationalist government and local modernizers. The school sponsored unprecedented modifications in childbirth practices; its staff promoted regular pre- and postnatal care, attended aseptic deliveries in a clinic or hospital, or less desirably at home, and gathered health statistics on mothers and infants. Its professors and graduates advised and taught at midwifery training programs around the country.

The founders and leaders of the school, and in fact the architects of much of the maternal and child health reforms in China during this period, were John B. Grant and his colleague and former student Yang Chongrui (Marion Yang 楊崇瑞) of PUMC (see chapter 10). Grant was instrumental in acquiring funding and approval from the Rockefeller Foundation for midwifery training, writing that the high infant mortality rate caused by tetanus neonatorum was "one of the outstanding public health problems" facing China, one easily controllable by creating midwifery training programs (RAC 1931a). With Grant's support, Yang helped to transform childbirth in China from a family-centered, unregulated event into a state-controlled institutional practice. Yang graduated in 1917 from the Women's Union Medical College, a precursor to PUMC, where she eventually specialized in obstetrics and gynecology. After completing a fellowship in obstetrics and gynecology at Johns Hopkins University and visiting several other countries, Yang returned to PUMC with greater knowledge of public health problems and programs worldwide, assuming a joint post as assistant professor of public health and head of the First Health Demonstration Station in Beijing, an urban experimental health center that included maternal and infant health work.

Among her patients, Yang repeatedly encountered cases of tetanus neonatorum and puerperal sepsis, two preventable diseases that greatly contributed to China's high infant and maternal mortality rates. She asserted that six million preventable deaths occurred in China each year, primarily among infants and childbearing women, and she blamed those deaths on the estimated four hundred thousand untrained midwives who were then the primary caregivers for parturient women and their newborns (Yang 1928a). Unfortunately, China had neither the money nor the number of physicians necessary to deliver all its babies in the manner that Yang and others saw as ideal, that is, in a clinic or hospital setting attended by a highly trained physician. She also recognized that prevailing birthing practices and traditional midwives would not easily be displaced. Thus Yang advocated reforming midwives themselves, and she recommended that "the development of midwifery practice in China should be an integral part of maternity and child health, rather than merely an obstetrical procedure as [is] the common practice in other countries" (RAC 1932). One component of her dual approach to midwifery reform consisted of lower-level training for traditional midwives in short midwifery courses of two and six months' duration that stressed the rapid training of many midwives in modern maternal and child health knowledge. Upon completion of this course, the traditional midwives (*jieshengpo*) were required to register with the government and apply for a license to practice. Yang promoted the training courses as an efficient way to quickly reduce the high death rates associated with childbirth. A second component consisted of a higher-level training program that provided more detailed training in midwifery and required an internship. Yang thereby hoped to create a midwifery profession with increased legitimacy that would eventually eliminate the need for lower-level training.

Alongside these prominent national-level efforts, childbirth reform was also driven by initiatives disseminated from several different places, both urban and rural. The National Midwifery Board established a Second National Midwifery School in the capital of Nanjing in 1933 as part of a citywide modernization program that included a nursing school and model districts similar to those elsewhere in the country. Shanghai, a major publishing center and home to a large foreign population, saw the development of countless private maternity hospitals and training programs. In many other cities as well, local notables established maternity hospitals, midwifery training programs, and child health projects as part of model sanitation districts (*weisheng mofan qu*) or experimental public health districts (*weisheng shiyan chu*). In rural areas, model mass education movement (*pingmin jiaoyu yundong*) districts like Jiangning county, Ding county, and Qinghe county included midwifery training programs and education classes for patients. Numerous other rural and county-level public health stations and hospitals were established, all of which nominally included a maternal and child health division, and most offered some sort of maternal and child health care and/or training. Medical missionaries also established hospitals and schools in remote areas. In many cases, the Chinese welcomed Western philanthropic involvement because it helped compensate for the lack of political stability and funding for public health projects. As with the case of the CMB's relationship with Shi Meiyu and Kang Cheng, these diverse efforts at medical modernization were not without internal tensions. While Marion Yang advocated that midwives, not nurses, should be responsible for childbirth, many of the medical and nursing schools countered that midwifery belonged under the purview of nursing, and they continued to train their nurses as modern obstetrical practitioners (Johnson 2011).

Despite all these reform initiatives, modern methods of childbirth reached very few people, and the vast majority of Chinese women saw few or no improvements in the safety of childbirth or in maternal and infant care. Most continued to employ a combination of religious practices and traditional Chinese medical techniques and *materia medica* as they had during the Qing. Furthermore, few had much faith in the young, newly minted, and unmarried modern midwives who had no personal experience with childbirth. Outside the sphere of the First National Midwifery School and cities like Shanghai and Nanjing with their private maternity hospitals and midwifery schools, childbirth remained very much the same as it had been in previous centuries. Nonetheless, the First National Midwifery School and Guomindang attempts at reform left an important legacy in the form of increased state control over reproduction and the use of a tiered training system that continued into the 1980s.

Maternal and Child Health in Wartime (1937–1949)

The Japanese invasion of northern China in 1931 weakened the Guomindang's tenuous control over China and effectively put an end to any wide-ranging plans for public health reform. The subsequent Second Sino-Japanese War (1937–1945) and civil war with the Chinese Communist Party (1945–1949) further hindered Guomindang efforts to implement its earlier policies. Schools and hospitals were closed or severely restricted and much of the medical personnel in all fields, including obstetrics and midwifery, were sent to help the war effort elsewhere. Nonetheless, even during the tumultuous period between 1931 and 1949, the First National Midwifery School and some Guomindang health-related ministries continued to function (see chapter 11).

Even more remarkably, during this time the Chinese Communist Party (CCP) also established midwifery training and childbirth reforms in some of the areas that it controlled, as part of a wider project to improve the health of rural inhabitants and gain their support. Since the establishment of its rural bases, the CCP implemented, or attempted to implement, intensive maternal and health projects, leading to popular support for the Communists. Health policies in these areas were a crucial part of their success. Between 1936 and 1949, maternal and child health were important components of health policies in the CCP-controlled border region in Shaanxi, Gansu, and Ningxia Provinces (Shaan-Gan-Ning), which encompassed thirty-five thousand square miles and had a population of 1.5 million people. Here, pregnant and postpartum women and their newborns received extra rations of meat, cooking oil, salt, vegetables, and cotton. The CCP utilized traditional Chinese medicine combined with aseptic birth practices, even providing free midwifery training for both traditional and new midwives in "people's schools" (*minban*), cooperative training programs administered by the people. Their goal was to have "a midwife in every village" (Minden 1979).

In rural Yan'an, the communist regime's wartime headquarters in northern China, the CCP also began to utilize and support traditional Chinese practitioners, denouncing Western medicine as imperialist. However, as Karen Minden and Kim Taylor have each noted, this policy was motivated by necessity, not only ideology: there were not enough modern physicians to serve this large rural area. The CCP set up short-term training programs for paramedical personnel, primarily traditional midwives or "young peasant boys" to establish medical cooperatives in their villages. One of the primary goals of the CCP rural health movement was to reduce infant mortality by training midwives in aseptic techniques, and by encouraging pregnant women to utilize trained midwives as their birth helpers. Anecdotal evidence suggests that CCP efforts did help to reduce maternal mortality rates in the Communist base region, although persuading women to become trained birth helpers, and to utilize such trained midwives, remained a difficult task (Minden 1979).

Maternal and Child Health in the People's Republic of China under Mao (1949–1976)

After the founding of the People's Republic of China (PRC) in 1949, improving maternal and infant health again became a national priority, though it was not at the top of the CCP's long list of improvements for the new nation. Combined with promoting "national physical culture," advancing maternal and infant health was notably included in the forty-eighth principle of the 1949 Chinese People's Political Consultative Conference (Zhongguo ren min zheng zhi 1949). Rather than relying on foreign philanthropy as Republican-era reformers had, the CCP worked with the national All-China Women's Federation and the Ministry of Health to establish a county-based public health system similar to the one begun during the Nationalist era.[2] In the early decades of the People's Republic, maternal and child health became explicitly politicized, as reproduction was targeted to fulfill national policy objectives. The PRC used maternal and child health efforts to improve the health of its people, to further national economic goals, and also to legitimate its rule by emancipating women from the dangers, and pain, of childbirth.

Beginning in 1949, the government implemented a two-tiered system of midwife instruction, similar to Marion Yang's program, to educate new, younger midwives as well as retrain traditional ones. The CCP, however, did not view traditional midwives as negatively as the Guomindang had. Instead, as in their rural outposts during the war, the CCP encouraged utilizing the experience and knowledge of traditional midwives, combined with a "new birth method" in order to improve the health of the population. This designated method was a series of aseptic procedures, largely for home births, that included washing hands, tying and packing the umbilical cord, and administering silver nitrate eye drops to prevent eye infections.

The new birth method was in fact not new at all, having begun in the 1920s at the First National Midwifery School. The curriculum and pedagogy of these PRC courses was also very similar to those used by the First National Midwifery School's old-style midwife retraining programs. Although they took place thirty years apart, both sets of courses focused on simple aseptic birth techniques, and both sought to generate support for modern midwifery by using scare tactics that utilized gruesome birthing stories and cited high maternal and infant mortality statistics among traditional births (Zhu 1949). Like their predecessors, the CCP government also had difficulties persuading women to enter public service as nurses and midwives. While the official rhetoric heralded these selfless women healers as builders of the new nation, in actuality the state glorified women's work as factory workers and toilers rather than health care workers (Goldstein 1998). As in the Republican era, national policies and local practices diverged considerably under the CCP.

The Chinese Ministry of Health at this time modeled its structure and programs on those of the Soviet Union. By the early 1950s, therefore, all formal undergraduate and post-secondary midwifery schools were closed, and secondary nursing and midwifery programs were eventually merged. In 1952 the PRC also began promoting the Soviet "psychoprophylactic painless childbirth method" that was to free women from the pain of childbirth without the use of chemical anesthesia or analgesia (Goldstein 1998). This psychoprophylactic method was a medical expression of the dominant political ideology: the CCP had liberated the Chinese people, and this freedom from oppression extended to women's birthing experiences. But while the party "liberated" women by granting them legal equality in the workplace and in the home, in reality these efforts fell short in many areas, not least with the promise of pain-free childbirth.

The Ministry of Health of the early 1950s was also decidedly pronatalist, as a socialist system was theoretically immune from Malthusian population pressures and food shortages. The ministry restricted access to contraception, especially sterilization and abortion (Greenhalgh and Winckler 2005). As the Guomindang had done in decades prior, PRC leaders targeted women in campaigns to encourage national motherhood that, according to Joshua Goldstein, "inject[ed] political incentives into domestic chores," making family life a measure of patriotic commitment (Goldstein 1998, 159). During the 1950s and 1960s, women were urged to be good mothers and housewives, creating healthy offspring and a clean and peaceful home, so that their husbands could in turn become more effective workers and producers. The pronatalist campaigns, however, were contradicted by the simultaneous calls for female labor and women's liberation from the shackles of patriarchal households and onerous housework (Manning 2006).

Initial ministry opposition to contraception gradually softened during the 1950s, though discussions of public health proved dangerous. In 1953, several female CCP members wrote to the All-China Women's Federation demanding contraception in order to participate in "socialist construction," and later, Mao Zedong publicly supported access to contraception at the 1958 Beidaihe conference (Greenhalgh and Winckler 2005). It was during this time, however, that Marion Yang was purged as a rightist for her support of demographer Ma Yin-chu, who had advocated limiting population growth via family planning and contraception (Lei 1990). Yang's political misstep resulted in her being erased from PRC history as the pioneer of modern birth practices; she was replaced by one of her former students and colleagues, Lin Qiaozhi (Khat'i Lim). Lin was deemed China's pioneer of maternal and child health, and she was appointed a longstanding member of the All-China Women's Federation and China's National People's Committee (Guo 1990). The way in which Yang was replaced by the more politically connected Lin Qiaozhi exemplifies the vagaries of politics and public health under the CCP.

After Mao accused the Chinese Ministry of Health of ministering only to 15 percent of China's population, referring to those with means and money to access health care, a new health care delivery system was implemented in 1965 (Lampton 1972). Rural cooperative medical systems and health centers were established nationwide, and training of paramedical personnel began in communes and brigades.[3] By this time, the PRC had attained the goal of one health center for each of the approximately two thousand counties nationwide (Lucas 1980). Like housing and food allotment, health care was controlled by one's work unit (*danwei*) and was managed by paramedical workers who covered many aspects of public health, including immunization, sanitation, and maternal and child health (Chen 1985a). Barefoot doctors and their counterparts in factories and urban areas, called Red Worker Doctors, Red Medical Workers, and Red Guard doctors, received instruction in modern techniques like prenatal screening, aseptic childbirth, postnatal care, family planning, and immunization. Midwives, often recruited from among traditional midwives, were (re)trained in three- to six-month courses to provide monthly or weekly prenatal examinations which, depending upon the parturient's condition, included blood pressure readings, urinalysis, estimating delivery date, auscultating fetal heartbeat, and determining fetal position (Sidel 1972). They were also taught to use aseptic birth techniques.

These paramedical workers were responsible for publicizing mass health campaigns and were especially important in propagating and recording contraception use. By the early 1980s, as China's family planning policies became more stringent, barefoot doctors were trained to perform vasectomies and female sterilization (Kane 1984; Greenhalgh and Winckler 2005). Paramedical workers also oversaw the implementation of national guidelines for protecting the health of mother and infant. Though policies differed by commune or brigade, after the fifth or seventh month of pregnancy women were assigned light work and shorter working days, and they received thirty to sixty-five days of maternity leave. Time off during the workday was given to breastfeeding mothers to feed their infants for the first twelve months (Hu and Zhang 1982).

The reproductive health programs of the CCP appear remarkably effective on paper, with drastic drops in infant and maternal mortality rates. According to Lin Qiaozhi, China's maternal and child health policies resulted in lower maternal and infant mortality rates nationwide, as by 1959 approximately 60 percent of rural births were attended by trained health workers; that number was 95 percent in large cities (Lim 1959). While such statistics are impossible to verify, there was undoubtedly unprecedented improvement in the overall health of the then six hundred million Chinese between 1950 and 1965 (Sidel and Sidel 1977). By 1980, the national infant mortality rate was estimated at fifty-six per one thousand, a considerable drop from the much higher rates of just two decades before. But a national survey in the mid-1970s revealed that age-specific death rates were still higher for women than for men in the twenty-five to thirty-five (childbearing) age group, reflecting sustained risk of maternal death (Kane 1984).

Shifting political goals continued to affect the delivery of health care, especially in rural areas. During the early People's Republic the new childbirth methods were largely resisted by the midwives themselves and the public they were meant to serve. Gail Hershatter's interviews of rural women in Shanxi Province in the 1990s and Li Xiaojiang's interviews of rural women in Henan and Yunnan Provinces, many of them of minority ethnicities, illustrate both the broad diversity of birth practices and the limited reach of the state (Hershatter 2008; Lai 2003). Despite the state rhetoric and the policies aimed at reforming midwives, few women utilized the state's orthodox procedures. Instead, they continued their longstanding local traditional customs regarding childbirth, even though Cultural Revolution proscriptions against Chinese superstition and religious practices circumscribed women's access to fertility deities like Guanyin. A three-year study completed in 1953 showed that only 5 to 10 percent of women availed themselves of the new birth method, a marked difference from the official figures (Zhonghua quanguo minzhu funü 1953). Interviewees also recalled that discussing personal issues like childbirth in public was considered offensive and crazy. Even among the midwifery students, detailed clinical diagrams of internal and external organs induced embarrassment and disgust (Goldstein 1998).

Nevertheless, these experiences show that childbirth in the Maoist era was colored by a continuation of Chinese state efforts to manage human biology, and by the creation of frameworks for more extensive efforts to manage the population, whether by increasing or decreasing it, or by generally improving its health. Early CCP campaigns demanded compliance with the new policies, beginning with the "one pregnancy, one live birth; one live birth, one healthy child" movement in the 1950s, and continuing in the early 1970s with the "later, longer, fewer" campaign that exhorted people to marry later, space children several years apart, and have fewer children (Chen 1985; Davin 1985). In this way, reproduction practices in the Maoist era were politically and ideologically nationalized through medical discourse.

Maternal and Child Health in the Reform Period (1978–Present)

Economic growth since 1978 has engendered a commoditized, commercialized economy of childbirth, and the resources that people can draw on to protect maternal and child health are greater than ever. Because most couples are limited to one child, they also invest heavily in the outcome of pregnancy (Johnson 2011). Modernized fertility clinics and hospitals boast state-of-the-art equipment, while other businesses offer a welter of products, paraphernalia, and services to help women "educate the fetus" or "do the month." The relaxation of Maoist ideology has also enabled the resurgence of popular and folk religion, including the veneration of female deities with the power to confer sons and cure pediatric illnesses (Fan 2003; Law 2005; Chau 2008).

The Ministry of Health, along with other government agencies, has initiated multifaceted campaigns to promote maternal and child health, with impressive results. From 1991 to 2004, the maternal mortality rate dropped from eighty to forty-eight per hundred thousand, and the mortality rate for children under five dropped from sixty-one to twenty-five per one thousand (Ministry of Health et al. 2006). China is a signatory to the United Nation's Millennium Development Goals to reduce maternal and infant mortality, and it appears that it will meet the targets with respect to infant mortality (Rudan et al. 2010). But China's overall rate of maternal and infant mortality is still higher than that of other countries with comparable levels of economic development. Researchers both inside and outside China have attributed this to a number of systemic challenges, rooted both in history and in the unintended consequences of China's economic reform policies.

First, China's prodigious economic growth has been unevenly distributed, exacerbating historical inequities between richer, coastal, and urban areas, on the one hand, and poorer, interior, and rural areas on the other. Because China's minority ethnic groups tend to reside in more inland, rural, and remote geographical areas, these inequities also manifest themselves as ethnic disparities. Simultaneously, the privatization of the health care system has intensified these inequities (Blumenthal and Hsiao 2005). During the 1980s, the Maoist commune system was dismantled, essentially eliminating the rural safety net. The central government also sharply reduced its funding for state hospitals and clinics, and the responsibility for funding them devolved to local governments. Poorer locales soon fell behind. Furthermore, the health care system became profit-driven: while physicians were required to provide standard medical care at state-determined prices, they were allowed to freely generate revenue on new technologies, procedures, and drugs. Economic reforms have thus weakened incentives to provide primary care and preventive services, including in the area of maternal and child health (Ministry of Health et al. 2006).

The resultant disparities in access to maternal and infant health care are evidenced in the vast differences in the maternal and infant mortality rates in different regions: in 2004, the rural mortality rates were 3.2 times higher than urban ones (Ministry of Health et al. 2006). The disparity is especially troubling because an estimated 75 percent of maternal and infant mortality is attributable to "avoidable deaths" that would not have occurred if the woman had had access to the necessary medical care (Ministry of Health et al. 2006). Unfortunately, lower-tier hospitals often do not have the equipment or personnel needed to manage obstetrical emergencies, and obtaining proper care can be logistically daunting for rural women (Gao et al. 2010). Current mortality rates also reflect inequities within urban areas, where migrant workers who have left their officially registered homes in the countryside have no right to access social services in the cities where they work and reside (Ministry of Health et al. 2006).

The intensifying medicalization of childbirth has also had negative consequences. Since 1995, a key Chinese government strategy for reducing maternal mortality has been to increase the percentage of births taking place in hospitals (Harris et al. 2007). The current government target is to raise rates of hospital delivery by the year 2015 to 80 percent in poor western regions, and 95 percent in the developed east (ZRGGW 2009). Alongside a host of incentives meant to encourage hospitals births, the government has actively sought to eliminate the practice of home births (Cheung et al. 2005; Gao et al. 2010; *China Daily* 2011). In the mid-1990s, midwife training programs were discontinued, and the Chinese press portrays midwife-attended home births as a backward, rural custom whose rapid disappearance is cause for congratulations (*People's Daily* 2001; *People's Daily* 2002). While hospitals may still have "midwives" on staff (including some trained prior to the mid-1990s) most are more properly described as labor and delivery room nurses with obstetrical training (Cheung et al. 2005; Cheung et al. 2009; Harris et al. 2009).

While such policies have indeed reduced the nationwide maternal and infant mortality rates (Liang et al. 2012; Liu, Yan, and Wang 2010), the limitations of this hospital-based strategy are also apparent. The lack of resources in lower-tier rural hospitals means the quality of obstetrical care is highly uneven. One study, for example, found that higher rates of hospital delivery in midwestern China led to a decrease in maternal deaths from obstetric hemorrhage, but an increase in deaths from infection (Liang et al. 2012). Furthermore, hospital births often include interventions that are unnecessary or that carry the potential for complications (Johnson 2011). In particular, the rates of caesarean section in China have increased dramatically, with one study estimating that C-section rates have quadrupled over the past three decades (Guo et al. 2007). While statistics vary, it is not uncommon for reported rates of C-section in urban hospitals to be well over 60 percent, with some as high as 80 percent (Wang et al. 2010). Some of this increase can be attributed to higher rates of hospital births and access to surgical technology. But research indicates that these increases are primarily driven by a growth in elective C-sections (Wang et al. 2010). Women who request C-sections see them as preferable to vaginal delivery, for reasons that include a desire to avoid pain or potential complications in labor, the desire to give birth at an auspicious time, and the belief that C-sections produce a more attractive and smarter child and that they result in less damage to the woman's figure and pelvic floor (Harris et al. 2007; Guo et al. 2007). Doctors are also willing to perform them because C-sections are more profitable than vaginal deliveries (Harris et al. 2007). However, C-sections also carry real risks for maternal and infant health (Wang et al. 2010; Lumbiganon et al. 2010).

Meanwhile, the focus on hospital births has led to a dearth of midwives. The result is that rural women with inadequate access to hospitals also lack access to other trained birth attendants. Health care professionals and policymakers have therefore called for more resources to be devoted to midwifery and the management of normal births (Hoekman 2010; Mander et al. 2010). Consumer demand for a more satisfying birthing experience may also eventually play a part in modifying practices. In the late 1990s, for example, hospitals from Inner Mongolia to Shanghai began offering "doula" (*daole*) services for women who wished to have one-on-one care during labor. The concept originated in Europe, where doulas are lay women who support the mother during labor and/or the postpartum period. An association with Western modernity has helped to make doulas popular in China. However, a recent study at a Shanghai maternity hospital found that its doulas were former or current obstetrical nurses and labor and delivery room midwives (Cheung 2005). For the moment, therefore, the woman-centered doula culture of the West is simply another form of hospital-based care in China.

Family Planning Policies and MCH

From 1978 to 1980, the Chinese leadership implemented increasingly restrictive regulations on childbearing, culminating in the codified, official policy that each couple would be allowed to have only one child, with very few exceptions (Greenhalgh 2008, 31–33). In a marked contrast with the pronatalist, anti-Malthusian orthodoxy of the early PRC, family planning advocates now argued that China could not develop economically if its huge population ate up its resources and inhibited its growth. The new Chinese Constitution adopted in 1982 subsequently affirmed that "the state promotes family planning so that population growth may fit the plans for economic and social development." To enforce these policies, officials deploy punitive bureaucratic measures, such as fines. But enforcement efforts have also included coercive measures such as forced abortion and sterilization, which while officially condemned are nonetheless used. Beyond the potential damage to women's health, the family planning policy has intensified historical tendencies to discriminate against female infants. China's sex ratio at birth (SRB) has increased continuously since 1982, and was estimated to be 120.5 overall in 2005 (the normal SRB is 106). Concurrently, there are high rates of excessive female mortality in children aged zero to four (Li 2007). As a result, China is estimated to have millions of "missing girls" (estimated at 40.9 million according to the 2000 census), namely, girls whom one would expect to be there, given normal SRBs and rates of infant mortality. Furthermore, SRB and rates of excess female infant mortality both increase sharply as birth order increases (Chen, Xie, and Liu 2007; Wu et al. 2003). In other words, parents whose first child is a girl are taking steps to maximize the possibility that subsequent births (or surviving children) are male, including the (illegal) use of sex-selective abortions. While Chinese government reports do not openly discuss the gendered effect of the one-child policy per se, they do point out that discrimination against girls is a major impediment to improving the infant and child mortality rate (Ministry of Health et al. 2006). The government has been enacting measures to mitigate discrimination against girls, including a recent crackdown on sex-selective abortions (*China Daily* 2012b). Chinese policymakers and social scientists have also been debating the future of the birth limitation policies, and the Chinese government recently confirmed that provincial officials are considering a relaxation of the one-child policy restrictions for urban couples (Greenhalgh 2008; National People's Congress 2011).

Finally, there is some evidence that women with unauthorized pregnancies may be less likely to use prenatal services or seek hospital births. Some of this is because excess births are most common in rural areas, where son preference is strongest and access to care is lowest. But some studies also suggest that women may avoid health care to avoid attracting official attention. Furthermore, because they do not receive state financial assistance for out-of-quota births, they may forego health care because it is too expensive (Klemetti et al. 2011). It thus appears that state family planning policies influence families' cost-benefit calculations as they decide whether to use prenatal or obstetrical care, and what level of care to give girl or boy babies.

Future Trends and Strategies

As in earlier eras, China today faces the challenge of caring for a huge and diverse population distributed over a vast land mass, a population that variously draws on healing methods ranging from folk religion to biomedical surgery. Furthermore, it is clear that the innate distortions of the current Chinese health care system will not resolve themselves. Thus, like their Nationalist- and Mao-era predecessors, today's leaders agree that state activism is crucial for continued improvements to maternal and child health (Ministry of Health et al. 2006). In particular, further reductions in maternal and infant mortality will require a reduction of socioeconomic inequality. For example, maternal education levels affect infant mortality rates, because educated women are more likely to employ health care services (Song and Burgard 2011; United Nations 2011). Similarly, inadequate access to prenatal care and worsening environmental pollution have been identified as factors contributing to a reported 70.9 percent increase in birth defects in China from 1996 to 2010 (Ministry of Health 2011a; *China Daily* 2012a). Besides increasing the availability of medical technology, therefore, China will also require broader reforms.

Chinese policymakers and health care professionals recognize the complexity of the problem, and they are actively seeking solutions. China's drive to build world-class scientific and educational institutions has enabled the creation of modernized systems of health data collection, dissemination, and analysis, thereby further facilitating information exchange and meta-analytical studies (Rudan et al. 2010). Interested Chinese parties also regularly collaborate with international researchers, agencies, and NGOs, and they are fully aware of global trends. As with any nation, however, China's ability to enact the needed reforms will depend on its ability to muster the necessary political will, financial means, and human resources. Its future successes or failures will matter not only to the nine hundred million or so women and children in China, but to the global community as well.

Notes

1. This section is taken largely from Tina Phillips Johnson, "National Reproduction in Republican China," chap. 4 of *Childbirth in Republican China: Delivering Modernity* (Lanham, MD: Lexington Books, 2011), with the permission of the publisher.
2. The China Medical Board was compelled to leave China in 1951, and PUMC and its affiliated organizations were placed under Chinese government control.
3. The first cooperative medical system was established in Union Commune, Henan, in 1955, with brigade health auxiliaries called barefoot doctors. These programs went nationwide in 1965. (See chapter 13 in this volume.)

4 Tobacco Smoking and Health in Twentieth-Century China

Carol Benedict

TOBACCO SMOKING HAS been pervasive in China for more than three hundred years. Introduced into East Asia from the Americas by the Spanish and Portuguese in the sixteenth century, tobacco quickly became a commercial crop grown along the South China seaboard. By the 1680s, when the conquering Qing dynasty finally consolidated its hold over China, tobacco cultivation was underway throughout much of the empire. For most of the Qing period (1644–1911), tobacco in the form of snuff or pipe tobacco was widely used in China by both men and women of all ages and social classes.

We now know what some Chinese physicians perceived as early as the seventeenth century: tobacco in any form is hazardous to health. The human cost of tobacco smoking and snuffing in late imperial China must have been great even if, in the absence of quantitative data, we cannot know tobacco's exact impact on Chinese morbidity or mortality before 1900 or even before 1950 or so. In the late nineteenth century, however, a particularly deadly form of tobacco—the manufactured cigarette—began to be sold in China. Machine-rolled cigarettes, filled with easily inhalable "bright" tobacco, were immediately popular in China just as they were elsewhere around the world. The Chinese cigarette market expanded spectacularly, with sales rising from about three hundred million sticks sold in 1900 to over eighty billion in 1937 (Cox 2000, 17). Still, China was a relatively poor country at the time and many smokers preferred locally produced pipe tobacco to more expensive cigarettes. As a result the per capita consumption of cigarettes in China remained relatively low before 1949, thereby muting somewhat the adverse health effects of cigarette smoke for many in the population, especially those who lived in the countryside.

After 1949, the newly established People's Republic of China greatly expanded the Chinese tobacco industry, making cigarettes more available and more affordable than ever before. As a consequence, there was an unprecedented increase in Chinese cigarette consumption between the 1950s and 1970s and an even more dramatic increase after 1978. The upsurge in cigarette smoking since 1978 has led to a sharp rise in smoking-related death and disease. More than three hundred million Chinese citizens currently smoke, constituting one-third of all smokers worldwide. Already one million deaths occur each year due to tobacco, and the annual number is projected to rise to about three million per year by 2050 (Peto, Chen, and Boreham 2009, 68). China is only in the early stages of a looming health crisis caused by cigarettes that will continue for many decades to come.

This chapter surveys the history of smoking and health in China over the course of the twentieth century. Organized roughly along chronological lines, it follows two interwoven thematic strands to make its central arguments. One theme concerns dramatic changes in tobacco usage that in the post-1949 period gave rise to China's current epidemic of smoking-related morbidity and mortality. A second theme addresses twentieth-century transformations in Chinese ideas about tobacco's physiological effects and the emergence of two distinct anti-smoking movements that sought to curtail cigarette use in China—one at the beginning of the century and the other at century's end. Like the popularization of the cigarette itself and the consequent surge in smoking-attributable disease, changes in Chinese medical thinking about tobacco occurred within a broader global context. The two movements to control tobacco were not unique to China but paralleled similar efforts underway in other countries. Although many Chinese and Western physicians recognized tobacco's harms before 1900, scientific confirmation that tobacco is deadly emerged only gradually as the century progressed. An international consensus to this effect did not form until the 1950s. In the first half of the twentieth century, opponents of tobacco in China utilized semiscientific medical arguments against cigarette smoking but theirs was fundamentally a moral and political crusade, not a public health campaign. In our own times, tobacco control efforts in China, like those elsewhere, are directed primarily at educating the public about the scientifically proven health hazards of smoking. Despite these important differences, a unifying thread linking these past and present anti-smoking movements is the conviction that a smoke-free society is a vital prerequisite for China's national strength and economic prosperity.

Chinese and Euro-American Conceptions of Tobacco and Health, circa 1900

In the early twentieth century, Chinese medical ideas about tobacco were in flux. Prior to 1900, many Chinese doctors working in the classical tradition recognized that excessive smoking could be harmful but they also believed tobacco could be a potent and beneficial medicine. From the 1620s on, those who wrote about tobacco consistently included cautionary notes about its potential dangers as well as recommendations for its medicinal use. Zhang Jiebin (1563–1640), a famous physician of the late Ming period and one of the first authors to mention tobacco, believed that it protected against a host of ailments, including malaria. But Zhang also warned that when used over a long period of time, tobacco could do grave bodily harm. He concluded, "People all like to use it but they do not yet see its damaging effects" (Zhang 1994 [1636], 639).

The fact that Chinese physicians recognized tobacco's hazards facilitated acceptance of Western chemical knowledge of nicotine and its negative health effects in the twentieth century. Articles using scientific terminology to discourage tobacco use on health grounds began to appear in Chinese newspapers in the 1890s and were published sporadically throughout the last decade of Qing rule (Liu 2009a, 2, 42–43). Although clearly influenced by Western medicine, these commentaries retained the flexible Chinese classificatory scheme that allowed tobacco to be both a powerful medicine and a toxic drug at the same time.

At the time there was as yet no consensus in Western medical circles about smoking's physiological effects. German scientists had established in 1828 that tobacco contained nicotine but this discovery actually stimulated interest in tobacco's potential therapeutic benefits. In part, the absence of a solid epidemiological framework impeded nineteenth-century doctors from recognizing tobacco's lethality: lung cancer, the first disease to be reliably linked to smoking, was rare before 1900. Some Victorian physicians were aware that pipe smoking caused mouth cancers but the first hypothesis that smoking contributed to lung cancer appeared only in 1898 and the first textbook mention of a possible correlation came only in 1912 (Proctor 2011, 18).

Given that many Western physicians at the turn of the twentieth century regarded moderate tobacco use as a relatively benign habit, it is hardly surprising that foreign doctors practicing in China also disagreed about smoking's effects. Some believed that tobacco smoke warded off malaria while others thought it exacerbated the deleterious effects of tropical climates on Euro-American bodies (Li 2010c, 114). Those who looked beyond the health of the foreign community to consider tobacco's impact on the Chinese population believed pipe smoking and snuffing, the predominant modes in use in China at the time, were relatively harmless. William H. Jeffreys and James Maxwell, authors of an early survey of disease in China, for example, believed that pipe smoking posed few health risks because "native tobacco is mild," although they predicted that the introduction of cigarettes would "change the conditions speedily" (Jeffreys and Maxwell 1911, 662).

The Anti–Juvenile Smoking Movement, 1890–1911

Jeffreys and Maxwell were correct in their assumption that cigarettes posed unprecedented health risks for Chinese smokers. Tobacco use had been prevalent in

China for centuries, but increased consumption of combustible cigarettes filled with flue-cured tobacco made smoking much more deadly. Prior to the introduction of manufactured cigarettes in the 1890s, all tobacco sold in China was either sun- or air-cured, processes that resulted in tobacco too harsh to inhale. Flue-curing, a method only developed in the United States in the 1830s, made tobacco smoke far less alkaline and therefore mild enough to draw deeply into the lungs (Proctor 2011, 31–35). After cigarette manufacturers began blending "bright" flue-cured Virginia leaf with Turkish burley leaf in the years just before and after World War I, the resulting smoother draw made easily inhalable cigarettes popular around the world.

By the 1920s, physicians in Europe and the United States began to notice a dramatic rise in lung cancer and some began to suspect a causal relationship between cigarette smoke and lung tumors (Proctor 2011, 150–151). This trend was particularly striking in countries such as the United States where cigarette smoking was widespread throughout the entire population, not just in urbanized areas along the coast as was the case in China. By the 1950s, an international consensus had formed among scientists that cigarette smoking was indeed a cause of cancer and other serious diseases.

In the early 1900s, decades before the devastating physiological effects of inhalable cigarette smoke were scientifically confirmed, anti-smoking activists in China, influenced by the international temperance movement, agitated for the abolition of cigarettes altogether. Like their counterparts elsewhere, these crusaders blended semiscientific knowledge—some evidence-based and some not—with moralizing rhetoric to advance their cause. Emerging within the context of the "new" imperialism characteristic of the late nineteenth century and influenced by the fresh intellectual currents of social Darwinism and eugenics, those opposed to tobacco tended to focus on the dangers that smoking represented not just for the individual smoker but for the Chinese nation as a whole. As in the United States and England, where the fin-de-siècle anti-cigarette movement got its start, Chinese reformers initially concentrated on eradicating smoking among juveniles, the group whose "physical deterioration," it was believed, placed the nation's collective health most at risk.

The specter of national degeneration brought about by cigarette-smoking youth in China first appeared in a set of translated physiology primers based on a curricular series sanctioned by the American Woman's Christian Temperance Union (WCTU) and used in the United States as part of an educational movement known as Scientific Temperance Instruction (STI) (Rogaski 2004, 120). These textbooks, designed for young children, identified alcohol and tobacco as the cause not only of ill health but of a host of social problems as well. They warned boys and girls not to smoke cigarettes on the basis that doing so would cause severe physical and mental deterioration, leading to delinquency.

Several STI texts, with their strong anti-tobacco message, were among the first science books translated from English into Chinese by John Fryer (1839–1928). Fryer was the premier translator of Western books for the Jiangnan Arsenal, one of the Qing dynasty's key institutions for military modernization in the late nineteenth century and an important gateway for the importation of Western scientific knowledge (Rogaski 2004, 109). Faithful to the original American schoolbooks, the translated primers linked juvenile smoking to delinquency, criminality, and moral degeneration (Hunt and Fryer 1893; Kellogg and Fryer 1896). Cigarettes were not blamed for all of China's woes—pride of place in that regard was given to opium—but they were singled out as a particularly pernicious poison for young people because they were said to inhibit proper skeletal, muscular, and brain development. The texts stressed that boys and girls who smoked would grow up deformed, depraved, ignorant, and totally incapable of serving the nation in adulthood, leaving China vulnerable to foreign incursion. For Chinese readers, this connection between smoking and national weakness was further emphasized by continual references to the "civilized" Western countries where anti–juvenile smoking legislation had already been passed (Kellogg and Fryer 1896, 50a, 60a).

Although highly controversial back home and not at all welcomed by many American educators, these books entered China with the "authority of Western science" and "the promise of enlightened governance," both of which were inordinately attractive to reform-minded Chinese intellectuals at the time (Rogaski 2004, 123–124). For example, in his commentary on the translated STI texts the influential political thinker Liang Qichao (1873–1929) placed the practice of personal hygiene, including abstention from tobacco, within the context of China's subjugation to imperialist powers. The connections between nonsmoking and the health of the nation continued to resonate for many physicians and social reformers throughout the twentieth century.

Several well-known Chinese doctors appropriated STI rhetoric into their own writings on tobacco. For example, Ding Fubao (1874–1952) and Yu Fengbin (1884–1930) both strongly opposed juvenile smoking. Ding, the classically trained scholar who made a name for himself as a translator of Western medical texts, denounced cigarette smoking among young people using language highly reminiscent of STI literature. In a hygiene primer published in 1903, Ding wrote, "If they [children] smoke cigarettes, then their bodies cannot grow strong. Their muscles will become soft and pliable and without strength they will not be able to move. They will not become skilled workers." Ding further underscored the importance of passing anti–juvenile smoking laws, pointing to Germany and Japan as models (Ding 1903, 19–22). Yu, a 1907 graduate of the medical school of St. John's University, a founding editor of the *National Medical Journal of China*, and eventual president of the Chinese Medical Association, promoted an explicitly eugenic agenda focused on the causal relationship between marriage and family hygiene. He warned against early marriage, arguing that having children too young would result in a sickly family and by extension a degenerating nation. Yu implored young people to protect future generations by refraining from the "race poison" of cigarette smoke (Yu 1930, 24).

In its waning years, the Qing dynasty promulgated its own regulations against juvenile smoking, prompted in part by the example of Japan, which passed an anti–juvenile smoking law in 1902. In 1907, the Qing Ministry of Education declared that students were forbidden to smoke because smoking "is not hygienic" (Liu 1998, 546). The following year, the Chinese imperial government ordered a ban on smoking among those under sixteen and also made it illegal to sell cigarettes to anyone under that age (Liu 1998, 544). After the collapse of the Qing in 1911, successive Republican-era regimes passed regulations aimed at reducing smoking among juveniles, although such legislation was not generally enforced.

Late Qing–Early Republican Anti-Cigarette Campaigns, 1910–1912

In the years just before and after the 1911 revolution, inspired by similar organizations established abroad, activists set up anti-cigarette societies in China. Some were sponsored by organizations such as the World Woman's Christian Temperance Union (WWCTU) or the Young Men's Christian Association (YMCA) (Liu 2009a, 80). Several foreign missionaries took up the eradication of cigarettes in China as personal crusades. Sarah Boardman Clapp Goodrich (1855–1923), for example, who became director of the Chinese branch of the WWCTU in 1910, launched an attack on the British American Tobacco Company and its stated goal of putting a "cigarette in the mouth of every man, woman, and child in China" (Benedict 2011, 216–217). Partially through her efforts, women's anti-cigarette associations, modeled on the American Anti-Cigarette League, were established in Beijing, Tianjin, and Shanghai (Liu 2009a, 75, 77–78). Edward Waite Thwing (1867–1943), a Presbyterian minister based in Tianjin, wrote a series of anti-cigarette articles that appeared in *Dagong bao* from January to July 1910, including a discussion of smoking's physiological harms (Liu 2009a, 27). In line with the dominant discourse of the times, he focused on juvenile smoking and the detrimental effects it had on a nation's preparedness for war, citing J. W. Seaver's study of Yale University students to underscore that smoking hindered youth development (Liu 2009a, 44). Although this study and others like it lacked scientific rigor, it was widely cited in temperance literature at the time.

Foreign missionaries were not the only ones concerned about the dangers of smoking for Chinese youth. In the period between 1900 and 1937, Chinese officials, progressive intellectuals, and social feminists concerned about China's future also took up the crusade against cigarettes. One well-known Chinese personality who got involved in the anti-smoking cause was the statesman Wu Tingfang (1842–1922). Wu, who studied law in England, was twice tapped by the Qing dynasty to serve as minister to the United States, Mexico, Peru, and Cuba. Upon his return to Shanghai from the United States in the spring of 1910, Wu declined any further governmental service and instead turned his attention to social issues, albeit ones with political overtones. Soon after his return, he took over as head of the Shanghai Anti-Cigarette Smoking Society, which was established in 1908 but did not achieve prominence until Wu reorganized it in the spring of 1911.

The society, which at its height had about three hundred members, was the largest anti-tobacco organization in China at the time. Its officers included some of the most influential figures in Shanghai political and business circles. Beginning in June 1911 and continuing into 1912, the organization prodded major Shanghai newspapers to print articles and editorial cartoons that highlighted the medical, moral, and economic harms of smoking. It also held public meetings to reach a broader audience, such as the one held on July 11, 1911, where a famous opera singer performed anti-cigarette songs before one thousand spectators (Liu 2009a, 103–114, 269–273).

Physicians Ding Fubao and Yu Fengbin, also members of the society, wrote numerous newspaper articles about the health hazards of smoking. For example, in an essay that appeared in *Shenbao* in May 1911, Ding stated that smoking "weakens the heart, contaminates the lungs, over-stimulates the digestive system, overburdens the kidneys, poisons the optic nerves, and enervates the brain" (Liu 2009a, 119). In a similar *Shibao* piece, Yu Fengbin described tobacco as a poison with "one hundred harms" and "absolutely no benefits" (Liu 2009a, 120). These articles, by stressing only the detrimental health effects of smoking rather than balancing harms with benefits, represented a clear break from classical Chinese medical ideas about tobacco.

Tobacco and Health in the 1930s New Life Movement

The critical discourse that regarded the elimination of cigarettes as an essential element in the construction of a hygienically modern nation was given concrete form as public policy during the New Life Movement of the 1930s. The New Life Movement fundamentally sought to mobilize the population to improve personal habits and public hygiene in order to strengthen China. Although ridiculed by many, the Nationalist government's efforts to transform the bodily habits of its citizens reflected the power of the "hygienic modernity" ideal for China's leaders in the early twentieth century (Rogaski 2004, 238). The ideological foundations of the New Life Movement mixed selective elements from Confucian morality with Protestant notions of disciplining the spirit through asceticism, and views of the supremacy of the state with the values of military discipline and order. Yet at its core was the idea, brought forward from the early twentieth century, that the "degeneration" of the Chinese "race" was the fundamental reason for China's national crisis (Dirlik 1975, 954–955).

Cigarette smoking was a target of the New Life Movement from the outset. While the Nationalist regime never attempted to stop cigarette production—the tax revenues generated from cigarette sales were too lucrative for that course of action—they did make efforts to curb cigarette use during the 1930s. Jiang Jieshi (Chiang Kai-shek, 1887–1975), leader of the Nationalist Party and the primary author of the New Life program, had a reputation as a nonsmoker although his American-educated wife, Song Meiling (1897–2003), famously smoked until shortly before her death at age 105. Jiang himself viewed smoking as one of the many vices that degraded China. From his perspective, smoking a cigarette in public was not only "undesirable and slovenly," but it, along with other behaviors such as indiscriminate spitting, undermined the essential project of national regeneration (Dirlik 1975, 950). "No smoking" was one of the ninety-six specific rules listed in the official movement handbook. On paper at least, throughout the 1930s, workplaces and public venues were to be made smoke-free.

Jiang highlighted cigarettes prominently in his inaugural address launching the New Life Movement on February 19, 1934. Echoing the late Qing efforts to stem juvenile smoking, Jiang explained how an incident a few days earlier had refocused his resolve to initiate a "movement to achieve a new life." After seeing a boy smoking a cigarette on the streets of Nanchang, Jiang said, he imagined how the boy would likely grow up to become an opium addict (Jiang 1975 [1934], 18). Jiang lamented that this kind of behavior was one of the main causes of China's inability to defend itself against foreign aggression.

Jiang's call for a nationwide end to smoking initiated a wave of anti-cigarette activism in many local communities, especially in the spring of 1934. Some branches of the Chinese WCTU organized anti-cigarette rallies as part of the New Life Movement. The YMCA and the Boy Scouts did the same. In some communities, the new regulations against smoking were taken as a sign that the government was prepared to back up civic activities already underway, such as boycotts of stores that sold cigarettes (Yang 2002, 905–907). In other counties, government officials took the lead in carrying out the anti-smoking mandate: some county executives prohibited cigarette smoking outright and even closed down shops that sold them. Soldiers and students patrolled the streets of some towns, insisting that smokers extinguish their cigarettes (Yang 2002, 908).

Chinese women who smoked were particularly singled out during the New Life campaign. It was around this time that cigarettes came to be associated with a particularly stigmatized type of "new woman" known as the "Modern Girl." Portrayed in popular culture and political rhetoric alike as hypersexualized, apolitical, and extravagant, the cigarette-smoking Modern Girl increasingly came to signify bourgeois decadence and insufficient national loyalty. These associations came forward after 1949, and served to make smoking by women a highly disreputable practice in the second half of the twentieth century (Benedict 2011, 222–239).

Association of cigarettes with the Modern Girl in the 1930s denormalized female tobacco smoking to the point that smoking prevalence (of both pipe tobacco and cigarettes) among women began to decline at mid-century. A recent birth cohort analysis finds that over 25 percent of Chinese rural women born between 1908 and 1912, who would have come of age in the 1930s, smoked tobacco (at ages fifty to fifty-four) but that smoking declined among subsequent cohorts (Hermalin and Lowry 2010, 9). By 1949, prevalence rates among women had greatly diminished. In the 1950s and 1960s, these rates sharply declined: whereas the proportion of women who smoked before age twenty-five was 10 percent for all urban women born before 1940, it was only 1 percent for those born between 1950 and 1964 (Liu et al. 1998). In contrast, smoking prevalence among men remained consistently high, with roughly seven men out of ten using tobacco at peak ages of consumption across the entire twentieth century (Hermalin and Lowry 2010, 12).

Changing Patterns of Chinese Tobacco Use and Anti-Smoking Activities, 1949–1976

Anti-cigarette campaigns in the first half of the twentieth century did little to reduce tobacco consumption, at least among men. But before 1949, relatively few Chinese men (and even fewer Chinese women) smoked cigarettes. Most smokers, especially those in rural areas, continued to smoke far less expensive pipe tobacco. Given that 80 percent of the population resided in the countryside, relatively low rates of rural cigarette consumption continued to keep national per capita consumption figures down even as cigarette sales in the aggregate soared. In 1931, the Nationalist government estimated that Chinese smokers annually consumed only two hundred sticks per capita, or half a cigarette per day (Lee 1934, 37). By contrast, U.S. cigarette consumption in 1931 was about 2.5 cigarettes per adult per day (U.S. CDC 2009). By 1950, mean U.S. cigarette consumption per adult was 10 per day but it was only 1 per Chinese adult per day in 1952 (Zhang and Cai 2003, 17).

The ascendency of the manufactured cigarette in China as an item of mass consumption in the countryside as well as in urban areas occurred largely as a result of economic policies and developmental strategies pursued by the Chinese government after 1949. After taking power, the Chinese Communist Party committed fully to building up the Chinese tobacco industry because tobacco cultivation and cigarette manufacturing supported peasant livelihoods, created factory jobs, and, as in the Republican era, generated significant tax revenue. In

1952, the CCP nationalized all tobacco companies and then deliberately boosted the overall supply of cigarettes by encouraging local production of tobacco leaf and establishing new cigarette factories in the interior. Notwithstanding annual fluctuations and more extended periods during the 1960s when production stagnated or declined, total domestic annual production of Chinese cigarettes grew from 80 billion in 1949 to 238 billion in 1958 and 392 billion in 1970 (Yang 2008, 17; Li, Hsia, and Yang 2011, 2469). Still, rural sales of cigarettes remained low throughout the Maoist period, largely due to continued lack of purchasing power on the part of farmers.

As the CCP was ramping up production of manufactured cigarettes in the 1950s, a new international scientific consensus about the deadliness of cigarettes was emerging overseas (Proctor 2011, 224–235). Building upon decades of underrecognized research, particularly that pioneered by German scientists in the 1930s and 1940s, English and American epidemiologists definitively established a link between smoking and lung cancer in the 1950s. This led in turn to the release in January 1964 of the U.S. surgeon general's report, the first declaration by an American official that cigarette smoking could be deadly. The flood of scientific studies on the hazards of smoking conducted since 1964 led many governments to regulate tobacco. In China, however, little was done in the way of tobacco control before the 1980s.

Chinese medical experts were not unaware of the mounting evidence linking smoking to disease in the 1950s and 1960s. Dr. Weng Xinzhi, often identified as the "father" of China's contemporary anti-tobacco movement, learned of the surgeon general's report soon after its publication. He credits it with having a catalyzing effect on his activism, which began in the late 1970s. According to Weng, virtually no one in China agitated publicly against tobacco prior to Mao Zedong's death in 1976 (Kohrman 2007, 90n19). Some tentative research on the relationship between lung cancer and cigarette smoking was carried out in China under the auspices of the Ministry of Health during the late 1950s as part of a broader research project on diseases of the respiratory system (Chen 1961, 168). These early studies found an increased incidence of lung cancer in China but concluded that cigarette smoking was only one among several contributing factors. The Cultural Revolution (1966–1976) brought such research to a halt, and it only gradually picked up again after 1978 when Deng Xiaoping's regime began reemphasizing science and technology as key to the success of China's economic reforms.

While Mao was still alive, specialists such as Weng Xinzhi who opposed tobacco on medical grounds not only had to contend with state policies that promoted smoking as essential for economic development, but they were also faced with powerful Chinese leaders, most famously Mao Zedong himself, who remained skeptical of smoking's harms. Mao was a lifelong chain-smoker who made no effort to conceal his habit from view. Indeed, he frequently called attention to himself as a smoker by lighting up when meeting with foreign dignitaries. At a party celebrating the eightieth birthday of Anna Louise Strong (1885–1970) hosted by Mao on the eve of the Cultural Revolution in November 1965, the chairman asked his foreign guests to raise their hands if they smoked: "The doctors say I should not smoke: I say I do. How many of you people smoke?" Mao, seeing that he was outvoted in the smoker poll, laughed and commented, "Well, it seems that in this too I'm in the minority." He went on to say, "Nevertheless I shall smoke and urge you to also." Beyond the subtle signals Mao was sending Chinese officials in attendance with this seemingly offhand yet politically loaded comment, his words reveal a certain nonchalance about his own health as well as that of others (Porter 1997, 252). On the other hand, Mao's personal physician, Li Zhisui, reports that Mao on occasion used cigarette holders because he believed they filtered out nicotine (Li and Thurston 1996, 67–68).

Whatever Mao's personal beliefs about the health effects of smoking, he and others in the CCP did little to educate the public about its harms. The lack of leadership from the center did not mean that there was no anti-smoking activism in the People's Republic between 1949 and 1976. Juvenile smoking remained a particular concern for many, just as it had in the first half of the twentieth century. Continuing the precedent that had been established during the Republican period, the Ministry of Education consistently prohibited smoking among secondary school students (Ngok and Li 2010, 101). Indeed, young people themselves on occasion attempted to prevent their peers from smoking. The Beijing No. 26 Middle School Red Guards, for example, listed smoking as one of the bad habits that "absolutely must not be cultivated" and they ordered "those under thirty-five to quit drinking and smoking immediately" (Schoenhals 1996, 220). There were rules against smoking among "sent down" youth during the 1960s and 1970s, although young men widely flouted them (Benedict 2011, 236). During the Maoist period, however, many young women refrained from smoking because by then female cigarette smoking was widely condemned as bourgeois.

China's Epidemic of Cigarette-Related Illness and Death, 1978–2010

After Deng Xiaoping launched his program of economic reforms in 1978, there was a dramatic expansion in Chinese cigarette consumption as higher incomes enabled urban smokers to buy more expensive brands and as large numbers of rural smokers switched from pipe tobacco to cigarettes. Total annual production of Chinese cigarettes grew from 852 billion in 1980 to 1.6 trillion in 1990, 1.7 trillion in 2000, and over 2 trillion in 2010 (Li 2011, 2469). The average number of manufactured cigarettes smoked per person per day (among current smokers) rose steadily from one in 1952 to four in 1972 to ten in 1992, a rate similar to that of the United States forty years earlier (Zhang and Cai 2003, 17). It remained at about fifteen cigarettes per day per smoker on average between 1995 and 2002, dropping to about fourteen per day per smoker in 2010 (Li, Hsia, and Yang 2011, 2469).

The increased availability of cigarettes since 1978 has led to significant health problems for millions of Chinese citizens. Four nationally representative surveys conducted between 1984 and 2010 indicate that the prevalence of cigarette smoking among those aged fifteen and older has remained high over the past thirty years, increasing from 34.45 percent in 1984 to 35.3 percent in 1996 and then decreasing to 31.4 percent in 2002 (Yang 2008, 16–17). The 2010 survey revealed that the current smoking rate among people aged fifteen and above has dropped to 28 percent but the total number of current smokers, most of whom are men, has increased to 301 million. Fifty-three percent of men aged fifteen and older currently smoke but only 2.4 percent of women do (Li, Hsia, and Yang 2011, 2469–2470).

The significantly higher prevalence rates among Chinese men than among Chinese women means that men bear the brunt of smoking-related mortality. By 1990, smoking was already causing the deaths of about 12 percent of middle-aged men, according to a prospective cohort study of 224,500 men (Niu et al. 1998). Recently Jiang et al., using data from a nationwide retrospective mortality study, calculated that tobacco caused 16 percent of total male deaths in 1987 and 3.7 percent of total female deaths (11.2 percent of total deaths) (Jiang et al. 2010, 7). This is a little higher than in earlier studies but it is lower than smoking-attributable mortality from developed countries such as the United States. The main reason for this discrepancy is likely that mortality due to smoking has not yet peaked in China, since more than two-thirds of adult smoking-related death occurs only later in life. Many Chinese who initiated cigarette smoking in the 1980s and 1990s are only just now entering middle or early old age, and their health problems associated with smoking will only materialize as they grow older.

Several trends suggest that morbidity and mortality associated with tobacco use will rise over time. First, between 1998 and 2003, the proportion of current heavy smokers (those who smoke more than twenty cigarettes per day) increased substantially overall and doubled in men, rising from 26 percent to 51 percent (Qian et al. 2010, 770). Second, the average age of smoking initiation has been continually dropping over the past twenty-five years. For men, the average age in 1996 was about nineteen, compared to twenty-two in 1984; for women, the age of smoking uptake dropped from twenty-eight to twenty-five across the same time period. By 2002, the average age at which men began to smoke was about seventeen and about nineteen for women (Yang 2008, 17). In 2010, more than half of daily smokers aged twenty to thirty-four years reported smoking before the age of twenty years (Yang 2010, 421). Increases in the average number of cigarettes smoked per day and the earlier age of smoking initiation will clearly have an adverse impact on current smokers as they age.

Diseases reliably linked to smoking, such as lung cancer, emphysema, heart disease, and stroke, are all on the rise in China. Nationwide, data from two large surveys demonstrated that modified mortality from lung cancer rose from 7.17 per one hundred thousand in the 1970s to 15.19 per one hundred thousand in the 1990s, an increase of 111.85 percent. Rates for men increased faster than for women (Zhang and Cai 2003, 19–20). The third national survey on causes of death in China conducted by the Ministry of Health in 2004–2005 revealed that crude death rates from lung cancer in China had risen 465 percent since 1973–1975 when the first such survey was done. Lung cancer is now the leading cause of cancer deaths in urban China (Chen et al. 2010). According to Gu Dongfeng et al., the population-attributable risk of lung cancer associated with cigarette smoking in 2005 was 50.6 percent in men and 14.8 percent of women. It was the leading cause of deaths attributable to smoking among men forty years or older, causing an estimated 113,000 male deaths in that year (Gu et al. 2009, 154–155).

Active smoking in China causes upward of one million deaths per year but another one hundred thousand Chinese die each year as a consequence of exposure to secondhand smoke. In 2010, an estimated 556 million nonsmokers (72 percent) aged fifteen years and older reported being exposed to secondhand smoke and 38 percent said they are exposed to secondhand smoke on a daily basis (Xiao et al. 2010, 434). Secondhand smoke caused more than 22,000 lung cancer deaths and 33,800 ischemic heart disease (IHD) deaths in 2002. Eighty-one percent of IHD female deaths and 74 percent of lung cancer female deaths in 2002 were attributable to passive smoke (Gan et al. 2008, 95–98). Jian-Bing Wang et al. found that in 2005 exposure to secondhand smoke at home was responsible for 5.2 percent of lung cancer deaths among nonsmoking women, and similar exposure in the workplace was responsible for 6.2 percent of the deaths among women who did not smoke (Wang et al. 2010, 963).

Tobacco Control Initiatives, 1978–2012

The ascendance to power of Deng Xiaoping in 1978 marked not only a departure from the autarkic economic policies of the past but also the beginning of a new approach to tobacco control. Grounded in evidence-based research and led by medical experts, many of whom were affiliated in one way or another with the Peking Union Medical College (PUMC), the late twentieth-century anti-smoking movement differed from its early twentieth-century antecedents in that it was concerned not only with the collective health of the nation in the abstract but also with the very real human toll being exacted by tobacco use. Based on sound medical science and enjoying institutional support from both government and nongovernmental organizations, the contemporary tobacco control movement has made considerable strides even as it continues to face significant challenges.

By the 1970s, the myriad health risks of smoking were well-established facts widely accepted by the international scientific community. Chinese physicians, cognizant of the scientific consensus regarding tobacco abroad and concerned about the worsening public health situation due to increased cigarette smoking at home, took the lead in early prevention efforts. Beginning in 1978, highly respected authorities such as Weng Xinzhi and Dr. Ye Gongshao not only headed up new studies on the health effects of tobacco but also publicly urged the Ministry of Health to address the burgeoning epidemic of smoking-related illness (Ngok and Li 2010, 101).[1]

Medical experts were also instrumental in the creation of the Chinese Association on Tobacco Control (CATC), the first national association set up to promote and coordinate tobacco prevention in China. Founded in 1990, CATC is an advocacy group composed of people from various professions who have volunteered to engage in tobacco reduction activities. Many members are prominent in the health field (Ngok and Li 2010, 106). Weng Xinzhi was executive vice president of the organization from 1991 to 1998, and the first president was PUMC graduate Wu Jieping (1917–2011), the well-known urologist and former vice chairman of the Standing Committee of the National People's Congress.[2] Subsequent leaders have generally been retired Ministry of Health officials.

CATC has achieved a great deal in terms of networking, scientific research, and health education in China since its founding. In 1996, together with the Chinese Academy of Preventive Medicine and in collaboration with the Johns Hopkins University School of Hygiene and Public Health, the organization carried out the third national smoking prevalence study (Yang et al. 1999, 1247–1248). In 1997, CATC successfully hosted 1,800 delegates from 114 countries at the Tenth World Conference on Tobacco or Health in Beijing. Chinese President Jiang Zemin's speech at the opening ceremony of the conference focused unprecedented official attention on the issue of smoking and health.

CATC, which is registered with the Ministry of Civil Affairs (MCA) and supervised by the Ministry of Health (MOH), has been a strong voice for tobacco control even when such advocacy has put it at odds with different departments of the Chinese government. For example, in 2008, the MCA was planning to confer the prestigious China Charity Award on six tobacco companies. Strong opposition from CATC members led to the withdrawal of the nomination. Similarly, in 2009 when the Shanghai Tobacco Corporation donated two hundred million renminbi to the Shanghai 2010 World Expo, twenty professionals affiliated with CATC wrote a public letter appealing the decision. The money was subsequently returned (Jun et al. 2011, 311). In December 2011, CATC vehemently objected to the election to the prestigious Chinese Academy of Engineering of a research scientist with ties to the tobacco industry. The professional credentials and credibility of CATC members ensure that such protests, even if unsuccessful as they were in the latter case, are widely reported by the Chinese and international press, thereby raising the profile of the anti-tobacco cause.

The Ministry of Health has been at the vanguard of tobacco prevention in China since the late 1970s. Together with the Ministries of Finance, Agriculture, and Light Industry, the MOH issued the first official policy document on tobacco control in China on February 28, 1979. The joint circular focused on reducing smoking initiation among young people and educating them about tobacco's harms (Ngok and Li 2010, 107). In the mid-1980s, the ministry began to recommend bans on smoking in public venues and the placement of warning labels on tobacco products. In the 1990s, such policy recommendations resulted in national legislation requiring the printing of health warnings on cigarette packs and smoke-free regulations aimed at reducing public exposure to secondhand smoke, as well bans on tobacco advertising in electronic and print media (Lee and Jiang 2008, 35–39).

In 2002, the National Tobacco Control Office (NTCO) was set up within the Ministry of Health. Part of the Chinese Center for Disease Prevention and Control (CDC), the office was headed for many years by Dr. Yang Gonghuan, who has also served as director of the PUMC Institute of Global Tobacco Control. The office has wide-ranging responsibilities, including providing scientific evidence for legislative initiatives, training health care professionals in tobacco control, promoting anti-tobacco programs, and interfacing with international tobacco control agencies (Lee and Jiang 2008, 36). However, since its establishment the office has been severely understaffed and underfunded.

Beginning in the 1980s, Chinese experts, CATC, and the Ministry of Health joined forces with international organizations to advance tobacco prevention in China. The Ministry of Health began to work with the World Health Organization (WHO) on this issue in 1979, and the WHO Collaborating Centre for Tobacco or Health was set up in Beijing in 1986. WHO also began to sponsor research on the health hazards of smoking in China. For example, Wu Yingkai (1910–2003), the former director of surgery at PUMC, served as the senior investigator for the WHO Multinational Monitoring of Trends and Determinants in Cardiovascular Disease (MONICA) survey in the 1980s and 1990s.[3] Tobacco reduction was a central focus of the disease prevention programs put in place as a result of the program's findings (Wright 2004, 575).

In the 1990s, tobacco control became an issue of global health governance as WHO spearheaded an effort to reduce smoking around the world. The organization's Tobacco Free Initiative, launched in 1998, led to the Framework Convention on Tobacco Control (FCTC), the first health treaty negotiated under the auspices of WHO. The FCTC entered into force in 2005 and now has 168 signatory countries, including the People's Republic of China. The FCTC was ratified by the National People's Congress in August 2005 and it took effect in China in

January 2006 (Lee and Jiang 2008, 44–45). The treaty's provisions include rules that govern the production, sale, and distribution of tobacco and also sets out specific steps for governments to control tobacco use, including bans on tobacco advertising, the creation of smoke-free work and public spaces, the placement of prominent health warnings on cigarette packs, and the adoption of tax and price measures to reduce tobacco consumption.

China has made some progress toward implementing FCTC requirements since its ratification in 2005. The good news is that health education is demonstrably having an effect on public awareness of tobacco's hazards. Among Chinese adults, more than 80 percent now recognize that smoking causes serious disease and more than 75 percent are aware that smoking causes lung cancer (Yang et al. 2010, 441). Well-educated urbanites are now smoking at somewhat lower rates (Kohrman 2010, 190S). However, many remain unaware of the specific health consequences of smoking and even fewer realize the dangers of secondhand smoke.

Despite some attitudinal changes, smoking remains very common among Chinese men. Quitting is rare and relapse rates are high (Qian et al. 2010, 771–772). Moreover, the number of cigarettes being produced and consumed in China continues to climb. Retail sales of cigarettes in China grew by almost 23 percent between 2005 and 2010, from 1.88 trillion sticks to 2.23 trillion. In 2010, the China National Tobacco Company produced 2.27 trillion cigarettes, or 40 percent of the world's total output. Less than 1 percent of cigarettes produced in China are exported each year, which means most are smoked by China's more than three hundred million smokers, many of them in the countryside where health education about tobacco's risks remains limited (Cui 2010, 252).

Exposure to secondhand smoke remains a serious problem. Since the 1990s, prohibitions against smoking in public have appeared as specific provisions in several nationally binding regulations but at present China has no comprehensive smoke-free law (Chen, Shin, and Beaglehole 2012, 779). Local jurisdictions have long had the authority to implement smoke-free policies and many cities have done so. But there has been wide variation among municipalities in terms of where smoking is allowed and where it is not (Jun et al. 2011, 310). Smoking in public areas remains common and no-smoking signs are widely ignored.

As health researchers are quick to point out, a major barrier to effective tobacco control in China remains the considerable economic and political clout enjoyed by China's tobacco industry. Government at all levels continues to benefit directly from tobacco: although the proportion of tobacco revenues has been declining since the 1990s the government still derives about 6 percent of its revenues from tobacco taxes. Tobacco is the only agricultural product to be taxed at the subnational level and this creates perverse incentives for local governments to encourage farmers to grow tobacco. In certain areas, particularly the southwest, agricultural taxes on tobacco leaf production remain a vital part of government financing.

In addition to economic barriers to tobacco control there are also political and institutional ones. To facilitate implementation of the FCTC, an interministerial body was set up in 2007 and oversight was granted to the Ministry of Industry and Information Technology (MOIIT) (Ngok and Li 2010, 102). As it happens, MOIIT is the agency that supervises China's State Tobacco Monopoly Administration (STMA). This administrative arrangement thus represents a significant conflict of interest because the ministry in charge of promoting cigarette production is also responsible for coordinating FCTC implementation efforts around the country (Jun et al. 2011, 309). Day-to-day management of FCTC implementation is delegated to the acutely short-staffed and underfunded NTCO in the China Center for Disease Control and Prevention (Cui 2010, 251).

In the past decade new sources of international funding for tobacco control in China have become available, primarily through the Bloomberg Global Initiative to Reduce Tobacco Use and the Bill & Melinda Gates Foundation. The Bloomberg Initiative and the Gates Foundation have supported new Chinese nongovernmental organizations such as the Kunming-based Chaoyi Jiankang (Pioneers for Health), which the first Chinese NGO specifically established to curtail tobacco use in China. Significant funding has also been granted to U.S.- and European-based institutes working on tobacco control in China, including the Johns Hopkins Institute for Global Tobacco Control, the CDC Foundation, the WHO Collaborating Centre for Global Tobacco Surveillance, the International Union Against Tuberculosis and Lung Disease, Emory University's Global Health Initiative, and the Campaign for Tobacco-Free Kids (Kohrman 2010, 194S). In 2009, the Bill & Melinda Gates Foundation also joined forces with the China Medical Board in an initiative that focused on encouraging smoking cessation among health care professionals and working closely with medical universities and their affiliated hospitals to create smoke-free campuses (Liu and Chen 2011, 1219).

Conclusion

The manufactured cigarette triumphed in China only after the establishment of the People's Republic of China in 1949. Introduced into China in the 1890s, cigarettes became increasingly popular after 1900 but many smokers, especially those in the countryside, simply could not afford them. As a consequence, the health risks associated with inhalable flue-cured tobacco smoke remained relatively low in the first half of the twentieth century. Only after the Chinese Communist Party nationalized the tobacco industry in the 1950s and deliberately boosted the overall supply of cigarettes by encouraging local production did manufactured cigarettes begin to reach all segments of society. The fact that cigarettes became widespread in rural China only after 1949 and especially after 1978 means that the main public health consequences of cigarette smoking in China are emerging only in the present century. If current trends persist, epidemiologists predict that tobacco use will kill perhaps as many as one hundred million Chinese citizens in the first half of the twenty-first century. This is nearly as many deaths as occurred due to epidemics, violence, and famine during the entire tumultuous twentieth century.[4]

Although the epidemiological effects of increased cigarette consumption have become fully evident only in recent decades, anti-smoking activism in China dates back to the beginning of the twentieth century. Those opposed to tobacco at that time were motivated above all by concerns over China's fate during an age when internal disunity and foreign imperialism threatened to dismember China entirely. Blending moral, economic, and medical arguments appropriated from the international temperance movement, anti-cigarette activists sought to eradicate smoking in order to strengthen China. As such, early twentieth-century health warnings about tobacco were part of a broader effort to construct a hygienically modern nation.

In China today, government health agencies and nongovernmental organizations lead a vibrant and scientifically informed tobacco prevention movement. Arguments against smoking are now firmly grounded in evidence-based research, and medical experts focus above all on issues affecting individual health and public health, not on the "evils" of smoking. Yet like their early twentieth-century predecessors, contemporary tobacco control advocates regard a smoke-free society as vital for China's future prosperity. They continue to leverage the Chinese government's aspirations to be a responsible participant in global health governance—as evidenced by the NPC's ratification of the Framework Convention on Tobacco Control—to push for policies (still unfulfilled) such as a national ban on smoking in public venues, tax increases that meaningfully raise the retail price of cigarettes, and graphic health warnings on all tobacco products.

To date, tobacco control efforts in China have focused primarily on reducing consumer demand for cigarettes rather than on limiting supply. But anti-smoking activists in China are increasingly holding cigarette companies accountable for selling deadly products, and efforts are underway to persuade Chinese officials that the short-term economic benefits conferred by tobacco taxes will soon be overtaken by long-term health costs attributable to smoking (Cui 2010, 252). The economic costs of tobacco use are already very high, accounting for 0.7 percent of China's GDP in 2008 ($28.9 billion). These costs, which rose by more than 300 percent between 2000 and 2008, will only increase over time as more and more Chinese citizens become ill and die as a result of smoking (Yang et al. 2011, 269). Chinese smoking prevalence rates are likely to remain high for many years to come but eventually medical and economic arguments against tobacco will prevail. Not only will the roaring expenditures and loss of productivity attributable to smoking become too great a burden for society to bear, but the projected loss of one hundred million lives will someday simply be too tragic to ignore.

Notes

1. Both Weng Xinzhi and Ye Gongshao were trained at the Peking Union Medical College. Weng Xinzhi studied at PUMC in 1941 and 1942 before it was closed due to war. An expert in tropical medicine who also carried out extensive research on COPD, Weng was the principal investigator on China's first national smoking prevalence survey, carried out in 1984. Ye Gongshao, a 1935 PUMC graduate, was a preeminent Chinese pediatrician who spearheaded the establishment of the field of maternal and child health in China. In 1981 she organized health professionals to investigate the smoking status of secondary school students in Beijing. Based on her findings, she and her co-author suggested that the government initiate an educational program in primary schools on the hazards of smoking.

2. Wu Jieping graduated from PUMC in 1942.

3. Wu Yingkai was a resident, research fellow, assistant professor, and lecturer at PUMC from 1933 to 1940. He was director of surgery at PUMC from 1946 to 1956.

4. See chapter 1.

.

PART II
DISEASE TRANSITIONS

5 Epidemics and Public Health in Twentieth-Century China

Plague, Smallpox, and AIDS

Xinzhong Yu

WHILE EPIDEMICS HAVE occurred throughout Chinese history, the contemporary understanding of public health is a recent import from the West, and these two topics are not necessarily related. But due to the fact that public health and the prevention of epidemics are so closely linked in our modern understanding, it has become common to discuss the two subjects as one in contemporary academic research. Chinese public health came into existence during the intensely rapid changes of the twentieth century, which was also a time rife with epidemics.

This chapter will focus on the relationships between epidemics and the evolution of public health in China, with particular attention to the plague, smallpox, and HIV epidemics. It asserts that the public health and hygienic movements often served the political purposes of the state rather than necessarily addressing the most critical medical problems.

A General Survey of Epidemic Diseases

Examined merely on the basis of extant historical records, the frequency of China's epidemics has seen a constant increase (Zhang 2008, 32–33). Based on statistics from available historical records through the year 1949, the Republican era (1912–1949) experienced the greatest frequency of epidemic outbreaks (Li 2004, 1). Our own statistical analysis of the modern period (1573–1949) also shows that the frequency of epidemics in the Republican era was much greater than in previous times, with 3.08 occurrences per year, while that number was only 1.09 for previous eras (Yu et al. 2004, 24–25). After 1949, owing to the increasing details and completeness of relevant medical records and statistics, there are no years without any reported epidemics. The emergence of this phenomenon in the modern period is certainly related to the fact that the occurrence and spread of disease was facilitated by such aspects of modernity as rapid increases in population, social mobility, and ever-increasing internationalization (Yu 2003, 340–344). More importantly, however, I fear that this apparent trend may also reflect the degree to which there now exists an interest in recording, maintaining, and preserving the most complete possible data. It is only from the twentieth century onward, after the creation of the Public Health Administration, that the practice of recording public health and mortality statistics became one of its key programs. Since then, statistics regarding epidemic diseases have obviously seen a steady increase in both quantity and detail, to the point where it has become impossible to separate the gradual increase in records on epidemics from the increasingly detailed statistics on health and life produced by public health administrations and research departments (Liu 1996 [1937], 441–446).[1] In the twentieth century, epidemic diseases—and acute infectious diseases in particular—have been an important factor in threatening the lives of the Chinese people and in influencing both the Chinese psyche and the social order. Both the epidemics themselves and the fact that their danger was ceaselessly recorded and emphasized also hastened and promoted the establishment of public health measures.

Although there were no years without epidemics during the twentieth century and the statistics regarding these epidemics are voluminous, these statistics primarily contain information regarding large-scale, fatal epidemics, and such epidemics don't appear to have been more numerous than before. Furthermore, socioeconomic developments and the establishment of more and more complete public health measures appear to have reduced the severity of such epidemics. In my humble opinion, the following are the key formative epidemics that influenced Chinese society: the cholera epidemic of 1902, which spread to numerous areas across the country (Shan 2008); the spread of the Manchurian plague in 1910–1911, which had global ramifications (Nathan 1967; Iijima 2000, 137–208; Deng 2006, 271–286); the outbreak of the plague throughout Shanxi and Inner Mongolia in 1917–1918 (Xian 1988, 126–128; Cao and Li 2006, 352–380); the cholera epidemic of 1919, which affected both northern and southern China (Iijima 2000, 237–261; Li 2004, 42); the national cholera epidemic of 1932 (Yu et al. 2004, 279–306; Deng 2006, 427–433; Liu 2007, 113–124); the 1947 plague epidemic in eastern Inner Mongolia and western Manchuria (Deng 2006, 412–418); the long-term schistosomiasis epidemic that affected the middle and lower reaches of the Yangzi River, the flood basin of Lake Taihu, and southeastern China;[2] the national epidemic of cerebrospinal meningitis in 1966–1967 (Deng 2006, 620–624; Xin Zhongguo yufang yixue lishi jingyan weiyuanhui 1988–1991, 3: 32–33); the hepatitis A epidemic that affected Shanghai in 1988 (Shao 1993, 1615; Cao 2008, 149–164); and the AIDS epidemic that has affected China since 1985.

In general, it is not difficult to see that acute epidemic diseases like cholera and the plague posed a significant threat to society in the first half of the twentieth century. In contrast, the epidemics that posed the greater threat during the second half of the century were the nonvirulent acute or chronic infectious diseases that arose in response to specific circumstances. Existing statistical data also demonstrates this point. Take, for instance, the plague: during the first half of the century, there were 1,162,643 reported cases (1,037,502 fatalities), while only 4,763 cases (1,468 fatalities) of the plague were reported during the second half of the century. This represents a 245-fold decrease (or a 707-fold decrease in fatalities) from the first half of the century to the second (Li 2002, 294). Regarding smallpox, with the exception of the higher rate during the initial outbreak in the 1950s (with an average of 11.22 cases per hundred thousand in 1950), the incidence of smallpox was generally lower, at less than 1 per hundred thousand, until the disease had essentially become extinguished by the 1960s (Lü et al. 1997, Deng 2006, 597–598). Regarding cholera, the ancient strains had disappeared by 1952, but a newly introduced strain spread to many places in the 1960s and 1970s. Nevertheless, the morbidity rate was still fewer than 10 per hundred thousand and the disease was essentially under control by the 1980s, with an incidence less than 1 per hundred thousand (Lü et al. 1997; Xin Zhongguo yufang yixue lishi jingyan weiyuanhui 1988–1991, 3: 42–43).

Furthermore, epidemic disease as a cause of death gradually decreased as well. Related to advances in China's modern epidemic reporting system, available research shows a continuous trend of increasing incidence of epidemic diseases prior to the 1970s, which reached an apex in 1970 but then began a steady decline. By 1994, in fact, this rate had decreased to an average of 203.68 deaths per hundred thousand. Deaths from acute contagious diseases among all causes of death dropped with each passing year; in the 1990s, such deaths fell to the eighth most prevalent cause of death regardless of differences between urban and rural areas, and in cities were no longer even one of the ten most prevalent causes of death (Lü et al. 1997, 38; Dai 1993, 20).

Regarding the type of infectious diseases, Fan Rixin's statistics have shown that the epidemic diseases with the greatest incidence in the 1930s and '40s were dysentery, cholera, typhoid fever, recurrent fevers, and smallpox (Zhang 2008, 61–62). By the beginning of the 1950s, "the primary infectious diseases were respiratory tract and insect-borne infectious diseases with high incidence and high death rates, such as measles, smallpox, kala-azar and malaria." After the 1980s, this situation gradually changed such that infectious diseases of the gastrointestinal tract, such as dysentery and viral hepatitis, which are marked by high incidence and low death rates, became more prevalent (Dai 1993, 20). Here it is important to note that while smallpox, cholera, the plague, and other virulent acute infectious diseases had a large impact on the general population due to their frequent occurrence and widespread nature during the first half of the century, in terms of the major causes of death among urban populations, they were actually not as significant as is generally thought. As Jia Hongwei's research on statistical data on causes of death in Nanjing, Beijing, Guangzhou, and other cities between 1932 and 1935 indicates, "the most threatening diseases that confronted the inhabitants of Beijing, Nanjing, and Guangzhou were actually not the legally designated infectious diseases on everyone's minds. Rather, tuberculosis, convulsive diseases, diseases of the upper respiratory and gastrointestinal tracts, aging, and stroke claimed a higher proportion of deaths than did legally designated infectious diseases such as typhoid fever, bloody dysentery, smallpox, cholera, diphtheria, scarlet fever, and measles" (Jia 2012).

The Plague and the Creation of Institutions of Public Health

Within the short span of less than twenty years at the end of the nineteenth century and the beginning of the twentieth, two large epidemics of plague had global effects: the plague outbreak of 1894 in Hong Kong and southern China, and the Manchurian outbreak of pneumonic plague in 1910–1911. Subsequent plague episodes occurred between 1917 and 1947, all but one of which were bubonic plague. Presumably because of its enormous impact and influence, no fewer than five monographs have been written on the plague in modern China (Nathan 1967; Benedict 1996; Iijima 2000; Cao and Li 2006; Summers 2012). Among these, Iijima Wataru investigates the process of the institutionalization of health care in modern China from the perspective of the plague. Several of these authors consider the management of the Manchurian plague by the Qing government to be the beginning of public health in China (Deng and Cheng 2000, 473). Under both the Qing and Republican governments, bureaus of plague prevention were established. The Central Office for Plague Prevention eventually became a central element of the Republic of China's Ministry of Health.

Since the history of the plague in China, the involvement of the Western powers, and the rise of China's public health institutions have been so well documented, we can see how the plague had an important stimulating effect on the establishment of institutions of public health and on health administration in China. Nevertheless, this acceleration could have only emerged against the background outlined below. On the one hand, the Great Powers continuously used health and epidemic prevention as an excuse to erode China's sovereignty and interests, while on the other hand Chinese society was facing a national crisis and in its efforts to strengthen and preserve the country also saw health care as a symbol for science, culture, and progress, which it pursued quite self-consciously (Hu 2008b, 214–232; Yu 2012, 47–64; Iijima 2000, 137).

Cleanliness, Epidemic Prevention, and the Hygiene Movement

While it is part of basic human nature to like cleanliness and dislike filth, the intimate connection between cleanliness and health care is a product of our modern age (Vigarello 1988). In traditional China, awareness of the close relationship between uncleanliness and the rise of epidemics existed early on, but cleanliness was still more a matter of personal preference than an important measure in the prevention of epidemics, and it was not a responsibility shouldered by state or local officials. In the modern period, however, the introduction of Western ideas and practices about hygiene and epidemic prevention caused a shift in attitudes. Cleanliness not only came to be seen gradually as the most important element of epidemic prevention and hygiene, but it became an important matter for individual health and national strength (Yu 2009, 63–78). Large numbers of China's elite were frequently pained by the lack of hygiene-related knowledge in China's general population. They went so far as to consider this "the greatest obstacle for progress in health care" (Zhang 2006a, 125–126). How to mobilize the masses to pay attention to hygiene, how to disseminate ideas about hygiene among the masses, and how to raise awareness of hygiene among the population therefore became the focus for the state and for society in their efforts to promote health. Against this backdrop, cleanliness as the basic appeal for a mass hygiene movement became the common thread running through all matters related to health care in the twentieth century.

There were many mass hygiene movements in the twentieth century, beginning with one organized by the Federation for Education in Chinese Medicine, an organization that was composed of the Chinese Medical Missionary Association, the Chinese Medical Association, and the Christian YMCA. From 1915 to 1916, this organization held meetings in more than twenty cities, including Shanghai and Changsha, to assemble China's first nationwide hygiene movement. Sponsoring speeches, hygiene-related exhibits, and media publicity, and issuing pamphlets and putting up posters, these movements disseminated information on the prevention of epidemics, advertised the benefits of hygiene for the individual and the state, and initiated vaccinations and efforts to stop smoking (Bu 2009a, 305–319). These kinds of activities were sponsored numerous times in various locations (Wang 2011, 18–20). In addition, nongovernmental organizations like the Chinese Anti-Tuberculosis Association and the Chinese Leprosy Association also sponsored numerous campaigns for hygiene education during the Republican period (Zhang 2006a, 132–134). These movements were primarily focused on publicity and education, and did not possess the government's capacity for mobilization.

After the Nationalist Government was formed in Nanjing, it began to take an interest in these mass hygiene campaigns. In May 1928, the Ministry of the Interior of the Nationalist Government in Nanjing adopted the Regulations for the Disposal of Waste, which stipulated that each city should organize a thorough cleanup twice a year, on May 15 and December 25. At the same time, the Outline for the Implementation of Mass Rallies for the Hygiene Movement also assigned these dates for each city to sponsor mass sanitation campaigns, which were to last for two days: the first day was to be focused on displaying examples and illustrations of hygiene and on inviting hygiene specialists to give lectures, and the second day was reserved for parades and for the thorough cleanup (Guomin zhengfu weishengbu 1928, 16; "Weisheng yundong dahui shixing dagang" 1928; Zhu 2009, 357–359). The year 1934 was a turning point for the hygiene movement in the Republican period: the Nationalist government initiated the New Life Movement throughout the entire country, and the hygiene movement subsequently became one movement under the umbrella of this New Life Movement. With the violent outbreak of the Sino-Japanese War, this movement also came to a halt, but recovered bit by bit in various locations after the conclusion of the war (Wang 2011, 60–61).

When the People's Republic of China was founded in 1949, it was impossible for the new regime to directly continue the Republican policies, but it managed to quickly initiate a movement with an almost identical character by a different method. In 1952 the central government responded to the perception that the United States had engaged in germ warfare in North Korea by launching a mass movement that became the Patriotic Hygiene Movement. This involved the entire population in efforts to clean up environmental sanitation in town and country, exterminate plant diseases and insect pests, and crush germ warfare. At the same time, it founded central and local Patriotic Hygiene Movement Committees. The specific content promoted by the Patriotic Hygiene Movement varied, but the most universal and common efforts centered on eliminating the four pests (rats, bedbugs, flies, and mosquitoes), waste disposal, and sewage management (Li 2007b, 211; Xiao 2003, 97–102). During the Cultural Revolution, this movement suffered destruction, but it recovered and then progressed gradually after 1976. For the first few years after the Cultural Revolution, the main focus was to get rid of the trash that had piled up like a mountain during the ten years of upheaval and to tackle waste management in a comprehensive fashion. Beginning in the 1980s, it turned in the direction of promoting a clean, green, and beautiful environment (Xin Zhongguo yufang yixue lishi jingyan weiyuanhui 1988–1991, 2: 30).

Throughout the entire twentieth century, the various hygiene movements were primarily centered on cleanliness. Even though their direct goal was health and epidemic prevention, the people who launched the different campaigns additionally had their own political agendas. The Federation for Hygiene Education in China, for example, used hygiene activities to expand its influence, while the hygiene campaigns associated with the New Life Movement had a very strong politicizing tendency, emphasizing that each individual in their acts of hygiene carried the responsibility to establish a modern and strong nation. Thus its ultimate goal was not the health of the individual body but was instead a way for the administration to display its legitimacy (Nakajima 2008, 43). Based as it was on the premise of countering germ warfare, the PRC's Patriotic Hygiene Movement also clearly had a highly politicized goal. On the one hand, it seized the opportunity to arouse patriotic feelings in the population and directed these feelings to benefit the trajectory of self-governance, using the power of the masses to supplement the government's inadequate ability to establish personal hygiene while also demonstrating the concern of the People's Government for the population. On the other hand, it also used this movement to strengthen its ability to mobilize the masses, giving legitimacy to this method of mass mobilization, and subsequently also achieving a sustained promotion of hygiene (Yang 2006, 350–354).

Prevention by Immunization and the Extinction of Smallpox

China is a country that started the practice of preventive inoculation very early. Current research shows that human smallpox inoculation appeared in southern regions like Anhui and Jiangxi from at least the mid-sixteenth century on and by the Qing dynasty had already spread north and south of the Yangzi River. After the cowpox vaccine was discovered in England at the end of the eighteenth century, it was quickly imported to China's interior via Macao and from there spread progressively from the south to the north, promoted by social forces and local government officials (Fan 1953, 106–153; Leung 1987, 240–246, 249–252). Even though vaccination with cowpox or smallpox was already quite common in the late Qing period, the actual inoculation rates were still limited because of the meager government financial resources for health care and the fact that vaccination was voluntary. The author's research has shown that in the late Qing period the vaccination rate for children in the developed regions of Jiangnan was at most 30 to 40 percent (Yu 2003, 247). In spite of this state of affairs, preventive inoculation was quite well-received in Chinese society.

From the beginning of the twentieth century, smallpox vaccination became one aspect of the government's health care administration (Yu 2008, 57–58). In the police regulations that appeared during the last few years of the Qing dynasty in a few areas, provisions regarding compulsory smallpox vaccination made their appearance (Iijima 2000, 75, 78). These kinds of rules were continued through the Beiyang period (1912–1928) (Deng and Cheng 2000, 313). When the Nationalist government was established in Nanjing, it promulgated the Smallpox Vaccination Ordinance on August 29, 1928, which stipulated that children must be vaccinated twice (between three months and one year, and at age seven to eight). If "parents, guardians, or other people responsible for child care" failed to vaccinate children according to this method, they would be punished (Zhang and Xian 1990, 35–36). In the following year, the government issued the Regulations for Provincial and City-Level Smallpox Vaccination Education (Deng 2006, 443–444).

In addition, the Central Office for Epidemic Prevention and other nascent public health institutions also adopted the research and manufacture of cowpox and other vaccines as one of their important tasks. From the time the Central

Office for Epidemic Prevention was established, it developed vaccines like small-pox vaccine, cholera serum, typhoid serum, and rabies vaccine, intensifying its efforts to develop and manufacture specific products for public use in response to each of the various epidemics that occurred (Deng 2006, 372–373). Summarizing the work that had been done in the area of health care during the previous ten years, Liu Ruiheng, director of the government's Health Administration, stated in 1937, "The local health offices in each province and city have in recent years made great efforts to conduct smallpox vaccinations and preventive injections for typhoid and cholera" (Liu 1996 [1937], 434). There is no doubt that these efforts contributed to the expansion of smallpox vaccinations, even though the lack of financial resources at the time meant that universal implementation was still a long way off, especially in the rural areas (Deng 2006, 444). And from today's perspective, even in the big cities the vaccination rate appears to have been quite unsatisfactory. The official statistics for vaccination rates in postwar Shanghai for the years 1946–1949, for example, were 15.2 percent, 57.3 percent, 47.4 percent, and 26.8 percent, respectively (Xin Zhongguo yufang yixue lishi jingyan weiyuanhui 1988–1991, 3: 98). Moreover, the limited effectiveness of other immunizations like cholera serum caused people to be suspicious, and preventive inoculation for diseases like diphtheria or scarlet fever failed to be implemented on a large scale (Jin and Xu 1991, 174).

After the founding of the People's Republic of China, prevention was firmly established as the primary strategy in dealing with epidemics, and the task of vaccinations was strongly emphasized. In 1950, six research institutes for biological products were set up in the major cities, and charged with the task of researching, developing, and manufacturing various biological vaccines. In the space of fifty years, these centers produced a large number of new products and technologies (Cai, Li, and Zhang 1999, 48–50). This was one factor that promoted the popularization of preventive inoculation. At the same time, to guide epidemic prevention at each level of government, new structures were established to initiate grassroots-level epidemic prevention stations. These launched large-scale mass vaccination campaigns for smallpox, plague, and cholera across the country and actively pushed for inoculation with the BCG vaccine against tuberculosis. They first implemented free smallpox vaccinations and then continuously increased the varieties of vaccines for preventive inoculation. By 1978, when this system of grassroots structures for epidemic prevention had gradually reached completion, the government began to implement a countrywide program of immunizations that involved issuing universal planned immunization cards to all children of the appropriate age. In 1982, the Health Department convened the first national conference on planned immunizations and published the Nationwide Regulations for the Task of Planned Immunizations and a "1982–1990 Plan for the Task of Nationwide Immunizations," which clarified the concept of planned immunizations and the vaccines employed, and unified the procedures

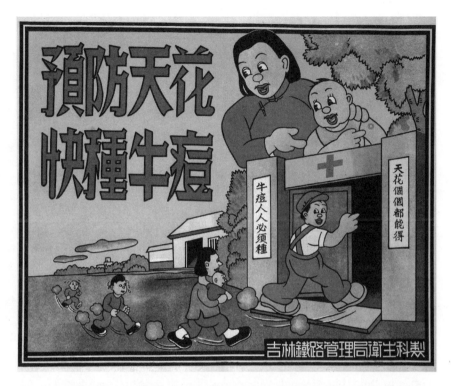

Figure 5.1. Jilin Railroad Hygiene Department poster: "Go to have smallpox vaccination." Circa 1956. *Source:* U.S. National Library of Medicine, National Institutes of Health, Chinese Public Health Posters. http://www.nlm.nih.gov/hmd/chineseposters/prevention.html.

for childhood immunizations. From then on, this task continued to be promoted consistently until the goal of disseminating childhood immunization through the entire country was reached in 1991 (Dai 1993, 66–69).

The effect of preventive immunizations, beginning with smallpox vaccinations, on the prevention of epidemics is beyond any doubt, with particularly clear results in the case of smallpox prevention and treatment. As Liu Ruiheng, the director of the Health Administration, pointed out already before the Sino-Japanese War, because of the dedication to the task of preventive smallpox vaccination, "in recent years the number of smallpox patients in every major city has shown a clear downward trend" (Liu 1996 [1937], 434). After 1952, the number of smallpox patients in the entire country began to drop sharply to the point where the disease was essentially eliminated after 1961 (Xin Zhongguo yufang yixue lishi jingyan weiyuanhui 1988–1991, 3: 97). Even though there are many reasons for the elimination of smallpox, such as the strengthening of quarantine and disease surveillance, the popularization of smallpox vaccination is without a doubt the most important factor (Xin Zhongguo yufang yixue lishi jingyan weiyuanhui 1988–1991, 3: 98–101). For the later part of the twentieth century, preventive vaccination became a fundamental factor affecting the pattern of the spread of infectious diseases in China.

Recent research shows that

> Infectious diseases with targeted preventive measures, such as smallpox, measles, polio, cerebrospinal meningitis, encephalitis B, malaria, and kala-azar disease, have all been eliminated or at least controlled, while the incidence rates for infectious diseases with no targeted preventive measures, like hepatitis, typhoid and paratyphoid fever, and dysentery, were actually sustained at rather high levels and their morbidity rates likewise remain serious (Lü et al. 1997, 38).

The targeted preventive measures in this quotation refer to preventive immunization.

Epidemics Under New Circumstances: The Prevention and Control of AIDS

AIDS, which stands for Acquired Immune Deficiency Syndrome, is a virulent infectious disease that is caused by the human immunodeficiency virus, commonly abbreviated as HIV and also called the AIDS virus. Its main channels for transmission are through sexual intercourse, through the blood, and from mother to child (Lin, He, and Wan 2004, 1). This disease first manifested in 1981 in the United States; by the end of the last century, depending on the estimate, the HIV virus had infected between thirty to forty million and one hundred million people worldwide (Fu and Yu 2000, 1). China discovered its first AIDS patient in 1985, and the disease has spread continuously since then. At the end of June 2001, the government formally announced that the HIV infection rate and the AIDS patient rate were 26,000 cases and 1,100 cases, respectively. According to estimates by relevant organizations and specialists, the actual infection rate for AIDS in China in 2003 had already reached 1,040,000, which included 200,000 fully developed cases, and the present AIDS infection rate lies at 840,000 people, with 80,000 among these suffering from the disease. Moreover, this rate increases yearly by 20–30 percent (Deng 2006, 657). Current research tends to divide the spread of AIDS into three periods: an introductory period of 1985–1988, a phase of expansion from 1989 to 1993, and a period of rapid growth from 1994 on (Lin, He, and Wan 2004, 7).

Even though AIDS is not highly contagious and the number of people who have fallen ill or died from the disease is negligible as a proportion of the number of actual deaths in China overall (Zhongguo weisheng nianjian bianji weiyuanhui 2000, 454), the number of infected people continues to climb because of the absence of any effective treatment methods. In addition, the group of people with a high risk of infection suffers from frequent discrimination, and it is relatively difficult for the state and for society to put into practice effective management practices. For these reasons, the panic and impact on society caused by AIDS is quite serious, to the point where some have elevated the prevention and treatment of AIDS to a matter of life or death for the Chinese people (Guowu yuan yanjiu shi keti zu 1993). As a direct result of its enormous influence on society, contemporary research has divided the spread of AIDS into three stages: first, the spread of the AIDS virus; second, the spread of AIDS as a disease; and third, the abnormal mental and psychological responses of infected or sick people as a result of the infection, as well as the range of responses from people in the social environment of infected or sick people (Wu, Qi, and Zhang 1999, 3). Such responses include not only fear, but also discrimination against infected persons. Before the turn of the twenty-first century, the government frequently referred to social virtues when it discussed solutions for this epidemic. Yuan Mu, for example, stated as follows in the preface of a book titled *Fearfully Guarding Against AIDS: For the Sake of the Survival of the Chinese People:*

> Regarding our approach to the problem of AIDS, . . . how can we bring into play the superiority of the socialist system, wipe out the manifestations of social vices like drug abuse and prostitution, and block the key channels for the spread of AIDS? . . . These issues all require urgent research and the creation of a plan for realizable countermeasures (Guowu yuan yanjiu shi keti zu 1993, 2).

In these kinds of formulations and in the popular understanding, AIDS patients were frequently closely associated with moral flaws. In addition, information about AIDS tended to be adulterated with racial and sexual discrimination and therefore wittingly or unwittingly aggravated the discrimination against certain racial or sexual groups (Hyde 2007). In actuality, the current problem of AIDS in China has some aspects that are caused by the special characteristics of Chinese society and its public health problems. The most representative example of this is the large groups of rural people in areas like Henan who have been infected with HIV as a result of contamination during the process of selling their blood for use in blood transfusions, as a result of which a heartbreaking AIDS village was formed (Gao 2005). The cause of this tragedy is obviously not only the poverty and hunger for money among China's rural population but also the excessive commercialization of medical enterprise in contemporary China and the lack of serious supervision of public health. As a result, there is not only a marketplace for blood collections that take place under conditions that lack measures to safeguard hygiene, but there are substantial risks, such the encouragement of local governments to cut corners in the blind pursuit of economic development (Shao 2010, 228–239).

Thus we can see that AIDS is a social problem, with obvious sociocultural and political factors. At the same time, even though the state and society have attached great value to the prevention and treatment of AIDS, and have taken various positive actions, the spread of AIDS is continuing (Ding 1993, 156; Deng

2006, 656–659). These factors have started to compel some scholars to contemplate the limitations and predicaments inherent in approaching the problem strictly from the angle of biomedicine and public health. Weng Naiqun, for example, addressed the problem of the sociocultural construction of AIDS quite early: "Because the spread of AIDS is closely connected to political, economic, and ideological and religious sociocultural factors, its actual prevention in society becomes particularly difficult" (Weng 2001). The research of Pan Suiming and collaborators has furthermore indicated that the "problem" of AIDS in China emerged on the tail of specific social problems. The conflict of scientific theories that was produced by the cognitive process of this "problem" influenced the formulation of relevant policies, and these in turn constructed the present conditions for the "problem" of AIDS. "In comparison with the harm done by AIDS per se," observe Pan, Huang, and Li (2006, 85–95) "the damage done to society by certain potential mistakes in the conception and implementation of AIDS treatment and prevention may be even larger." Or in other words, the problems that have manifested as the result of AIDS and its prevention and treatment are to a very large extent due to preexisting problems in society and not created by AIDS per se. Pan, Huang, and Li also raise the issue of authority over health in the context of preventing and controlling epidemics, claiming that in the process of prevention and treatment we should introduce such factors of modern culture as "a sense of responsibility of the individual toward society, a respect for human life, a spirit of tolerance, and the rational acceptance of the diversity of society" (85–95). And most recently, in the discussion at the end of the report *Analysis of Policies to Prevent and Cure AIDS,* based on the research conducted by Zai Zetian, all the commentators additionally draw attention to the issue of respect for the right to life and the question of how to avoid the expansion of government authority by means of the prevention and treatment of epidemics (Zhang 2010).

The above discussion demonstrates that academic circles in China have become aware that problems of public health are not only problems of science but also problems of society and culture. They have launched critical self-reflections on the cognitive mode of "hygiene—economy (race)—state" that was universally accepted early in the twentieth century and are proposing an alternative cognitive mode of "hygiene—health—right to life." At the same time, they have expressed concern over the fact that the state has continuously expanded its authority in the process of the modern construction of public health (Yu 2011a, 9–12, 20; Yu 2011b, 48–68) and have raised the need for establishing pluralism, so that the government should not bear the sole responsibility for preventing and controlling disease but should permit and encourage more and more nongovernmental organizations to participate. Undoubtedly, these are extremely important and eagerly awaited directions in the construction of public health in contemporary China.

Twentieth-Century Epidemics and Public Health

Current research on public health, and discussions of hygiene in the prevention of epidemics in particular, are still almost always launched around epidemics, especially virulent infectious diseases. This approach is of course not unreasonable, considering that the violent outbreaks of epidemics in the first place directly stimulated the development of some efforts concerning hygiene and epidemic prevention. And as we will see from an examination of a great many statements and legal regulations on public health in the twentieth century, the vast majority of cases take epidemic prevention as their most important and fundamental concern. Wu Lien-teh (伍連德), for example, was one of the key contributors to the work of public health in China during the Republican period, and his primary target in a relatively early article proposing the implementation of hygiene methods is clearly infectious diseases (Wu 1915a, 6–10). In the numerous discussions on public health from the Republican period, epidemic prevention is always the most important or primary task at hand (Zhong 1931, 24–27; Zhang 2008, 259–264). Moreover, the laws promulgated quite early in this same period regarding medicine and hygiene were also mostly related to the prevention of epidemics (Zhang and Xian 1990).

When we get to the Communist era, this situation remains basically unchanged. In 1950, for example, Zhou Enlai explored the role of medicine and hygiene in a report on the government's work, stating, "At the same time that the People's Government is leading the people in the struggle against ignorance, it is also leading the people in the fight against disease. In the past year, the People's Government has already launched a large-scale struggle for the prevention and treatment of epidemics" (Zhou 1984 [1950], 48). This sort of mentality demonstrates clearly how universally people at that time took epidemic prevention as the center of health care. Even in 1988, Li Tieying, then a member of the State Council and director of the Central Patriotic Hygiene Committee, still talked first about the problem of the violent outburst and spread of epidemics when he discussed what aspects to emphasize in the work of disease prevention (Li 1992c, 94).

Nevertheless, we must not forget that the connection between epidemics and public health is not a necessary one, and that public health is obviously a recent import from the West. Even though many epidemics, and acute infectious diseases in particular, imperiled the health of the Chinese population and influenced Chinese society, in the large majority of cases the epidemics that people paid most attention to in the early part of the twentieth century, such as plague, smallpox, and cholera, were not after all a particularly significant cause of death for the population as a whole. That public health authorities were so fixated on acute epidemics is doubtless related to the panic they caused and the impact that these diseases had on society. In other words, while the focus of public health was related to protecting health, at the same it was perhaps even more concerned with social stability and the public's impression of the government. The examples discussed above show clearly that the motivating factors in the construction of public health were often social and political, and their implementation frequently had aspects of politicization, to the point where we can say that a number of health-related affairs were ultimately political affairs.

At the beginning of the twentieth century, for example, the first health-related tasks carried out by the Qing court and local officials were not connected to epidemics per se. During the Manchurian Plague in the late Qing era, the primary motivating factors in the Qing government's exhausting all its resources on epidemic prevention were the pressure of international opinion and the government's attempting to prevent the erosion of national sovereignty by the Great Powers. Consequently, the "plague prevention" efforts were placed under the direction of the Ministry of Foreign Affairs (Hu 2008b, 214–232; Yu 2012, 47–64).

Regarding the hygiene movements, even though their direct primary goal was cleanliness for the sake of epidemic prevention, their background also included the intention of the state, on the one hand, to increase its control over the bodies of the population (Lei 2011), and, on the other hand, to seize the opportunity to demonstrate the legitimacy of state power itself. When the government mobilized to launch the large-scale schistosomiasis campaigns in the 1950s, the influence of schistosomiasis on the health of soldiers and the sources of troops was certainly a factor. But perhaps more importantly, the launching of such a large-scale prevention and treatment program for this longstanding disease was the ideal tool for displaying the superiority and legitimacy of the new China. And to go even further, by means of this movement the government was able to find an absolutely perfect reason to continue the mass mobilization and to further push for the collectivization of society.

In reality, these movements, while directed at the health of the masses, nevertheless often showed a lack of necessary respect for the desires of the people and their human rights. For the sake of faster, better, and more efficient results, the government popularized a number of untested or immature prevention and treatment methods, to the point of turning the masses into experimental animals (Sun 2007, 105–112; Xin Zhongguo yufang yixue lishi jingyan weiyuanhui 1988–1991, 3: 251). We have seen how epidemic diseases were used in many cases as pretexts for political action, and how the rise of a large number of public health projects is consequently not something that can be explained entirely by a superficial statement about safeguarding the health of the masses. More important were successive governments' manipulations of health-related social ideologies and public opinion to safeguard and convey the legitimacy of their rule.

Clearly, whether we are discussing epidemics or public health, neither of these is a phenomenon that can be explained and grasped entirely by science alone; rather, both include profound social, political, and cultural factors. While this point is still rarely emphasized in mainstream academic research, it is even more absent at the level of actual implementation. Nevertheless, the AIDS crisis that emerged in the 1980s, because of its very particular characteristics, has propelled researchers and health care workers to begin paying attention to the nonmedical factors of epidemics and public health. It has also prompted social questions regarding the process of epidemic prevention, related to such issues as the fair distribution of health-care-related resources, the vilification of a disease, and social discrimination. On a deeper level, it has also stimulated reflections on such questions as the right to health and life and the excessive expansion of state power and authority. In other words, people have already begun to critically examine the twentieth-century myth of the modernization of health care. Regarding the purpose of health care, they focus no longer on ethnic and national strength and prosperity and on economic interests, but more frequently on ensuring the rights of the individual. At the same time, they no longer regard the state's expansion and implementation of functions in the domain of health care and the concomitant expansion of authority as inherently appropriate and a matter of course.

Finally, when we scan the development of public health in the twentieth century, we can see that in the early period, the creation of structures for the administration of health care and cleanliness was primarily a function of transformations taking place in systems of management. The establishment of research and development facilities like the Central Office for Epidemic Prevention demonstrate that the construction of public health was relying more and more heavily on the power and progress of science. Arriving at the end of the twentieth century, the appearance and continued expansion of AIDS has impelled people to begin to reflect more and more critically on the cognitive model of resolving health care problems solely from the angles of biomedical science and public health. Instead they advocate that we draw on social and cultural aspects of epidemics and public health, base ourselves in society, and use multi- and interdisciplinary, multidirectional, and cooperative approaches to solve problems of health care.

Notes

1. After 1949, although the health department kept some statistics, they are not as comprehensive as those that had been recorded in the 1980s in *Zhongguo weisheng nianlin* [Yearbook of hygiene in China].

2. See chapter 6 in this volume.

6 Schistosomiasis

Miriam Gross and Kawai Fan

Farewell to the God of Plague

Mao Zedong

While reading the June 30th edition of the *People's Daily,* I found that Yujiang County has rid itself of schistosoma. With my mind racing, I could not sleep. A light breeze brought its warmth, as the rising sun approached my window. Looking at the southern sky in the distance, I happily set my pen to paper.

I.

Crystal-clear water
And emerald hills
Are many,
But of what use?

Even Hua Tuo, the legend,
Was helpless
Before this little bug.

In thousands of villages
Bursting with weeds,
Men are dying.

Tens of thousands of homes
Are abandoned. Demons
Sing there.

Walking daily for many miles
Among these desolate dwellings,
Following Heaven and wandering,
I see a thousand Milky Ways.

When the Cowherd inquires of
The God of Plague, be sure
To tell him, in joy or grief,
That he has passed away
In the tides.

II.

So many poplars and willows
Dangle in the spring wind.

The people of China
Number six hundred million,
Each one as great as Shun or Yao.

Under our command,
Red rain flows like waves,
Whirling in the wind.

With great effort, we can turn
Green mountains
Into bridges.

Heaven links the Five Ranges,
While silver-colored hoes dig.

Along the Three Rivers,
Arms like iron swing,
Exploding like an earthquake.

May I ask, God of Plague,
Where you intend to go?

The bright flames
Of paper boats
And candles lit
Scorch the skies.

Translated from the Chinese by Joshua Bocher

Introduction

Since the construction of the Three Gorges Dam basin (1994–2006), schistosomiasis, a water-borne and snail-transmitted parasitic disease, has garnered increasing notice in China as a critical public health issue (Zheng et al. 2002, 147–156). The disease has grown to epidemic proportions since 2001. The return of schistosomiasis has larger implications than just the resurgence of a horrible parasitic disease. Chairman Mao's historic anti-schistosomiasis campaign is widely considered by the Chinese government and most Chinese people as one of their preeminent and most well-run health crusades. It became a symbol of government care for the people, brought international attention to the Chinese public health model, and still serves as an important model for current campaigns against SARS, avian and swine flu, and AIDS.

It is time to reassess this crucial campaign. This chapter aims to recapture the legacies of the Republican era (1911–1949) and the Japanese impact on the famous Maoist campaign. The campaign never achieved Mao's goal of complete elimination, an almost impossible standard for endemic parasitic diseases like schistosomiasis and malaria. Amazingly, it did succeed in bringing the disease under control. Although this campaign is famous for its prevention arm, which purportedly eliminated the disease during the Great Leap Forward (1958–1961), in fact the most important work was control efforts via the treatment arm during the Cultural Revolution (1966–1976) and shortly after. Today, Maoist-era successes have been eroded. It is unclear whether the government will provide the resources necessary to once again bring the disease under control.

While accurate numbers are hard to find, in 1949 schistosomiasis infected approximately 10.6 million people, with another 100 million at risk (Cheng 1971, 26). The species of schistosome most common in China, *Schistosoma japonicum*, is prevalent along and to the south of the Yangzi River. Historically, it affected eleven provinces—Anhui, Fujian, Guangdong, Guangxi, Hubei, Hunan, Jiangsu, Jiangxi, Sichuan, Yunnan, and Zhejiang—as well as the suburbs of Shanghai (see map 6.1).

Most humans and mammals contract schistosomiasis when they touch contaminated water during everyday activities. The microscopic parasitic worm passes through the skin and ends up in the intestines. After a few weeks, the worms start producing massive numbers of eggs. Some eggs remain cluttered in people's bodies, causing an immune reaction; others are expelled in excrement. Once egg-laden feces reaches water, the eggs hatch, and each produces a free-swimming miracidium, a first-stage worm, which infects a single type of snail, the one-centimeter-long *Oncomelania hupensis*. The snail emits cercariae, a second-stage worm, capable of infecting mammals and restarting the life cycle (see figure 6.1) (Davis 2003, 1431–1469). The disease can be prevented by reduc-

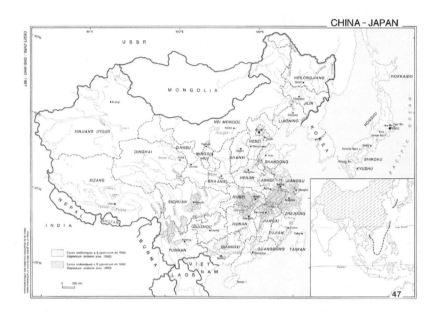

Map 6.1. Regional distribution of schistosomiasis in China in 1950 and 1980. *Source:* Reproduced, with the permission of the publisher, from J. P. Doumenge et. al., *Atlas of the Global Distribution of Schistosomiasis* (Geneva: World Health Organization, Parasitic Diseases Programme, and Université de Bordeaux, Centre de Recherche sur les Espaces Tropicaux, 1987) ("47 China—Japan," http://www.who.int/schistosomiasis/epidemiology/en/china_japan .pdf, 9).

ing the snail population, avoiding contaminated water, and ensuring good management of excrement. When people first catch the disease, the strong immune reaction causes dangerous spiking fevers and occasional death. The disease then settles into a long chronic phase whose main symptoms, lethargy and diarrhea, are rarely recognized as stemming from schistosomiasis. In the end stages the disease can cause massive fluid retention in the stomach (its most recognizable symptom), enlarged spleen and liver, cerebral lesions, infertility in both sexes, and dwarfism in infected children.

Schistosomiasis has at least a two-thousand-year history in China. In 1973, *S. japonicum* eggs were found in the remains of a Western Han dynasty (206 BCE– 9 CE) female aristocrat in Mawangdui, Hunan Province. A Han dynasty tomb in Hubei's Fenghuang Mountain also contained remains infected with *S. japonicum* eggs. Given that aristocrats probably had less contact with infectious environments than ordinary farmers did, it seems likely that the disease was fairly

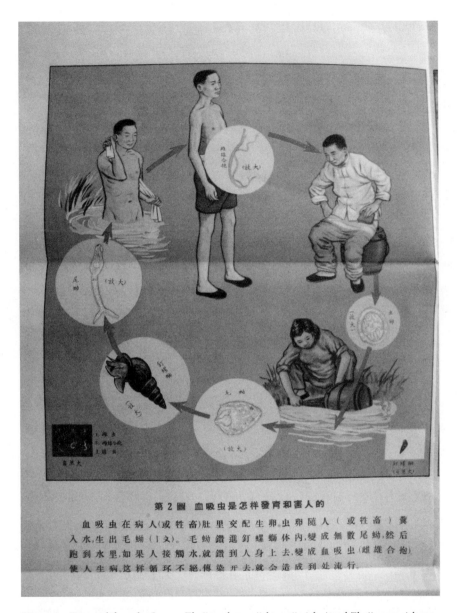

Figure 6.1. Disease life cycle. *Source:* Zhejiang kexue jishu puji xiehui and Zhejiang weisheng shiyanyuan (1956).

common in Hunan and Hubei Provinces during this period. The two provinces are still highly endemic today. As of now, fifteen ancient corpses have been found infected with the disease. Among them, two were from the Song dynasty (960–1279), and six were from the Ming dynasty (1368–1644) (Li 2006, 16–23).

Although the name for schistosomiasis, "xuexichong bing," is a modern medical term, by comparing the disease's symptoms and transmission with ancient medical texts, medical experts and historians have discovered that the Sui dynasty (581–618) medical classic *Zhu bing yuan hou lun* (Treatise on causes and symptoms of diseases), by Chao Yuanfang, recorded diseases similar to schistosomiasis. One, *gubing,* which means worms in the belly, is described as being acquired through contract with river or lake water in southern regions, and includes having a big belly (Li 2006, 16–23; Fan 1954, 862–864). Although schistosomiasis is a common disease in south China, because it is mainly asymptomatic until the late stages it is only in the last hundred years that it has been widely recognized.

Discovery of Schistosomiasis Japonica

The first variant of schistosomiasis (*Schistosoma haematobium*), which is also called Bilharzia, Snail Fever, and Big Belly disease, was discovered in 1851 by Theodore Bilharz in Egypt. However, scientists were unable to delineate the disease's complicated life cycle until Japanese researchers succeeded in 1913. In 1904, Dr. Fijiro Katsurada first discovered the Far Eastern variant of schistosomiasis in Japan and named it *Schistosoma japonicum*. In 1909, Akira Fujinami and Hachitaro Nakamura discovered that cows, dogs, and cats were infected by contaminated water, confirming that schistosomiasis infects the body through the skin. Keinosuke Miyairi and Minoru Suzuki first unraveled the disease's life cycle in 1913 when they discovered that snails could be infected with schistosomiasis. They also deciphered the larvae's life cycle inside the snail and determined which species of snail was the disease's intermediate host. In 1914, Robert T. Leiper, director of parasitology at the London School of Tropical Medicine, organized a team of specialists to investigate in the Far East. The team brought back a large number of snails, confirmed that *Oncomelania hupensis* was the intermediate host, and clarified the disease's life cycle (Farley 1991, 66–67).

While Japanese and British scientists unlocked the disease's life cycle abroad, medical missionaries spearheaded the first work in China. In 1905, the American doctor and missionary O. T. Logan examined a patient in Changde county, Hunan Province, and found schistosoma eggs in the patient's excrement. After comparing his findings with Katsurada's research report, he published a November 1905 article in the *China Medical Journal* (Logan 1905, 243–245). This first confirmed Chinese case opened up China-based medical research on the disease.

Schistosomiasis Work in China, 1900–1949

Discovering schistosomiasis in China turned out to be the easiest part of the problem. China's potentially vast infected terrain and population, limited health infrastructure, minimal number of Western-trained physicians, lack of knowledge about the disease, bankrupt governments, and disunited territory made addressing this slow-acting rural disease almost impossible.

According to Wu Zhongdao et al. and Kenneth Warren, during the Republican era almost all Chinese articles on schistosomiasis research focused on two areas: national disease distribution and case reports that included an exploration of signs and symptoms, testing methods, and treatment strategies. A smaller number of articles examined prevention, the intermediate host snail, and the disease's life cycle (Wu et al. 2006, 42–52; Warren 1988, 123–140; Berry-Cabán 2007, 45–53). In 1910, the medical missionary James Maxwell first reported that schistosomiasis was endemic in Hankou, Hubei Province. In the book, *The Diseases of China,* he described both the endemic conditions in China and the impact infection had on the human body (Jefferys and Maxwell 1910, 156–164). In 1924, with support from the Rockefeller Foundation's China Medical Board, the American physicians Earnest Faust and Henry Meleney from the Peking Union Medical College published *Studies on Schistosomiasis Japonica,* the first treatise to explore all aspects of the disease in China. Faust and Meleney also began to map the disease's endemic areas by sending questionnaires to doctors in areas they suspected were infectious. They discovered that nine provinces were endemic and divided the downstream area of the Yangzi River into six key endemic zones (Farley 1991, 94–96; Faust and Meleney 1924). By the early 1930s, all eleven endemic provinces were discovered. The number of endemic counties rose every year, especially in Zhejiang and Jiangsu Provinces and in Shanghai, perhaps because there were so many investigators located there.

The national government was first able to contribute to ongoing research by medical missionaries, private research institutions, medical schools, and urban hospitals in 1928 when the Nationalists established their government and inaugurated the country's first national Ministry of Public Health. Because the Nationalists did not control most of China, the "national" ministry had little actual power. Each province that established a provincial department of health acted independently and was expected to provide its own funding. At best, the national ministry could make suggestions for departmental organization and focus. Most provinces established a health center and a diagnostic laboratory at the provincial capital, and focused on maternal and child health, schools, health education, and data collection, with occasional efforts to mitigate large epidemics (Yip 1995, 48, 49). Very little of this work affected rural areas, where schistosomiasis was primarily located.

Like most researchers, the national and provincial governments focused on the disease's distribution. In addition, they established health infrastructure, trained medical and public health practitioners, and set up a research establishment, all of which were essential precursors for post-1949 work. Of particular importance was the national ministry's new field site in South Central China, which included a Department of Parasitology that made schistosomiasis a primary concern. The field site sent an anti-schistosomiasis unit to a newly established Zhejiang test site that worked from 1932 through 1949 to pioneer treatment and prevention methods applicable to rural areas, rather than hospital settings. Zhejiang would remain a key model schistosomiasis test site during the People's Republic (Kan and Yao 1934, 323–326; Kan and Kung 1936, 449–456; Yip 1995, 57, 105, 110, 111; ZGDE n.d.b).

From 1937 to 1945, war with Japan and increasing levels of government indebtedness made rural outreach impossible. From 1945 to 1949, despite civil war, the national and provincial governments built up infrastructure and started some important schistosomiasis work. For example, in 1946 the Jiangsu Health Department established the Southern Jiangsu Disease Prevention and Treatment Clinic (*Sunan difangbing fangzhi suo*) in Wu county to do schistosomiasis work. In April 1947, the Central Health Laboratory of the national Ministry of Health collaborated with this clinic on schistosomiasis research. The clinic investigated local disease distribution, engaged in clinical examination and early diagnosis, developed treatment and prevention methods, and began initial efforts at education (Shi 2010, 24–29).

Communists located in southern base areas such as Jiangxi and Hunan also recognized the disease in the 1930s and began to work on it, particularly since it had such a debilitating effect on their troops' fighting ability. Before the Fourth Field Army, led by Lin Biao (minister of defense, 1959–1971), marched south in 1949, the Health Bureau produced a medical handbook that taught how to avoid and treat five diseases common in the southern provinces—cholera, bacterial dysentery, malaria, foot ulcers, and schistosomiasis (Di si ye zhan jun hou qin weisheng bu 1949).

Republican-era work on schistosomiasis by foreign researchers, medical missionaries, private practitioners and institutions, the Nationalists, and the Communists all left a key legacy for the People's Republic. Although the barriers to wide-scale treatment and prevention activities were impossible to surmount, work during this period provided many essential prerequisites for the famous Maoist-era campaign. Researchers discovered many of the key infectious areas in China and made solid estimates about human disease demographics. Doctors' case reports investigated the parameters of the disease and explored treatment methods, while fieldwork described the disease's life cycle. Many young scholars who studied the disease would form a research establishment that provided many of the crucial developments for the Maoist campaign. Finally, test sites were established to begin the challenging work of developing treatment, prevention, and education methods that would work in the rural arena.

A Surprising Campaign Choice

On October 1, 1949, Chairman Mao announced the start of new China, a China that would finally stand on its own two feet, successfully modernize, and become an international powerhouse. This glowing vision was very far from reality. Instead, decades of war had devastated the economy. Large numbers of refugees, mass malnourishment, and limited prior health care made the prevalence of disease, particularly dangerous epidemic diseases, very high.

Out of this plethora of problems, it is astonishing that Chinese leaders chose an almost unknown, slow acting, rural disease as one of their first health efforts. At a time when the government needed early, rapid successes, schistosomiasis, a typically recalcitrant endemic disease, would repeatedly prove to be an unfortunate choice. Despite this, the government sponsored a campaign peak during the Great Leap Forward (1957–1958), completely revived the campaign during the Cultural Revolution (1969–1971), and in some places had a third campaign peak during the 1990s.

The government's initial support for schistosomiasis work seems strongly linked to early military security rather than public health. After liberating Shanghai in May 1949, CCP leadership was already considering how it could conquer Taiwan. But since the close to thirty-seven thousand Northern Chinese crack troops had no aquatic experience, they were sent to Shanghai's suburbs to learn marine invasion skills. In only a couple of weeks they started coming down with unidentified skin rashes. Some were sick enough to be hospitalized. It took months for the disease to be identified and even longer for it to be treated. Over fourteen thousand troops, 38 percent of the top soldiers in China, were incapacitated due to schistosomiasis. While it is unknown how this affected the putative attack on Taiwan, clearly forward momentum had been lost (SMA 1950a; SMA 1949–1950).

Military leaders soon realized that controlling the disease's impact was not a one-off affair. Throughout South and Central China large numbers of potential enlistees were deemed unsuitable because of schistosomiasis. For example, in 1954 in greater Shanghai, 33 percent of enlistees had schistosomiasis (SMA 1955b). Impediments to enlistment were a large concern, especially given the high mortality rates from the recent Korean War. Leaders of the East China Military District, which included the Shanghai region, were among the first to engage in schistosomiasis work. They set an example where the disease had both military and political connotations, rather than being framed as just a health campaign (Huang and Luo 1989, 154).

As leadership transitioned in 1954 from military districts to the government and party, rare discussions about schistosomiasis tended to focus on economic rather than military security. Leaders were concerned with the impact of parasites on worker productivity rates at a time when agricultural productivity was the main variable in gross national product. But schistosomiasis was not included as a high priority and, arguably, may never have become one without high-level CCP involvement (Fan and Lai 2008, 178).

The entire tenor of prior haphazard schistosomiasis work changed in late 1955 when Chairman Mao got involved in the work. According to Su Delong, one of China's top schistosomiasis experts and Mao's personal advisor on the campaign, Mao had previously dealt with so many ill villagers and soldiers that when the crack troops were discovered to have the disease in 1949, he became particularly interested in it (Warren 1988, 123–124).

Mao's focus on the disease was combined with great dissatisfaction with the Ministry of Health, which he accused of concentrating solely on cities, exhibiting indifference toward the masses, excluding Chinese medical doctors, and placing professional or scientific goals above party directives. The supposed mishandling of schistosomiasis provided the final lever to oust the deputy minister of health, He Cheng, in November 1955. In fact, the ministry had been working on schistosomiasis, but in addition to a grave funding shortage, it lacked personnel, materials, infrastructure, medications, and the power to do most rural public health work. Given the many diseases with a higher mortality rate, the ministry had decided to continue Republican-era strategies by focusing on test site areas, surveying, training personnel, and improving treatment regimens and snail elimination methods (Lampton 1974, 36, 46–49, 62). Mao nonetheless extracted the campaign from ministry control and emphasized its importance and independence by creating a new nine-person schistosomiasis leadership small group (LSG) directly under the Party Central Committee. In his December 1955 "Seventeen Articles on Agricultural Work," which determined priorities in the agricultural arena, Mao listed schistosomiasis as the disease most harmful to people and livestock. Other important documents at the time similarly highlighted schistosomiasis. Suddenly this easily overlooked disease skyrocketed to national importance. Throughout the campaign's history, the intensity of activity would rise or fall depending on Mao's attention. After Mao's famous 1958 poem "Farewell to the God of Plague," valorizing the first county to eliminate the disease, the campaign became so associated with Mao that even an intensification of the Mao cult during the Cultural Revolution was enough to help revitalize the campaign (Kau and Leung 1986, 688, 691; Kau and Leung 1992, 31).

Researching Schistosomiasis

From 1949 to 1955 the Ministry of Health mainly concentrated on research. Despite Mao's condemning the ministry for its scholarly focus, its decision not only played to its strengths, but had the added benefit of following Soviet advisors' injunctions. Unfortunately, because Soviet experts such as Tikhon E. Boldyrev (1900–1984) had no practical experience with this southern disease, their prescriptions tended to be vague or dependent on resources, both material and professional, that China lacked (Boerdeliefu 1956, 3–4). Since doing more research and surveys were among their nebulous recommendations, the politically battered ministry was able to continue prior policies while taking shelter under Soviet guidelines.

Utilizing the many researchers trained during the Republican era, the Institute of Parasitic Diseases (IPD) was established in 1950 in Shanghai with 220 staff divided into divisions studying schistosomiasis, malaria, filariasis, hookworm, and kala-azar. While other parasitic diseases mainly had a single working group, schistosomiasis had four, dedicated to prevention and control, diagnosis, clinical medicine, and pharmacology. The ministry also organized fifteen subinstitutes of parasitology or schistosomiasis, one in each province that had one or more endemic parasitic diseases. Both the provincial parasitic institutes and local subunits of provincial health departments began mass surveys and established test sites ("Report of the American Schistosomiasis Delegation" 1977, 428–429; Hsu and Hsu 1974, 348; Mao 1983, 117–125; Lampton 1977, 64; Lampton 1974, 36, 66).

After Mao took the newly launched campaign away from the ministry, he continued sponsoring schistosomiasis research. The original fifteen provincial-level parasitic institutes grew to forty-two research organizations. In addition, thirty-eight hospitals or big prevention units and some medical colleges had dedicated clinical research units and over two hundred disease-specific hospitals were created. All these institutions presided over a publishing boom that peaked after Mao's famous 1958 poem lauding the campaign suggested research on schistosomiasis would be well received: from 1924 to 1958 there had been fewer than 200 articles; from 1958 to 1960 close to 350 articles were published (Shen 1961, 3; Warren 1988, 127–129, 131; Lampton 1974, 51–56).

During the 1960s, the schistosomiasis research establishment experienced the same highs and lows as other professionals. Many institutes reconstituted themselves from 1961 to 1965 after the end of the Great Leap Forward and attempted to make science rather than politics the benchmark for their work (SMA 1963–1964). This effort fell apart during the Cultural Revolution, when unprecedented numbers of professionals were sent long-term to the countryside. Most campaign leaders, including the scientifically oriented Wei Wenbo, the head of the nine-person LSG started by Chairman Mao, were purged and deemed "political gods of plague." By 1972 the campaign's lead research agency, the IPD, was closed down (Lampton 1974, 19–22; Wang 1988, 5, 17, 36, 127; SMA 1972a; SWSMM 1971; SMA 1972b). The IPD had to wait until the end of the Cultural Revolution to reopen and rebuild its research efforts.

Campaign Activities

While the quality and later the quantity of professional research plummeted during the Great Leap and Cultural Revolution, campaign activities peaked. Campaign work was divided into two arms: prevention and treatment. Worldwide, controlling endemic parasitic diseases has proved to be extremely difficult, and eliminating them almost impossible. The schistosomiasis campaign garnered great national and international acclaim for its supposed achievements in preventing the disease (Horn 1969, 94; "Report of the American Schistosomiasis Delegation" 1977, 431; Sandbach 1977, 27). Prevention activities involved either altering personal hygiene habits or eliminating the disease's intermediate host, the miniscule *Oncomelania* snail.

In terms of personal habits, the campaign focused on two fundamentals: water and excrement. Campaign personnel encouraged large-scale well-digging to increase clean water sources. They tried to get fishermen and farmers to don protective leggings made of bandages. Personnel also constructed large numbers of village, field, and dock toilets to decrease the amount of fresh, egg-laden night soil pervading the environment. Since night soil was a major source of fertilizer, it normally was collected and dumped directly onto the field. Personnel encouraged people to move excrement vats away from water and to create a collectivized night soil center whose manager would ferment the night soil, a natural process that improved the fertilizer and killed off parasitic eggs (see figure 6.2) (*China Reconstructs* 1968, 16; Reed 1979, 163–165; Faust and Meleney 1924, 257; Wang 1988, 76–77; SQDA 1951).

While in theory these activities were worthwhile, they proved hard to implement. Rural people tended to find them expensive, uncomfortable, unnecessary, and, worst of all, a waste of time. In many cases they seemed an urban conceit. As one peasant put it, "How can people who till the soil be particular about things like city folks?" (Yu 1984, 71).

Faced with widespread resistance and difficulties in enforcement, campaign personnel decided that killing snails sounded easier. This decision was greatly influenced by the two-month, 1956 delegation led by the renowned Japanese scholar Yoshitaka Komiya, from the Japanese Society of Parasitology. Komiya was a Communist who had worked in China in the 1930s in the Shanghai Institute for Natural Science, where he began his lifelong interest in parasitology. He returned to Japan after World War II before coming to China in the 1956 delegation. Komiya advised Chinese leaders to focus on prevention rather than treatment, but to switch from feces management to snail elimination. Komiya suggested that snail burial, an elimination strategy not used in Japan, was China's best option because it was cheaper and required less technical sophistication (Iijima 2008, 56–63; Iijima 2007–2009, 14–21; Komiya 1957, 461–471; SMA 1952).

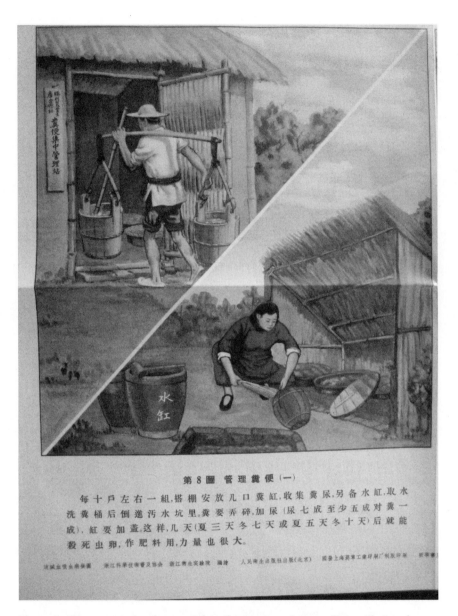

第 8 圖　管理糞便 (一)

　　每十戶左右一組,搭棚安放几口糞缸,收集糞尿,另備水缸,取水
洗糞桶后倒進污水坑里。糞要弄碎,加尿 (尿七成至少五成对糞一
成), 缸要加蓋。这样,几天(夏三天冬七天或夏五天冬十天)后就能
殺死虫卵, 作肥料用,力量也很大。

淀減血吸虫侮保圖　　浙江科学技术普及協会　浙江衛生实驗院　編绘　　人民衛生出版社出版(北京)　　圖旁上海装卓工業印刷厂制版印刷　　

Figure 6.2. Poster promoting the new night soil management system. *Source:* Zhejiang kexue jishu puji xiehui and Zhejiang weisheng shiyanyuan (1956).

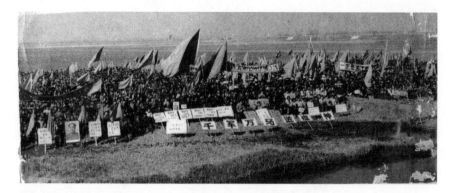

Figure 6.3. Mobilization for a mass snail elimination campaign, Dantu county, Jiangsu Province, 1960s. *Source:* Photo from the collection of Kawai Fan.

Localities all over China started experimenting. While a few could afford factory-produced molluscicides and flame-throwing machines that annihilated snails on vertical surfaces, most had to make do with homegrown methods. These included lime and tea cake, which had some ability to kill snails, and a wide variety of labor-intensive strategies such as dumping boiling water on snails, snagging them with chopsticks, and, most commonly, Komiya's method, suffocating them to death. The last method became the campaign's most famous activity (JSDA 1951–1957; SWSMM 1956; SQDA 1956; SQDA 1957).

Initially dubious, many people were willing to try since the CCP promised that one all-out effort would eliminate the disease forever (see figure 6.3). Unfortunately, even if around 80 percent of an area's snails are killed, they replicate so fast that ten months later they return to their former abundance (Reed 1979, 44–49). When campaigns prioritized speed over quality, as they almost always did, snails were sometimes buried under only a small amount of earth and popped right out again. Local leaders also did not want to sponsor snail campaigns since they took labor away from production. This led to a downward spiral whereby popular interest in snail campaigns waned and leaders assigned their least able workers. This led to perfunctory work, which in turn led to snails' returning even faster, justifying people's apathetic performance and leaders' designating few resources to the task (JSDA 1956b; SQDA 1957; SWSMM 1973). The result was that when snail campaigns became a political necessity, leaders staged a brief, flashy snail campaign and deemed their work on schistosomiasis prevention done for the year.

The campaign's treatment arm involved a different set of problems. It was hard to pin down the number of sick people because schistosomiasis is mainly an asymptomatic disease (or has symptoms readily ascribable to something else).

In addition, the test for the disease, stool samples, failed to pick up many of the cases. Many rural people were confused, and especially in women's cases, mortified at the idea of handing in stool samples. Oxen and water buffalo play a major role in spreading this disease, but it was even harder to procure accurate stool samples for them (Wang 1988, 89).[1]

Once sick individuals and animals were identified, campaign leaders had to contend with grave shortages in medicines, medical infrastructure, and equipment; limited funding for mass treatment; and, most importantly, insufficient numbers of trained personnel, whether doctors or veterinarians, who could safely use antimony, the disease's dangerous medicine. Small teams of experienced doctors were dispatched to the countryside, but most treatment was accomplished by retraining local Chinese medical practitioners to give antimony injections. County-level schistosomiasis treatment stations were established and ramshackle rural wards constructed from decrepit buildings and temples. Eventually, in the 1960s, the schistosomiasis research establishment developed oral versions of antimony and experimented with shorter medical regimens, which facilitated rural people's getting treated (Mao 1992, 33; Wang 1988, 45–46; SMA 1955a; JSDA 1956a).

Despite the disease's devastating nature, treatment personnel had large problems filling wards during the 1950s and even had patients running away mid-course. Patients' resistance seems to have stemmed from three factors. First, treatment was scary, due to multiple painful and dangerous injections. Second, because most asymptomatic people did not think they were sick and the available drugs only had a 60 percent cure rate, treatment looked like a scam. Finally, and most importantly, it was expensive. For most of the early campaign the government provided little or no treatment subsidies (Wang 1988, 45; JXDA 1957; JXDA 1953; JSDA 1956a).

The entire tenor of treatment changed in 1966 when the CCP made it completely free. Barefoot doctors, who emerged in 1970, and professional doctors sent long-term to the countryside greatly increased the number of practitioners and the expertise of medical care. Helped by new, easier oral treatment, the observation that few people died, and free treatment, many previously unwilling people flocked to get treated (Wang 1988, 46; JXDA 1966). Between mass Cultural Revolution treatment work and short-term intensive snail campaigns, the level of environmental infectivity greatly diminished, leading to a tipping point in many areas that brought the disease under control.

Fostering the Campaign

Educational outreach was a core part of the campaign. Campaign personnel tried to educate people, popularize campaign activities, and instill appropriate admiration for Chairman Mao and the CCP's efforts at transforming society.

While some education exploited successfully treated peers turned grassroots activists, most formal education focused on conveying the scientific rationales for campaign activities. Most scientifically oriented posters were headed by a large "Schistosomiasis must be eliminated" slogan, and by Mao's poem. This was followed by simple text and pictures explicating the disease's life cycle and linking it to prevention activities. Personnel soon discovered that many educational tools, particularly lectures, books, and posters, were ineffective because they were boring, villagers were busy, they required basic literacy, and many local people could not understand the specialized scientific terms. As a result, movies, plays, and slideshows became the preferred forms of education.

One of the most popular campaign-oriented movies was the 1961 film *Ku mu feng chun* (Getting a new lease on life), which combined campaign information with technological novelty via mobile film projection units dispatched deep into rural areas, where it was shown free of charge. In 1964, it was presented 850 times in Suzhou, where nearly one million people saw it; and 57 times in Nanjing, where 58,000 people saw it. Nanjing authorities sent mobile film projectors into infectious rural areas. In Anhui Province the local government presented movies related to schistosomiasis prevention a total of 5,400 times between 1964 and 1985 (Suzhou 1997, 141; Wang 1995, 152–153; Anhui sheng 1990, 206).

In the film, the main character, Kumeizi, is a child bride of the Fang family, destined to marry their son Fang Dongge. Because of civil war, the prospective couple loses touch, and after 1949, Kumeizi marries a man who dies of schistosomiasis. Finally, the couple is reunited at a schistosomiasis prevention station. Unfortunately, Kumeizi has also contracted the disease, but Fang refuses to leave her. After being treated by both Chinese and Western doctors, she eventually recovers. Fang and Kumeizi get married and enjoy a happy family blessed with children. The film showcases the transformative changes occurring in new China under the guidance of Mao and the CCP while castigating the Nationalists for neglecting the disease. It also educates people on how to eliminate the snails, suggests the importance of Chinese medicine and the need to integrate it with Western medicine, encourages people to think that despite not being medical experts, they, like Fang, can make major contributions to the campaign, and tries to instill the belief that a disease-free future is possible.

The strategy that health personnel favored most was on-site demonstration using microscopes. Each villager would get the novel pleasure of handling the machine and looking through its lens. Unfortunately for prevention personnel, "seeing is believing" only works if one shares a similar knowledge base. The villagers' understanding of the world did not include microscopy, pathogens, or the notion that a specific causal agent triggers a disease. This made the sight in front of them impossible to decode. Many villagers accused personnel of "playing tricks and demonstrating magic just to try and scare us" (Pan 1957, 9; Li 1992, 133).

Although education efforts sometimes went awry, the rhetoric and structure of mass mobilization campaigns helped enforce compliance. Campaign work was framed as a military campaign against "the enemy," who was "staging an armed rebellion." Workers assigned to shoveling were "soldiers" organized in a military structure of battalions, platoons, and brigades. They were ordered to use strategies stemming more from warfare against fellow humans than those best employed against mollusks. This approach helped generate feelings of obligatory patriotism and gave the work value beyond eliminating a few more snails (Yang 1992, 17–18; Yu 1992, 3–4; Mao 1992, 37; Li 1992, 101).

Another strategy was to infuse the campaign with competitions and community pressure reinforced by the need to save face. Leaders pitted individuals, small groups, and whole communities against each other to win community acclaim for killing the most snails or achieving the cleanest village. According to a 1957 Jiangxi report, competition "smashes conservative thinking and stops a self-satisfied attitude." Competition was even employed to spur people to get treated. In Qingpu, recalcitrant villagers "who kept making excuses that they were too busy" were told that "people from other villages are running here to get treatment even though they are busy too." Embedding intense competition into the campaign led to increased output without coercion or "motivated people's activism" (JXDA 1957; SQDA 1954; SWSMM 1957).

At the same time that pressure was applied, campaign propaganda also offered huge promise. When exceptionally ill patients were cured and villagers made infertile by the disease managed, post-treatment, to have children, the campaign and the party's successes were entirely evident. Unfortunately, there was no comparable phenomenon facilitating the campaign's prevention arm, where the constant reappearance of snails made people doubt the mass mobilization campaigns. The result was that treatment activities received frequent positive reinforcement while prevention activities waxed and waned based on people's trust in the party or Mao and their level of revolutionary fervor.

While at the grassroots level education seems to have played a less important role in promoting the campaign than structurally based encouragement, peer endorsement, and successful treatment, at the upper levels of the CCP, education appears to have been the primary approach. Upper-level education also had different messages. At the county level and below, prevention activities were linked to concrete scientific knowledge; treatment was marketed to people (but mainly men) as a mechanism to increase their work output and thus their work points, and to women as a method to reverse their disease-based infertility in order to have babies.[2]

In contrast, upper-level cadres' education ignored details about disease life cycle and focused on science as an ideology, a transformative power that—once wielded by the party and integrated with socialism—would motivate societal reconstruction, legitimize party leadership, and bring respect on the international stage (SMA 1955a).

This rhetoric, domestically and internationally, assigned a special role to Chinese medicine, which ideally would transform medical science. Though traditional doctors were used heavily by the campaign, they frequently employed Western medicine since Chinese medicine lacks a cure for schistosomiasis. While the need to substantively incorporate Chinese medicine was a frequent topic of high-level meetings, at the ground level Chinese medicine was rarely the focus. Instead, propaganda defined good medical care as cheap, effective, accessible, and speedy, irrespective of national origins.[3] The divergence of educational messages appears to have matched the needs of the respective audiences. Local cadres and educators needed to give villagers specific rationales for extra work and demonstrate that it would have personal benefit; upper-level leaders needed dramatic language proving that this ostensibly unimportant campaign was worth losing scarce political capital and resources and that advantages went beyond curing an unknown rural disease.

Reform-Era Schistosomiasis Work

The work carried out during the Cultural Revolution campaign peak made a crucial contribution to the control of schistosomiasis, but it was only in the late 1970s and 1980s that many places eliminated the disease. Just as China entered the Reform era, the global protocol for best addressing schistosomiasis shifted. Due to the creation of Praziquantel, an effective new medicine, in Germany during the mid-1970s, control work changed from disrupting transmission, which concentrated on snail elimination and some treatment, to controlling morbidity, which focused almost entirely on treatment. This new strategy has been effective. Unlike most countries, however, China has chosen to retain snail elimination as a core part of its control effort (Utzinger et al. 2005, 74, 86). Speculatively, this may be because it would be politically difficult to jettison the most famous part of this campaign or to imply that the years of backbreaking labor to kill snails under party guidance were unproductive.

During the Reform era in China, there have been improvements in both the organization of the work and the technical aspects of prevention and treatment. Starting in the 1980s, campaign workers and the Ministry of Health improved record-keeping to track the population's past treatment history. In addition, professional expertise at all levels came to the fore in decision-making. Finally, work was transferred to small, specialized groups rather than continuing with mass mobilization campaigns, which has led to better quality control (Wang 1988, 54, 116–117; Huang and Luo 1989, 158).

In terms of snail elimination, molluscides have become more affordable. Chemicals have also been used with greater efficacy due to increased knowledge about the snail's life cycle and the ability to let this information alter practice on the ground. There have also been vast improvements in locating snails utilizing geographical information systems and remote sensing (Zhou 2001, 97–106). However, these advances have sometimes been stymied due to lack of funding, particularly in more impoverished provinces. For example, in Jiangxi Province during the late 1970s and 1980s, work was limited to small-scale chemical use and some tractors. Prevention personnel only had enough resources to clear about one-seventh of the snail-covered territory annually. By the late 1980s the infectious area was actually increasing again (Zhong 1989, 69).

The reason a major epidemic did not arise, particularly in poorer places, appears to be outstanding changes in treatment. Previous treatment was impeded by poor testing methods, dangerous treatment drugs that required medical supervision, and low cure rates. During the Reform period, more successful testing methods were developed, and Praziquantel gained widespread use in 1980. Praziquantel is cheap, requires taking pills for a day or two, cures most cases of the disease, has few side effects, and even reverses some of the organ damage caused by the disease. It is so readily available and inexpensive that many people self-medicate. Of concern is that there are no clear alternatives if schistosomiasis ever becomes resistant to this medicine. Technical improvements were also made in cattle treatment. More concerted efforts to treat cattle, fewer cattle due to their replacement with machinery, better testing methods, and Praziquantel, which also works in cattle, have all increased the efficacy of this part of the campaign.

The World Bank ran a decade-long schistosomiasis project from 1992 to 2001 that loaned China seventy-one million dollars on the condition that China supply matching funds. This money alleviated funding shortages and prompted a third campaign peak that left more areas controlled, but it did not eliminate the problem everywhere (Chen 2005, 43–48). Some places, such as the area surrounding the snail reservoir Poyang Lake in Jiangxi Province, will probably never eliminate the disease because snails cannot be removed without destroying the whole aquatic ecosystem.

Since responsibility was handed back to the government in 2001, a dramatic increase in case rates has been observed. In addition to limited funding and lack of public awareness, the catastrophic 1998 flood of the Yangzi River and the Three Gorges Dam basin have created large new infectious areas. Global warming may also be contributing to the disease by increasing snail habitat (Utzinger et al. 2005, 70). These immediate and long-term threats have not been met with analogous increases in treatment, prevention, and education. Today there are thought to be 865,000 people infected with the disease, and the annual cost of schistosomiasis treatment has risen to four billion renminbi. This explosion of cases includes both new areas and regions known to still have the disease, and places like Shanghai that supposedly eliminated the disease in 1985 (Lee 2004). However, in 2004 China recategorized schistosomiasis as one of its highest communicable disease priorities. Li Keqiang, China's vice premier, stated the importance of controlling and preventing schistosomiasis at a September 7, 2010, national anti-schistosomiasis meeting, indicating there may be a renewed government commitment in the future (Utzinger et al. 2005, 76; Li 2010).

Conclusion

China's schistosomiasis campaign was an impressive accomplishment. Few other developing countries with limited resources have ever addressed an endemic disease on this scale. Despite every possible barrier, after the disease's discovery in 1905 the many actors involved in public health mapped out the parameters of the disease and created a research establishment that was essential for forward progress. Due to its advanced schistosomiasis work and willingness to provide assistance, Japanese scientists played a key mentoring role in research during the Republican era and in campaign directions during the early PRC campaign. The fact that the CCP and Chairman Mao chose an unknown rural disease as one of their earliest health efforts, and then continued the work despite many obstacles, greatly redounds to their credit. Although this campaign is famous for its prevention accomplishments during the Great Leap Forward, this chapter finds that the most effective campaign activity was treatment work during the Cultural Revolution (1966–1976). During the Reform era the campaign has often been neglected, but the disease has been partially contained due to technical and organizational improvements and work by the World Bank. Disease incidence has been rising rapidly since 2001. It is unclear whether the government will back up its revived concern with sufficient funding.

In some ways the schistosomiasis campaign has been radically rewritten in popular memory. The government portrays schistosomiasis work as a preeminent model of patriotic participation in a well-loved campaign. Today, schistosomiasis has little impact on the growing urban population, and rural people's situation is not well known. This, anecdotally, leads many urban people to claim that the disease was eliminated in 1958. Some urban dwellers also lament the loss of the innocence, hard work, and goodwill that supposedly reflects the way rural people threw themselves into the Maoist-era campaign. The archives portray a much more complex pattern of resistance and partial assimilation. Future campaigns may be the victim of prior success. Few people realize that the disease has reemerged, that resources need to be dedicated to this campaign, and that most rural people and local governments were unexcited about the campaign but were still able to make a transformative difference. Without this knowledge it is questionable whether people will be willing to advocate for the campaign in the future.

While the schistosomiasis campaign's future is in question, the model provided by the campaign is not. Current health campaigns, particularly those in the rural arena, appear to be revitalizing methods developed and refined in this and other campaigns during the Maoist era; the SARS campaign provides a particularly good example. Like the schistosomiasis campaign, the SARS campaign operated by mobilizing the entire population, using Maoist-era health propaganda education methods, tropes, and imagery; reviving traditional mutual household surveillance networks; and reconceptualizing the campaign from an attempt to manage pathogens to an all-out people's war by citizen soldiers against enemy germs. Finally, the takeover of the SARS campaign by top party leadership, like the schistosomiasis campaign, led to a purge of Ministry of Health leaders (He Cheng in 1955 and Zhang Wenkang in 2003) and signaled that the campaign was a top political priority that trumped normal administrative practices and patron-client relationships. Together these changes turned the tide against the SARS epidemic (Balasegaram 2006, 73–85; Hanson 2008, 1457–1458).

Perhaps the current interest in revitalizing the Maoist public health model is that mass mobilization health campaigns were fast and inexpensive, and did not require much health infrastructure or medical personnel. As China's countryside becomes increasingly depopulated of medical professionals, workable hospitals, and health funding, the allure of mass mobilization campaigns appears to be shining once again.

Notes

1. Collecting manure was difficult because illiterate workers had to be willing to gather samples out of the paddy fields, remember which animal they came from in a collectivized herd, and carry them around all day as they worked (JXDA 1957; SQDA 1952).

2. Since men were the main people sick, they constituted most of the infertile population. However, campaign propaganda never acknowledged this and instead specifically linked female treatment with increased fertility.

3. For example, in 1957, a peak treatment year, only 6.6 percent of the 74,544 people treated in Jiangsu Province used Chinese medical treatment; .7 percent used a mix of Western and Chinese treatment; and the rest used Western treatment (SMA 1955a; JSDA 1957).

7 Tuberculosis Control in Shanghai

Bringing Health to the Masses, 1928–Present

Rachel Core

Tuberculosis (TB) was one of the most widespread and deadly diseases in China in the early part of the twentieth century. The Chinese people had a saying about turning pale at mention of the disease, which they believed killed nine out of ten of its victims. This may have been an exaggeration; however, in the first half of the twentieth century, China's TB mortality rates were much higher than those in Europe, North America, and other Asian nations. Throughout the century, scientific discovery advanced TB control efforts worldwide, but given China's massive population, developing a system to bring scientific advances to the wide population presented a special challenge. In Shanghai, the speed of the city's urbanization, and the resulting size and heterogeneity of the population, amplified these challenges.

This chapter examines eighty-five years of efforts to control TB by connecting the population to the health and public health system in China's largest city. The chapter is based upon archival documents and interviews with providers and recipients of health care. The archival documents include clinic reports and numerous documents from government archives such as the Shanghai Municipal Archives (SMA). Interviewees included thirty-five providers of health care, including six retired doctors who attended medical school in the 1950s, and fifty-three recipients of health care, including forty-five TB patients at a municipal-level facility. Health care providers were identified through snowball sampling and care recipients were identified through respondent-driven sampling.

The chapter is divided chronologically into three sections, each of which co-incides with a different model of TB control. The first section considers limited success in bringing primary and tertiary TB prevention to affected individuals prior to the 1949 Communist victory.[1] The second section examines widespread efforts to bring the disease under control after 1949. After factories and other workplaces were socialized, TB control programs became systematized in 1958–1978, with district prevention and treatment stations overseeing efforts within individual workplaces. The relationship between district stations and individual workplaces, which provided an effective link ensuring that scientific advances could reach the masses, continued through the 1980s. The final section covers the period from 1992 to the present, and discusses China's adoption of the World Health Organization's Directly Observed Therapy, Short-Course (DOTS) TB control program after 1992. During this period, Shanghai has experienced wide-scale in-migration and the workplace-based urban health insurance system collapsed, so bringing TB control to the masses has proven challenging.

Prelude to Public Health Linkages, 1928–1949

Primary and Tertiary Prevention Efforts during the Nanjing Decade, 1928–1937

Shanghai sits on the Huangpu River. This final tributary joins the Yangzi River as it empties into the Pacific Ocean. Due to the city's strategic location near the confluence of these rivers, the 1842 Treaty of Nanjing following the Opium War designated Shanghai as a treaty port; foreigners carved out an International Settlement and French Concession and appointed municipal councils to govern these extraterritorial holdings. Over the course of the next century, Shanghai became China's leading port, its financial capital, and its industrial center. Workers flocked to the city, and during the first half of the twentieth century, Shanghai became one of the largest cities in the world. Shanghai's population exploded from around 1.5 million in 1925 to over 5 million in 1950 (MacPherson 1987).

Prior to 1949, Shanghai had more private, light industrial factories, and particularly textile factories, than any other city in China. Young female workers with nimble fingers staffed the looms, which ran twenty-four hours a day. TB was particularly prevalent among workers who lived and worked in close quarters with little ventilation, such as in the cotton mills (Honig 1986). These workers feared that taking time off to nurse a cough might result in contract adjustments or pay deductions, but their plight was much better than that of the urban poor, who did not have stable work. Before 1949, the ranks of urban poor in Shanghai had swollen to one million, many of whom had come to Shanghai to escape poverty in the countryside. They lived in crowded shantytowns near the river's banks and eked out an existence, often through informal work. In the 1920s and '30s, these urban poor included one hundred thousand public rickshaw pullers and thousands more private rickshaw pullers, fifty to sixty thousand dock workers, and twenty to twenty-five thousand professional beggars (Lu 1999). Finding stable factory work was the shanty-dweller's dream because many could not afford the deposit required to begin a starting position or an apprenticeship.

Such crowded conditions, with exploitive or unstable work, provided ideal conditions for the spread of infectious diseases such as tuberculosis. According to one survey, seven of every ten of Shanghai's millworkers suffered from TB, due to the grueling hours entailed by alternating day and night shifts (Honig 1986). Because effective antibiotics for controlling *Mycobacterium tuberculosis* did not exist prior to the 1940s, workers had a slim chance for survival if they contracted TB and the disease progressed to an advanced stage. In 1934, the *China Press* reported that nationally, TB was responsible for one-fifth to one-quarter of all deaths, including 30 percent of deaths of people ages sixteen to sixty (SMA 1935–1939). TB caused 1.2 million deaths per year throughout the nation (Li 1934). China's TB mortality rates were among the highest in the world; in 1935, TB mortality in China was estimated to have been four hundred per hundred thousand. This figure was eight times New Zealand's rate, five times the United States' rate, four times England's rate, and more than twice the rate in Japan (SMA 1935–1939).

Certainly, data on TB mortality from this period is not great. After the Nationalist (or Guomindang) government was established in 1928, it began to build a National Health Reconstruction program, which saw China's first concerted efforts to create and monitor health statistics based on infectious disease notification at the national level. According to a 1928 Ministry of Health directive, doctors were required to report diagnoses of several prevalent infectious diseases to authorities within twelve hours (Yip 1996). Despite its prevalence in the urban population, TB was not among the infectious diseases requiring notification in the initial 1928 directive. Consequently, the data that does exist for TB is incomplete, and in some cases is available only for the International Settlement and French Concession; however, the data that does exist suggests that TB mortality rates were declining even prior to the discovery of effective antibiotics in the 1940s (Zhang and Elvin 1998). While Thomas McKeown's influential thesis suggests that much of this decline can be explained by improvements in living and working conditions, I have found little evidence of systematic improvements in such conditions prior to the 1950s. At the same time, there were efforts to increase knowledge of disease transmission means and to reduce exposure to infection, which did affect mortality rates. I will examine these efforts and their limitations in the paragraphs below.

The governments of Shanghai developed no comprehensive plan to battle the city's leading infectious disease. Government documents from 1935 claim government avoidance of the TB problem, owing to the costs (SMA 1935–1939). Leading doctors, including Yan Fuqing (顏福慶), Wu Lien-teh, and Li Ting'an (李廷安), instead took up the challenge of TB control. In October 1933, they founded the Chinese Anti-Tuberculosis Association (CATA, 中國防癆協會), whose Shanghai branch, the Shanghai Anti-TB Association (SATA, 上海防癆協會), was founded five years later, in October 1938. CATA and SATA were the only organizations active in the 1930s and 1940s dedicated to elimination of a single disease. Their anti-TB efforts included both preventive and treatment programs.

In the area of prevention, CATA's public health activities included week-long educational campaigns, radio talks, and public lectures. In 1934, six doctors spoke on a radio station, one every two weeks for three months. According to CATA's *First Annual Report*, in 1934, fifty public lectures, with an estimated total attendance of 7,500, were given on Saturday nights and in colleges and schools (SMA 1935–1939). CATA conducted its first anti-spitting week from March 28 to 31, 1935.[2] More than one hundred people attended the opening ceremony of the campaign at ten o'clock in the morning at the Metropol Theatre on March 28. CATA had posters and handbills printed for the campaign and sent them to various government health officers to assist with distribution. The metropolitan police also granted CATA permission to have boy scouts distribute the handbills at intersections (SMA 1935–1939). The campaign included days with educational programs for students, merchants, and factory workers.

Certainly, these campaigns and lectures were better than nothing, but their scope and effectiveness were limited. The effectiveness of handbills and posters depends upon there being a literate public, but prior to the 1950s, only about 34.5 percent of workers had attended elementary school (Gardner 1969). Literacy rates among the urban poor, such as peasant migrants, were even lower. Most Shanghai residents would not have understood a 1938 flier titled "Unforgivable Mistakes," which educates the reader on the danger of microbes contained in the sputum of people who spit "just anywhere" (NLM 1938). The flyer's message becomes clear as one reads its text, but it would not have been clear to the urban poor, who lived in conditions that made them susceptible to TB. The efffectiveness of TB-week outreach activities, such as public lectures, depends on whether lecturers present material in an accessible way and the audience pays attention. Even if lectures in schools and factories achieved a boost in knowledge, these lectures missed large swaths of the population. School campaigns missed children who did not go to school. Factory campaigns missed those without stable factory jobs. While radio campaigns aim to reach a wider audience than public lectures, their effectiveness depends on consistent access to electricity, radios, and broadcasts in dialects and vocabulary understandable to laypeople.

In the area of TB treatment, CATA founded clinical facilities to help increase the number of TB treatment beds throughout the city. Prior to the widespread distribution of effective TB antibiotics in the 1950s, treatment generally involved improved nutrition and rest in isolated facilities where doctors encouraged patients to go outside to reap the healing benefits of sunlight and fresh air (Wu 1934; SMA 1938–1942b). In the 1910s and 1920s, government and private actors built a few TB treatment facilities on the outskirts of town to minimize sufferers' interactions with the rest of the population. Government facilities included the Municipal Council's thirty-six-bed sanatorium, founded in 1928. That facility did not meet the acute need for beds; relatives of TB sufferers sent pleas to the commissioner of health requesting that beds be made available (SMA 1913–1944; SMA 1930–1940; SMA 1929–1942; SMA 1913–1941). In June 1933, the Chinese government built the Chengzhong Sanatorium in a garden in the northern suburb of Jiangwan. This facility became the largest in the city, with 120 beds and space for patients to amble around its grounds. In 1934, private sources established the Hongqiao Sanatorium in the western suburbs (ZYHJF 1997).[3] The Hongqiao Sanatorium had 75 beds, including 10 beds for patients who could not afford to pay for medical services. CATA also established the first clinic at Nantao, which saw 634 patients between its opening on June 1 and December 31, 1934 (SMA 1935–1939).

During the years following the Guomindang (GMD) government's rise to power, the government of Shanghai did not have a systematic plan to battle China's deadliest disease. Certainly, the government did not prioritize TB education. CATA tried to make up for the government's lack of public health outreach by running programs, but these programs had only limited scope and effectiveness. The government did found some sanatoria to isolate TB patients, but more facilities on the scale of the Chenzhong Sanatorium were needed, as were additional beds for patients who could not pay for treatment themselves. TB mortality within Shanghai did improve, but these improvements were not sustained.

Backsliding during the War Years, 1937–1945

Conditions in Shanghai worsened during the Japanese occupation. The Japanese bombing commenced in August 1937, and for the next several months, hundreds of thousands of mostly Chinese people became refugees when their homes were destroyed by these bombs (SMA 1938–1942a; SMA 1938–1942b; Henriot 2006; Ristaino 2008). Many refugees lived in crowded, unsanitary conditions, which contributed to the spread of infectious disease. An early 1939 brochure called "The Birth of SATA" describes the "intense suffering" of refugees who flooded into the city, "laden with their meager belongings." The refugees included "sick, carried upon doors," living "huddled together" with healthy individuals in camps, sewing the "insidious seeds of TB" (SMA 1938–1942a).

During the war years, TB was on the rise and SATA's general secretary predicted the epidemic had not yet peaked. In 1939, the 2,759 deaths from TB in the city of Shanghai approached the combined total of 2,819 deaths from seven other diseases: smallpox, cholera, typhoid, diphtheria, scarlet fever, influenza, and meningitis (SMA 1938–1944a). In 1940, the number of deaths from TB exceeded the combined total from the seven other diseases. In 1941, the 4,503 deaths from TB exceeded the 3,548 deaths from other diseases by more than 25 percent. This increase in TB occurred at the same time that the number of TB beds in the city declined. Japanese bombs hit the Municipal Council and Chengzhong Sanatoria, forcing them to close. Government documents describe the evacuation of "patients, staff, and their effects" from the Municipal Council Sanatorium just before eight o'clock at night on August 12, 1937 (SMA 1930–1940).

SATA began its clinical work in response to the closure of these facilities as well as the growing need for care among refugee patients. In 1938, SATA surveyed the number of hospitals with TB wards, found only 529 designated TB beds in nineteen facilities, and decided to establish two facilities of its own (SMA 1938–1940). On October 20, 1938, SATA established a Tuberculosis Hospital with 100 beds devoted entirely to charity TB cases (SMA 1938–1942a). Beds in the hospital were supported by companies, nonprofit organizations, and individuals, including the Shanghai International Red Cross and a New York–based NGO called China Child Welfare. Bed sponsorship allowed the hospital to expand and by October 1940, the hospital had 230 beds, including a children's ward with 52 beds (SMA 1938–1942a). Pictures from the Tuberculosis Hospital's children's ward depict young patients lined up to be weighed to document that their health had improved. SATA also founded a self-sustaining facility for paying patients. On January 1, 1939, the Second Red Cross Refugee Treatment Hospital became affiliated with SATA and was renamed the Shanghai Hospital. The Shanghai Hospital had 60 beds: 6 for first-class patients, 14 for second-class patients, and 40 for third-class patients (SMA 1938–1942b).

Despite the many efforts to develop and staff TB treatment facilities, many TB sufferers received no hospitalization until their disease had progressed to an advanced stage. This meant that they required longer stays, with reduced chances for successful treatment. The Tuberculosis Hospital had extremely high mortality rates. During its first twenty months, the hospital admitted 1,361 patients, 560 of whom died (41.15 percent). TB cases admitted to the Shanghai Hospital also required long stays; however, mortality rates there were not nearly as high as those at the Tuberculosis Hospital. In 1939, more TB patients were discharged from the Shanghai Hospital with improved, arrested, or apparently arrested disease, than died from the disease. At the Tuberculosis Hospital that same year, twice as many patients died from the disease as were discharged with apparently arrested or improved disease condition (SMA 1938–1942a). Better chances for survival among patients at the Shanghai Hospital were due in part to the fact that they were paying patients with better access to nutritious food and health care throughout their lives than were patients at the Tuberculosis Hospital.

These two facilities increased the number of TB beds in Shanghai by over 50 percent, but demand was still far greater than the number of beds available. In meetings and publications, the supervisor of SATA's Tuberculosis Hospital emphasized that these beds were always full: "Cry for more beds is so great that we could without doubt double this amount for destitute TB patients if we had the resources" (SMA 1938–1942a). The superintendent of the Shanghai Hospital reported similarly, "A number of patients had to be turned away daily" (SMA 1938–1945; SMA 1938–1942a). To remedy this, SATA launched a Hospital Building and Equipment Fund Campaign to raise funds for additional facilities and equipment. This campaign took place from November 15, 1941, to February 28, 1942, and raised over one million dollars in national currency. It allowed SATA to purchase the former Municipal Council Sanatorium and move the Tuberculosis Hospital to this site in 1942 (SMA 1938–1944b; SMA 1943). That same year, SATA founded an additional hospital and clinic (SMA 1938–1944a; SMA 1938–1942a).

During the Japanese occupation, conditions in Shanghai worsened, which led to increased disease at the same time that some facilities were forced to close. SATA did its best, but the 290 additional beds it added were far too few for the scale of the epidemic. More resources and a feasible plan would be needed to bring the epidemic into check.

Postwar Recovery, 1945–1949

Despite continuing civil war between the Guomindang and the Communists, late-1940s Shanghai was more stable than it had been during the Japanese occupation. This relative calm and the vision of one pulmonologist would help to set the direction of TB control in Shanghai for the next five decades. Wu Shaoqing (吴绍青, 1895–1980) studied at the Xiangya Medical College in Hunan, graduating in 1921. Around 1930, Wu himself contracted a light case of TB and was sent to rest at a sanatorium; his TB recurred in 1937 (Zhongguo fanglao xiehui 1980, ZYHJF 1997). Throughout his career, Wu strove to include both patients and doctors in discussions of the disease. In 1946, Wu moved to Shanghai and became professor at Shanghai's First Medical College and director of the Pulmonary Department at the affiliated Zhongshan Hospital. Wu led the formation of the Shanghai Coordinating Committee for Tuberculosis Control from twelve civic and medical bodies, including SATA and the Shanghai Medical College. On March 10, 1947, the coordinating committee opened a TB Clinical Center at the site of today's Huashan Hospital. This clinic received 11,750 patient visits before the end of the calendar year (SMA 1947). The Coordinating Committee also helped to recover the Chengzhong Sanatorium and saw expansion of the number of designated TB beds in Shanghai to 841.

CATA and SATA's efforts in the 1930s and 1940s had succeeded in drawing attention to the problem of TB; however, prior to 1949, Shanghai failed to develop an effective grassroots infrastructure to systematically implement TB control. CATA and SATA largely failed to adequately pitch the prevention message to common people, such as illiterate workers, and failed to develop effective methods for treating the masses of suspected TB patients. Consequently, care was often left in the hands of the individual and the family. In the years following the

Japanese occupation, the Shanghai Coordinating Committee for Tuberculosis Control started to work with the government to develop a comprehensive plan for bringing developments in TB control, such as BCG vaccines, mass radiography, and antibiotics, to the masses, through workplaces and schools. Development of a new urban social and economic system would make these plans a reality.

Building and Systematizing the Link, 1950–1990

In 1949, decades of fighting between the GMD and the Communists came to an end when the Communists seized control of the Chinese mainland and the GMD fled to Taiwan. In 1950, Shanghai was a city of more than 5 million people, approximately 85 percent of whom had been born outside the city (Feng, Zuo, and Ruan 2002). The 1950–1957 period was one of large-scale in- and out-migration, with in-migration exceeding out-migration (Gui and Shen 1992). According to the 1953 census, the city's population was 6.2 million. The city also experienced geographical expansion during this time. In 1958, Shanghai expanded its boundaries to include ten counties that were previously part of neighboring Jiangsu Province. Ash (1981) estimates that if these countries had already been part of Shanghai, the city's population would have been 7 million in 1949, and almost 10 million in 1957. After 1958, Shanghai's population growth decelerated, then stagnated. Between the 1964 and 1982 censuses, Shanghai's population growth rate averaged only 0.5 percent per year—from 10.82 million to 11.86 million (Zhu 2008). This population stabilization came about largely due to creation of the urban work-unit system.

In the early 1950s, the government adopted policies to stabilize the population and socialize the economy. The government encouraged public and private institutions to extensively absorb the unemployed. Socialization of enterprise took place in three steps during the First Five-Year Plan, 1953–1957. First, the government persuaded capitalists, such as the owners of cotton mills, to turn over their firms. Second, it organized petty capitalists—dockworkers, noodle sellers, bicycle repairmen, etc.—into collective enterprises. Finally, it encouraged housewives and other unemployed people to pool their talents and resources and establish small factories and workshops within their neighborhoods (Whyte and Parish 1984). Expansion of schools also occurred as the government hired unemployed intellectuals to be teachers and administrators in secondary schools, starting in 1950 (U 2007). Between 1950 and 1957, all urban employment places, including transportation centers, banks, offices, hospitals, and other health infrastructure, were reorganized as "work units" (*danwei*). As an end result of these processes, in 1957 all urban adults were expected to be employed in a work unit.

Creation of the work unit established a system of urban workplace–based entitlements that became known as the "iron rice bowl." In addition to salaries, work units distributed food coupons, subsidized cafeterias and housing, provided day care or schooling for workers' children, and provided pensions. In the

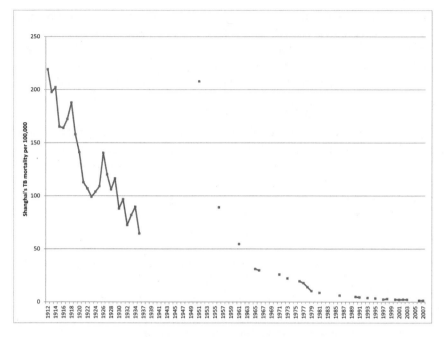

Figure 7.1. Shanghai's TB mortality per 100,000. *Sources:* For pre-1949 mortality rates, data from SMA (1913–1944; 1935–1939; 1938–1945). 1950–1979 mortality rates are from Sun (1981). Post-1990 mortality rates are from *Shanghai tongjing nianjian* 1992–2008.

realm of health, the Chinese Communist Party (CCP) built the work unit into a link between individuals and the public health and medical infrastructure. Work units provided medical insurance and primary care, and served as the workers' channel into the medical system. Socialization of hospitals also took place in the 1950–1957 era and resulted in an array of facilities ready to receive workers from factories, schools, and other workplaces.

The Work-Unit System and TB Control

Shanghai's TB mortality rates were declining as CATA and SATA began their work; however, postwar mortality rates showed that war undid some of these early advances. In 1951, Shanghai's TB mortality rate was 208 per 100,000, the worst it had been since 1914. TB mortality then declined dramatically until 1965 and less dramatically after 1965 (see figure 7.1). Before 1956, TB was the first or second leading cause of death in the city; by 1983 it was the tenth leading cause of death (ZYHJF 1997). How was this decline in mortality achieved and sustained? Declining disease was undoubtedly the result of a combination of factors, including steadier employment, more stable food supply, and medical advances. In the sections below, I examine how the work-unit system allowed medical and public health advances to reach the population by linking population members to the health care and public health system.

In the process of TB control, the relationship between district-level prevention and treatment clinics and work units was crucial. In 1957 and 1958, Shanghai built seventeen of these clinics, as well as one for the railroad industry (ZYHJF 1997). Many of these clinics had been built from previously existing facilities. For instance, SATA's Shanghai Hospital became a private facility again, after SATA established larger facilities in 1942 and 1943. This hospital was socialized in February 1956, and in September 1958 it became the Xuhui District Prevention and Treatment Clinic. In the realm of TB control, district TB prevention and treatment clinics played a central role in facilitating the type of access to population that Wu Shaoqing envisioned because district clinics maintained relationships with both municipal-level disease control facilities and grassroots doctors in workplaces. District clinics trained workplace doctors to execute primary, secondary, and tertiary TB prevention. These workplace doctors were similar to the barefoot doctors who would execute basic preventive and curative services in China's countryside in the 1960s and 1970s. District clinics reported progress to the municipal TB control centers, which had absorbed SATA in the early 1950s. District clinics also sent staff to municipal-level hospitals to receive advanced training, and clinics provided medical training for residents being trained at municipal-level hospitals attached to medical schools. As an example, the relationship between the Xuhui District Clinic and Wu Shaoqing's department at the Zhongshan Hospital was particularly close. Because the facilities were located only a few blocks apart, clinic doctors could easily consult with hospital doctors and attend workshops at the hospital.

Primary and Secondary Prevention Advances

In the years immediately following the 1949 founding of the People's Republic of China, the Communist Government prioritized prevention. Earliest Communist efforts included promotion of the Bacillus Calmette-Guérin (BCG) vaccine, which is prepared from a weakened strain of bovine TB. In the years following World War II, governments worldwide promoted BCG. As with many vaccines, BCG is given in infancy and childhood because it protects people who have not been exposed to the disease; it stimulates the production of antibodies, protecting against future infections. On January 16, 1950, the *People's Daily* reported that the Health Department of the Central People's Government promoted free BCG vaccination for children under five, young workers, students, and soldiers. The article encouraged families to bring young children for immunizations. Workplaces and school health personnel ran these free immunization clinics for young workers and students. According to the work report of the Shanghai Municipal Patriotic Hygiene Campaign, 53,791 people received the BCG vaccine during the

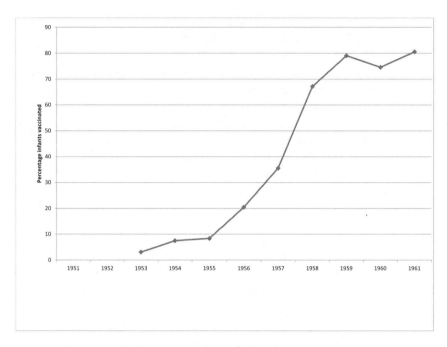

Figure 7.2. Percentage of infants vaccinated. *Source:* SMA (1963).

first ten months of 1952 (SMA 1953a). In 1953, 20,000 people took BCG orally and 67,437 received injections in Shanghai (Zhongguo fanglao xiehui 1954). After the socialization of industry, schools, and hospitals, number of immunizations and proportion of children immunized in Shanghai increased even more dramatically (see figure 7.2).

In addition to BCG, Shanghai's government promoted both enhanced and active case finding, that is, the finding of active cases of disease in order to bring people with active disease to treatment and avoid secondary infection (Toman 1979). Two types of case finding began to be used worldwide for TB control in the middle part of the twentieth century. Enhanced case finding (ECF) uses publicity and education to make the population aware of disease symptoms and promote voluntary reporting to disease control facilities. Active case finding (ACF) employs mass radiography—i.e., the use of mobile X-ray units—to meet three objectives: identifying high-risk suspects for future monitoring, isolating active cases in order to reduce transmission, and detecting cases early to reduce disease mortality (Golub 2005).

Preventive education materials from this era have less text and more didactic pictures than the materials distributed during the 1930s. Expansion of schools during the era also helped to raise literacy rates, but much of the preventive education in the workplace was presented in formats that illiterate people could understand. Preventive education included lectures and slide shows led by health professionals and trained workers. SATA's 1952 annual report includes lists of the type and place of these health education sessions: SATA held lectures in twenty-three work units, including twelve schools and seven factories. Six of those schools and one factory also held TB prevention slide shows. This programming reached 16,354 individuals (Shanghai fanglao xiehui 1953a). The number of workers and students reached through educational programs expanded rapidly in the next few years. According to a report by the Shanghai Municipal TB Prevention Committee, during the final three quarters of 1956, TB prevention work advanced to seventy-nine factories, reaching 114,445 workers (SMA 1950b).

While counts of attendees do not indicate whether those attendees actually understood materials being presented, SATA publications also contain guidelines on how to mobilize workers. In a 1953 article subtitled "Initial Results of TB Prevention Work at the Fifth National Cotton Factory," Song Yandong advised that after seeing traveling anti-TB exhibits, workers should give reports in small group settings (Song 1953). One of my interviewees who completed medical school in 1953 and used to go to factories to do anti-TB work corroborated that TB education was done this way. Instead of having a panel of doctors at the front of a large auditorium, health educational programs split doctors and workers into smaller groups to maximize workers' understanding and participation.

After their founding in 1957–1958, district clinics continued wide educational programming. For instance, in Yangpu—a district with many large factories—the district clinic showed fourteen movies to 11,200 workers in twelve factories in 1959. That same year, district clinic workers presented 195 TB prevention slideshows to audiences totaling 155,000 people at the Hudong Workers' Cultural Palace, and showed 1,855 posters in factory exhibits. In 1960, 23,500 people attended the clinic's thirty-eight movie screenings; 47,000 people attended 1,265 slide shows; and the clinic developed seven factory exhibits (Yangpu qu jiehebing fangzhi suo 1992). The other seventeen prevention and treatment clinics throughout Shanghai also did similar work.

With respect to ACF, Wu Shaoqing noted that with an estimated citywide prevalence rate of 5 percent, it would have been ideal to screen the entire population, but the city did not initially have enough equipment or personnel. To make up for this, initial ACF targeted workers and students because prevalence of the active disease was estimated to be 5–9 percent among these groups (Wu 1952). From 1950 to 1956, the equipment and personnel expanded and the total number of persons screened in Shanghai was 742,619 (SMA 1956). The China Medical Association claims that as the decade progressed, more than a million people were checked in an average year (ZYHJF 1997). This implies that 16–20 percent of the population was checked in a city of five to six million. Such a high number of screenings would be credible because by the end of 1953, the city had 115 facilities using X-rays, 788 personnel who worked with X-rays, eighty-one X-ray machines, and 151 TB specialists throughout the city (SMA 1953b). After 1958, the district clinics did checkups in factories throughout their districts. For instance, the Xuhui district clinic alone performed X-rays on 123,595 people in 1959 and 140,788 in 1964 (Mei, Zhong, and Wang 1991). Staff from this clinic and from individual workplaces then looked at X-ray slides together to identify suspected cases of TB; suspected patients had lungs with lots of cavities that looked like "painted opera faces."[4]

How was this push to find active disease received by young workers and students? I have found little evidence of resistance to health checks, but there is some. For instance, the SATA 1952 work summary notes increasing prevalence among factory workers, from 5.71 percent in 1951 to 5.8 percent in 1952. SATA explained this increased prevalence in the following way: "Last year, not all persons participated; perhaps those who knew they were ill did not participate. This year was stricter, so persons who wanted to avoid checkups due to illness could not" (Shanghai fanglao xiehui 1953b). Why would people who knew they were ill not want to participate? SATA's work summary does not delve into the reasons for this, but it is not difficult to imagine how people with little prior experience with the health system might have been afraid to go for a checkup. Given that TB had been a death sentence for most sufferers in the late 1940s, some people might not have wanted to know that they had the disease. Perhaps they feared being fired or blocked from future employment opportunities. Perhaps these individuals were afraid of the cost that treatment would entail. To avoid the phenomenon of workers' skipping checkups, SATA asked factory unions to divide workers into groups and explain how treatment would work for people found to be infected.

Tertiary Prevention Developments

Case-finding results in a reduction in transmission of active disease only when commitment to provide chemical treatment follows. Such commitment can only be met with adequate medical personnel, facilities, and resources. Along with the expansion of personnel noted above, Shanghai began to expand the number of TB beds available in various types of facilities between 1949 and 1953. In 1949, Shanghai had 841 designated TB treatment beds (ZYHJF 1997). Wu Shaoqing estimated that with a 5 percent prevalence rate for a city of five million, the resulting 250,000 cases would need approximately 30,000 TB sick beds (Wu 1952). New and expanded facilities included two specialized TB treatment hospitals: the Municipal Hospital, with 414 beds, and SATA First Hospital, with 160 beds. Thirty-two general hospitals in Shanghai also had 711 designated TB beds. Workplaces, including the Ocean Shipping Bureau, also built sanatoria designed to treat a host of diseases; in 1953 these facilities had 175 designated TB beds throughout

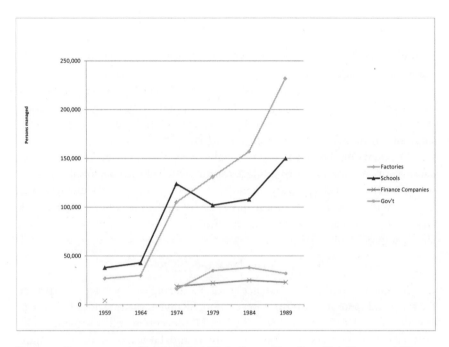

Figure 7.3. Persons managed by the Xuhui Clinic. *Source:* Data from Mei, Zhong, and Wang (1991).

the city (SMA 1953b). Finally, nineteen individual workplaces, including Jiaotong, Tongji, and East China Normal Universities, the *Liberation Daily* newspaper, and the Fifth National Cotton Factory, built TB convalescent rooms, with a total of 655 beds. These facilities increased the number of designated TB beds in Shanghai two-and-a-half-fold, from 841 in 1949 to 2,115, in just four years.

But simply providing personnel and facilities without improved commitment to covering treatment costs was not enough. The central government passed a resolution to provide health insurance for workers beginning in May 1951 (NLM 1953–1954). Cost of care would be covered through the workplace. This entitlement represented a major change in workers' lives and gave them access to the new TB treatment drugs—streptomycin S, para-amino-salicylate sodium (PAS), and isoniazid (INH)—which began to be distributed worldwide during World War II and the years immediately following.

One of my respondents contrasted the type of care he had received prior to 1949 with the care his factory provided when he was found to have TB in the 1950s. He was born in 1928, and when he was a child, four of the ten children in his family—two brothers and two sisters—died from illnesses. His family was so poor that his mother used ashes from the Buddhist temple mixed with water or lotus tea as medicine. As a child, when he had a kidney infection, a doctor wrote a prescription, but his family could not afford the medicine. Eventually, after his family appealed to the doctor regarding their financial situation, he received the medicine for free. At that time, he wanted to be a doctor so that he could save people's lives. After the 1949 revolution he instead learned to fix cars and worked in a diesel factory for thirty-three years, including thirty years as a quality control inspector. His factory had ten thousand employees, all of whom had a card for health insurance. "If the doctor in your factory clinic had no way to help you," he said, "they would send you to a hospital." In 1957, he discovered he had TB because of an examination by a mobile X-ray unit that had been deployed to his factory. He went to the hospital and then the sanatorium for one year, during which he took both Western and Chinese medicine. With the exception of meals while he was hospitalized, his factory paid for the entire cost of treatment, something clearly unprecedented in his life.

Better Management and Reduced Disease after 1949

Despite episodic political turbulence in China during the 1958–1961 Great Leap Forward and 1966–1976 Cultural Revolution, Shanghai made strides in TB control after 1949. During this period, district TB prevention and treatment clinics targeted young workers and students in their anti-TB work. As figure 7.3 illustrates, the number of people managed by the Xuhui District TB Prevention and Treatment Clinic increased dramatically between 1959 and 1989. The most dramatic increases were among industrial workers, school employees, and students. Schools under district clinic management included both primary and secondary schools, as well as universities and medical schools such as Jiaotong University and Shanghai Medical College. In the thirty-five years between 1958 and 1992, the Yangpu District Clinic inoculated 1,786,574 infants; took 3,152,215 X-rays in factories; and received 1,197,355 outpatient visits (Yangpu qu jiehebing fangzhi suo 1992). Widespread use of BCG helped to lower prevalence rates, and widespread use of effective antibiotics helped to improve mortality and lower incidence by preventing secondary infections. Figure 7.4 illustrates changes in TB prevalence in Yangpu district during the clinic's thirty-one-year tenure, from 1958 to 1990. In the first few years of the district clinic's existence, prevalence rates among students, workers, and the district's residents all rose as the clinic struggled to get a handle on the epidemic. Once TB control became systematized, prevalence for all groups declined steadily starting in the 1970s.

Breaking the Link and Building a New System
Demographic, Economic, and Institutional Changes

After twenty years of strict restrictions on population movement to urban areas, Shanghai began marketizing its economy in 1978. In the past thirty years,

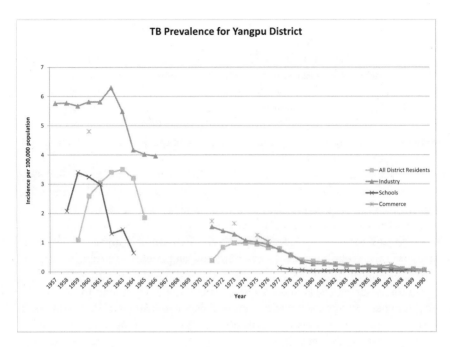

Figure 7.4. TB prevalence in Yangpu district. *Source:* Data from Yangpu qu jiehebing fangzhi suo (1992).

the city's population has more than doubled, with migrants largely driving this growth. Population was 11.86 million in the 1982 census, 13.34 million in the 1990 census, 16.41 million in the 2000 census, and 23 million in the 2010 census. While secondary industry accounted for 77.4 percent of the city's GDP in 1978, by 2000, tertiary industry accounted for half (50.6 percent) of GDP (Zhu 2008). The spectrum of migrants includes educated workers who move to Shanghai to work in financial services and foreign firms, factory and construction workers who work on a contractual basis, and illiterate migrants who cobble together an existence through day labor and other informal work.

For these migrants, as well as for the Shanghai residents who once staffed the city's state-owned and collective enterprises, guaranteed employment with benefits such as health care no longer exists. Starting in the 1990s, the work-unit system was dismantled throughout China, resulting in mass layoffs and lost benefits. According to official data, between 1998 and 2002, twenty-five million layoffs occurred in urban China (Bramall 2009). The majority of these job losses occurred in the manufacturing sector, and Shanghai's textile industry was particularly hard hit. In 1996, the municipal government began to replace the urban insurance system with one in which employers contribute to pooled funds and employees contribute to their own health insurance accounts; however, coverage is not complete. The health sector has also undergone marketization and has seen a shifting emphasis from preventive to curative services, for which higher fees can be charged. Many urban dwellers have had to pay rising costs out-of-pocket. How to continue to serve the masses after the workplace-based system declined has become a huge question for TB control and public health generally in the new era. The Shanghai government has responded to this question in two ways: by adopting parts of the World Health Organization's Directly Observed Therapy, Short-Course (DOTS) strategy and by establishing the Shanghai Municipal Center for Disease Control and Prevention (CDC).

With a $58.2 million loan from WHO, China began to implement the DOTS strategy in thirteen provinces between 1992 and 2001 (Wang, Liu, and Chin 2007). WHO developed the DOTS strategy, and the subsequent Stop TB Strategy, in response to the worldwide TB epidemic, which WHO viewed as a "global public health emergency" (Glaziou et al. 2011). Between 1995 and 2009, 127 countries used the program to treat forty-nine million patients. When a government agrees to implement DOTS, it commits to providing adequate financing for the program, ensuring a safe and adequate supply of TB drugs, and to monitoring program performance, often with technical expertise from WHO. Program performance monitoring uses two indicators: case detection rate and rate of treatment success. At the local level, governments provide free sputum smear and liver function testing and a free six-month standardized, supervised course of first-line antibiotics to TB patients.

Established in 1998, the Shanghai CDC modeled itself after the U.S. CDC and was the first CDC in China, preceding even the national CDC. Its establishment responded to both changing disease patterns and structural changes, such as the dismantling of SOEs and the ensuing crisis in preventive health (Peng et al. 2003). The Shanghai CDC has a three-tiered policy for TB control. Shanghai's central CDC guides TB policy and maintains records of the number and status of cases throughout the city. District-level CDCs undertake some of the tasks once handled by district prevention and treatment clinics, and also provide educational programming in schools and deploy their mobile X-ray units to factories and schools. Designated district-level treatment hospitals set the course of treatment for individual patients. Neighborhood-level community health centers (CHCs) have replaced clinics in individual workplaces. CHCs oversee patient compliance with treatment regimens, as workplace doctors once did.

Today's TB Control Challenges

Despite efforts to publicize the DOTS program and its free benefits to patients, between 1995 and 2002 the country's case detection rate—i.e., the ratio of reported cases to estimated incident cases—stagnated at around 20 percent (Wang, Liu, and Chin 2007). The fact that migrants could only receive DOTS benefits in the place of their official household registration, and consequently chose to forego care in their receiving areas, contributed to low detection rates. Lack of a centralized reporting system also contributed to low case notification. In the early years of DOTS, it also became clear that China had a disproportionate share of the world's multidrug-resistant (MDR) TB cases. The rise in MDR-TB suggests inadequate patient education. Patients did not take their drugs according to the prescribed course, either because they did not understand why doing so was important or because they failed to understand how the reimbursement program worked. When DOTS was originally established, patients paid for the entire six-month course of drugs out-of-pocket, then sought reimbursement only after they had completed the six-month course. The financial cost of paying up front for a six-month course of drugs proved burdensome for some poor patients. Reimbursement procedures were sometimes unnecessarily complicated, requiring multiple sets of documentation and trips to different offices (Wei et al. 2009). After these problems came to light, the national government increased its financial commitment to public health by 72 percent between 2002 and 2004 (Wang, Liu, and Chin 2007).[5] This increased financial commitment has helped to provide better coverage for migrants, but coverage is still far from complete.

The intensive interviews I conducted with forty-five TB patients from December 2010 to July 2011 brought several problems to light. One twenty-nine-year-old man from Harbin had been in Shanghai, where his family owns a machinery rental shop, for ten years. He originally had TB when he was seven years old. He started coughing again in 2005 and self-medicated with anti-inflammatories and Chinese medicine. He did not think much of the cough; when it was severe, he simply took more over-the-counter medicine. When his chest started hurting he realized it might be TB, saw a doctor, and took medicine for eight months from late spring 2006 to early 2007. During this time his health deteriorated, and it became clear that he had contracted a drug-resistant strain of TB. Throughout his treatment, all expenses associated with his illness, including three hospital stays, have been out-of-pocket, totaling more than 70,000 RMB (more than ten thousand dollars). Because he has extremely drug-resistant TB (XDR-TB) he had spent around 130,000 RMB (twenty thousand dollars) on the second- and third-line TB drugs, which he had been taking for four years at the time of our interview.

Certainly, this man's experience is not the norm—he required longer, more costly treatment than most of the patients I interviewed—but his experience of coverage gaps is typical. This man and his family had already lived in Shanghai for four years when he started coughing, but neither the municipal insurance scheme nor DOTS covered any of his care. Long-term migrants were not covered under the municipal insurance scheme until 2008; this often caused patients to delay seeking care. The extremely drug-resistant strain of TB he contracted required second- and third-line drugs; however, when he was diagnosed, DOTS only covered a standard, six-month course of first-line drugs. While all districts in Shanghai now cover the second- and third-line drugs, benefits cannot be extended retroactively.

Even people with official residence in Shanghai experience coverage gaps. For instance, a thirty-one-year-old female doctor I interviewed took TB drugs from July 2009 to August 2010. I interviewed her after a follow-up checkup, and she was so happy to be healthy that she was moved to tears. Despite the fact that she was enrolled in Shanghai's insurance scheme, she found that she quickly exhausted the funds in her health insurance account. Because she had not worked for very long, the account contained only a few thousand renminbi. She estimated that she paid around twenty thousand renminbi (more than three thousand dollars) out-of-pocket for illness-related expenses, including a month-long hospital stay. She reported that this experience changed her illness behavior and helped to inform her patient outreach.

In addition to the expansion of treatment benefits, recent years have seen a reinvigoration of TB educational campaigns, with district CDCs largely leading these grassroots efforts. Large-screen flash advertisements from the central and district CDCs play in public spaces such as shopping centers. The Changning CDC provides calendars with TB prevention slogans to children when they visit schools, and the Putuo CDC distributes magnetic bookmarks with the popular Chinese cartoon character Pleasant Goat. District CDCs also distribute seasonal marketing items, such as fans and umbrellas. Each year, targeted, week-long public education campaigns coincide with International TB Awareness Day on March 24. Local newspapers print articles to make the public aware of TB's symptoms, with instructions on where to receive free treatment. In honor of International TB Awareness Day, universities hold lectures and university hospital staff table to raise students' and employees' TB awareness. The Songjiang CDC participates in university efforts by holding contests in which students earn monetary prizes for designing educational campaign materials. These programs aim to bring TB prevention knowledge to the masses, as district TB prevention and treatment clinics did in workplaces and schools from the 1950s to 1992.

Conclusions

This chapter has examined eighty-five years of TB control in Shanghai, from pre-1949 efforts that only reached a sliver of the estimated caseload, to the Communists' expansive program, to the current program, led by the CDC. When the GMD came to power in 1928, TB was one of the most widespread and deadly diseases in China, yet the government had no comprehensive plan for disease control. CATA and SATA aimed to raise awareness of the disease and provide hospitalization for the most severe cases, but the scale of their activities did not match the scale of the epidemic. After the Communist Revolution, the creation of the socialist work-unit system allowed TB control to reach the masses on the scale that pulmonologist Wu Shaoqing envisioned. Nearly all urban residents were part of this system. The system allowed the BCG vaccines to reach newborns, children in schools, and young workers. To ensure that active cases made their way into the health care system, district prevention and treatment clinics worked with workplace doctors to target workers and children for educational campaigns and X-rays. Work units also guaranteed payment for treatment. This ensured that workers and their dependents had access to new TB antibiotics being developed in the mid-twentieth century and that they would not discontinue treatment due to inability to pay. All of these efforts contributed to declining TB rates. In 1992, the WHO program replaced the previous TB control program; however, in the early years of this program, migrants were excluded, except at the place of their official residence. In recent years, district CDCs have expanded DOTS to include migrants, and to cover second- and third-line drugs to combat multidrug-resistant TB. Today, the Shanghai CDC plays a key role in designing and implementing national TB control policies. Throughout these eighty-five years, bringing health to the masses has been a goal.

Notes

1. Interventions designed to prevent the body from being infected by the TB bacillus are known as primary prevention. Those aimed at early detection are known as secondary prevention. Tertiary prevention refers to treatments to stop the progression of active disease and prevent death.

2. While modern epidemiologists recognize that TB is actually transmitted through *Mycobacterium tuberculosis* present in droplets when persons with active TB cough, in the 1930s–1950s, indiscriminate spitting in public places was thought to be a primary culprit. Indeed, dried spittle might be kicked up and inhaled.

3. Today, the Chengzhong Sanatorium has become the Shanghai Pulmonary Hospital. The Hongqiao Sanatorium moved in 1937 and again in 1983 to the site of the present-day Xuhui Central District Hospital.

4. Interview with health care provider no. 18 (2011).

5. In 2002, China also received a $104 million loan from the World Bank and a $48 million grant from the Global Fund to Fight AIDS, Tuberculosis, and Malaria.

8 The Development of Psychiatric Services in China

Christianity, Communism, and Community

Veronica Pearson

THE STORY OF the introduction and growth of psychiatric services in China is by no means a linear progression toward the achievement of practices based on science. The narrative is one in which culture, foreign intrusion, economics, familism, and politics (especially politics) all form part of the framework within which the goal of providing accessible, affordable, and effective psychiatric care for all of China's citizens who require it is pursued. As we shall see, it is a goal that has not yet been achieved, although the efforts to do so continue. The chapter's content that covers the development of formal institutional care for psychiatric patients from 1898 is built around material from medical missionary sources prior to 1949. For the later periods the discussion is structured using formal policy documents (where available) and published analysis and research, supplemented by the author's own experiences and observations in China over three decades. We start, however, with a consideration of the question at the core of understanding the development and structure of psychiatric care—epidemiology.

The Epidemiology of Mental Illness in China

In order to understand the challenges involved it is necessary to have some idea of the numbers requiring services. Attempts to answer the deceptively simple question "How many people are there in China with a mental illness?" did not begin in earnest until 1982, which is where we will start.

Epidemiological Data

The first major epidemiological survey of the prevalence of mental illness in China was known as the Twelve Regions Survey and was carried out with the help of the World Health Organization in 1982 (12DQJ 1986). Despite some reservations about the methodology used, this survey was of profound importance. It was the first serious attempt to garner information that would permit rational planning of psychiatric facilities and resource distribution. The sample was based on five hundred rural households and five hundred urban households. At this time 75 percent of the population was defined as living in rural areas, so the equal distribution of survey sites between urban and rural areas almost certainly led to a bias in the results. The survey found a point prevalence rate for schizophrenia of 6.06 per thousand in the urban areas and 3.42 per thousand in the rural areas, translating into a total of 3.7 million people with schizophrenia nationwide. However, there is such variation in the rates within the twelve urban and twelve rural sites as to cast doubt on the accuracy of the results (Cheung 1991), Even so, the prevalence rates were roughly comparable with those in Western countries and Taiwan (Jablensky 1988). However, the prevalence rates for affective disorders, ranging from 0.37 to 0.89 per thousand, were much lower than elsewhere. This finding was almost certainly because of a tendency for Chinese psychiatrists to underdiagnose depression (Yan et al. 1984; Cheung 1991).

In 1987 a National Survey of the Disabled was carried out under the aegis of the China Disabled Persons' Federation and the Ministry of Civil Affairs (Wong 1990). This was the first time that serious efforts had been made to collect reliable data on the number of people with a disability. The results indicated that there were 51.64 million people with a disability in China, affecting 18 percent of all households. The prevalence of schizophrenia in this survey was 1.63 per thousand of population, or approximately 1.69 million people disabled by schizophrenia (Tian et al. 1994). The differences between these two surveys in relation to the most serious of the mental illnesses—schizophrenia—and thus the one that is hardest to hide from data collectors, suggests caution should be used in assessing their accuracy.

Currently, the prevalence figures that are most commonly used by the authorities in China are based on epidemiological research carried out by a team led by Dr. Michael Phillips (Huilongguan Psychiatric Hospital, Beijing) and Xue Zhang (Peking Union Medical Hospital), supported by a grant from the China Medical Board in New York (Phillips et al. 2009).[1] They point out that in low- and middle-income countries like China the disease burden attributable to neuropsychiatric conditions exceeds that for infectious, cardiovascular, and neuroplastic disease and are already the most significant causes of illness in women and men. Their sampling frame incorporated 113 million adults—12 percent of China's population—and included rural and urban areas. Screening was conducted for 63,004 adults, using an expanded version of the General Health Questionnaire administered by trained nurses, and 16,577 of those went on to have a diagnostic interview with a psychiatrist using a Chinese version of the Structured Clinical Interview for Diagnostic and Statistical Manual (DSM-IV) axis I disorders. The adjusted one-month prevalence rate of any mental disorder was 17.5 percent. Among individuals with a diagnosable mental illness, 24 percent were moderately or severely disabled by their illness, 8 percent had sought professional help at any time, and 5 percent had seen a mental health professional at any time. Of those with psychotic disorders, 85 percent were judged to be moderately or severely disabled by their condition and more than 70 percent of them had sought professional help of some sort at least once, but not necessarily from a specialist in the treatment of mental illness. In short, the projection of the results of this research to all of China suggests that 173 million adults in the country have a mental disorder and 158 million of these have never received any type of professional help for their condition. As the authors point out, while neuropsychiatric conditions and suicide account for 20 percent of the burden of illness in China, only 2.35 percent of the government's health budget is spent on mental health and less than 15 percent of the population has heath insurance that covers psychiatric illness.

Whatever the variation in numbers among the three surveys presented here, it is apparent that the number of people with a serious mental illness greatly exceeds the resources available to offer them treatment and rehabilitation. This is nothing new, as we shall see from the following discussion of the historical development of psychiatric care in China.

In the Beginning

Chinese medicine has a history dating back many thousands of years. During that time theories were formulated about psychiatric disturbances and doctors treated patients accordingly, leaving meticulously observed case histories. *The Yellow Emperor's Classic of Internal Medicine* (*Huangdi neijing suwen*), compiled during the second and first centuries BC, describes a condition known as *kuang* which is generally accepted as acute psychotic excitement, although a differentiation between mania and psychosis is not made (Tien 1985). Somewhat later, another psychiatric disorder, *dian,* was also recognized, the associated symptoms being lethargy and apathy—what today would probably be diagnosed as depression (Tseng 1973). There appear to have been few books specifically on mental disorders. What are now interpreted as symptoms of mental disorder were seen as an integral part of general medical practice and were treated in the same ways. Nor was there any tradition of institutional care for mentally ill people in imperial China. Needham (1970) reports that a few general hospitals were in existence before the Ming dynasty but the concept never really took root. Thus the introduction of asylums for the insane was essentially an alien form grafted onto Chinese society rather than an indigenous product. Asylums met two needs: they represented the Holy Grail of scientific medicine for doctors and met the desire of families in particular and society in general to tuck seriously disturbed people out of sight. As we shall see, asylums became the dominant model of formal psychiatric care from the nineteenth century through to the present day. As we shall also see, almost all of the care offered to those suffering from psychiatric disorders is, was, and always has been provided by their family members.

For Good or Ill: The Introduction of Psychiatric Institutions into China

The first recorded psychiatric hospital in China was opened in Guangzhou in 1898. It is possible that there may have been an earlier one in Foshan in the same province, but no records remain. The hospital was located in an area of Guangzhou called Fangcun (Fong Tsuen). It was commonly known as Kerr's Refuge for the Insane, after its founder, John Kerr. Dr. Kerr was an American medical missionary who had spent most of his adult working life in Guangzhou as the physician-in-charge at the Canton Hospital, the first hospital to be opened by missionaries in China in 1853 (Spence 1980; Tucker 1983).

For many years Kerr had been—unsuccessfully—trying to persuade the members of the Board of Missions of the American Presbyterian Church, which funded the Canton Hospital, to permit him to open a hospital for the mentally ill. They told him that he was already too overcommitted. In reality, it is much more likely that they were concerned that their medical services would be tainted by such a close association with insanity. Dr. Seymour Wenyon, the senior British medical officer in Canton, expressed this viewpoint clearly in two letters to the *British Journal of Medicine* in 1891. In the second he wrote,

> A missionary lunatic asylum is more likely to be a hindrance than a help to the great spiritual results which is [*sic*] our first business as missionaries to secure.
> . . . It was necessary to beware of the false sentiment which would divert us from our true mission and by increasing popular prejudice against us would sacrifice the spiritual well-being of thousands for the physical comfort of the few. (quoted in Kao 1979, 24)

His view was commonly shared among the medical missions (Yip 1995; Hillier and Jewell 1983), but Kerr lived closer to ordinary people, was fluent in Cantonese, and understood how wretched the lives of the mentally ill and their families could be and how extreme some of the measures were that were taken in their increasingly desperate efforts to cope. Patients were shackled, caged, occasionally deliberately crippled, and in extreme cases killed (Kerr 1898; Ingram 1918; Selden 1905; McCartney 1926; Woods 1929). The retelling of these incidents on the part of medical missionaries is not necessarily wholly disinterested. Yet, even if only partly true, they still speak of the misery and despair that were the lot of many mentally ill people and their families.

Undeterred, Kerr was sufficiently convinced of the importance of his cause to use most of his life savings to buy four acres of ground on which to build a psychiatric hospital some years before he retired from the Canton Hospital. With the aid of a donation from an anonymous Chinese citizen he was able to erect two buildings, by which time he was in his mid-seventies. He died soon after, and his work was continued by another medical missionary, Charles Selden. Martha Noyes Kerr, John Kerr's third wife, continued to work at the hospital. It is a mark of the esteem in which the hospital was held during this period that, when she retired on December 9, 1923, on her eighty-fourth birthday, Sun Yat-sen, founder of the first Chinese Republic, sent her a note through his secretary. Dr. Kerr had been Sun's instructor and mentor for one year at the Canton Hospital, when Sun was a medical student, and the two had been close. The note expressed his "gratification to learn that you attain today the great age of 84 years" and sent "his best wishes and in the name of our people, thanks you for the good work that you have done in our midst" (Szto 2002, 294).

Under Selden's regime, treatment at the Refuge—at least in its formal statements—consisted of a humanitarian approach (occupation, recreation, freedom within the grounds, respect for patients) combined with drugs. Specifically mentioned were hyoscine (a sedative and antispasmodic which may also have had antidepressant properties), paraldehyde (a sedative), and Erlenmeyer bromide (potassium bromide, an anticonvulsant and sedative used before the discovery of phenobarbital in 1927). Cold baths and ingenious devices of his own invention for physical restraint with minimum discomfort were also much used. From thirty beds the hospital expanded to seven hundred by 1933 (Lamson 1935), and since about 1904 had been taking in "police cases" paid for from the public purse. At least in the Refuge's early years, the Hong Kong authorities had an arrangement to transfer Chinese psychiatric patients there until a hospital for their care was provided in Hong Kong (Pearson 2008). All this suggests that the Refuge was meeting a need and that although it was not indigenous, institutional care had been shown to be acceptable.

Psychiatric Provision outside Guangzhou

Lamson (1935) reported that, other than Kerr's Refuge, there were no separate psychiatric institutions in China, although there were psychiatric wards attached to general hospitals in Suzhou, Beijing, and Shanghai. He claims that the Ministry of Justice announced its intention in 1930 to erect "lunatic asylums" in various large cities, but there is no evidence that this policy was ever carried out, although the fact that it was proposed by a government department concerned with law and order rather than health and treatment is itself of interest. The announcement of this intention was greeted by a scathing editorial in the *China Critic* on April 3, 1930, which remarked that it was easier to draw up such schemes than to carry them out. Expert services to the court and insane asylums required people trained in abnormal psychology and psychiatry, it said, pointing out that there were only two such people in China and one of them was abroad.

Lin (1985) states that by the time the Chinese Communist Party (CCP) came to power in 1949 there were psychiatric hospitals and a small core of psychiatrists in Beijing, Changsha, Chengdu, Guangzhou, Harbin, Nanjing, and Shanghai. All of these places had large foreign populations or significant foreign influence. Xia and Zhang (1981) offer a slightly lengthier list: Beijing, Chengdu, Dalian, Guangzhou, Nanjing, Shanghai, Shenyang, Siping, and Suzhou. Overall, the situation of mentally ill people seems to have been wretched, a view confirmed by a Chinese psychiatrist with experience working in China in the 1930s (Wong 1950).

In an address to the American Psychiatric Association in 1948, Dr. Karl Bowman reported on a three-month visit to China which he had undertaken on behalf of the World Health Organization to plan for the development of psychiatry and mental health there (Kao 1979). He observed that China had very little psychiatry, and estimated that there were approximately six hundred psychiatric beds and fewer than fifty psychiatrists for a population of approximately 450,000,000. Treatment methods at the time of his report included insulin shock therapy, which he said was in use in virtually all psychiatric hospitals visited, as well as metrazol (to induce chemical shock in the treatment of schizophrenia; it was similar to insulin but much more violent in its effects) and what he referred to as "electroshock treatment" (presumably electroconvulsive therapy). Bowman described China's psychiatric facilities in the following terms:

> Psychiatric hospitals in China are poorly equipped and in a bad state of repair and are giving largely simple custodial care. Lack of money seems to be the most important reason for this condition and the psychiatric hospitals merely reflect the generally impoverished condition of China. The teaching of psychiatry in medical schools is badly handicapped by the fact that there are almost no teachers available. There is great interest in psychiatry and a desire to develop it in every way possible. (quoted in Kao 1979, 47)

According to Tsung-yi Lin, a professor of psychiatry at the University of British Columbia and the PRC government's first honorary advisor on mental health in the reform decade of the 1980s, Western-style psychiatry did not take root in China in the same way that was true for surgery, or even medicine. He attributes this to (1) the greater language skills needed, (2) the fact that at the time there had not been breakthroughs in the treatment of mental illness similar to those that other branches of medicine had enjoyed, and (3) psychiatry's being more culture-bound in its understanding of the human psyche and therefore in its treatment and practice, and correspondingly less transferable (Lin 1985).

Professional Development

From its inception, the Kerr Refuge had a policy of training local doctors. In 1910 Andrew Woods was appointed a visiting neurologist and psychologist at the Canton Hospital and then in 1919 he became the first professor of neurology and psychiatry at the Peking Union Medical College (PUMC). The first full-scale academic program in psychiatry was established at PUMC in 1932 by Dr. Robert Lyman, who stayed at PUMC until 1937. Lyman had a profound effect on the graduate training of psychiatrists at PUMC. Many of the most senior and influential psychiatrists from the 1950s to 1980s were taught by Lyman or his students (Kleinman 1986). Lyman encouraged the teaching of social work and sociology in his department at PUMC (Lyman 1937; Lyman, Maeker, and Liang 1939), and under his leadership, departmental staff were at the forefront of academic research on neurology and psychiatry in China before 1949. The Chinese Society for Neurology and Psychiatry was formed in 1931 by two professors at PUMC (Kao 1976). In Shanghai, the work of Dr. Fanny Halpern, trained in psychiatry in Vienna under Alfred Adler (and therefore the first modern psychiatrist in China), led to new initiatives in teaching, research, and practice (Westbrook 1953). For instance, she pioneered the use of insulin shock therapy in the treatment of schizophrenia in China (Halpern 1940). Yet psychiatry was still an unpopular subject. Kleinman (1986) points out that, despite Lyman's success in the postgraduate training of psychiatrists at PUMC, only one graduate out of the 116 produced between 1924 and 1933 went into psychiatry. With regard to training, Lin states that "few medical students chose to specialize in psychiatry and even some of those who chose to do so had to overcome the strong objections of their parents to enter the speciality, which arose from their families' fear that mental illness would be transferred to their members who intended to enter psychiatry" (Lin 1985, 5).

Xia Zhenyi and Zhang Mingyuan, professors of psychiatry in Shanghai, comment that in pre-Liberation China,

> psychiatry was influenced by foreign schools. At the time exchange of experience within China was rare, so it was difficult to say which school predominated. For instance, north-eastern China was deeply influenced by the German-Japanese school e.g. Kraepelin. In Shanghai Dr. Su Zonghua had studied with Dr. A. Meyer, so diagnosis and treatment of mental disorders under him were based largely on the theories of the psychobiological school. In Nanjing, Beijing, Chengdu and other places, Freud's theories had considerable influence; but possibly because of the differences in social environment and economic status of Western countries, Freud's psychoanalytic therapy was never very popular in China. (Xia and Zhang 1981, 278)

The pursuit of the "Johns Hopkins model" of scientific medicine, and the standard public health approaches (which achieved so much success in China in the control of endemic and epidemic diseases) dominated medical training and service provision at this time. Neither approach had a great deal to offer those with a severe mental illness for decades to come (Yip 1995; also see chapter 1 of this volume).

The People's Republic, 1949–1966

In the ten years prior to 1949 China had been ravaged by the Japanese occupation and civil war between the Nationalists and the Communists. Chaos took its toll at many levels. This was exemplified by the deterioration in Kerr's Refuge in Canton (Mo 1957; Selden 1937). The only possible way was up, and the decade following 1949 was one of enthusiasm among those engaged in psychiatric work, perhaps because, in the new world they were creating, anything was believed to be possible. The Chinese Society of Neurology and Psychiatry was formed in 1954, and in 1955 it began to publish the *Chinese Journal of Neurology and Psychiatry*. Patriotic enthusiasm is evident in this declaration by the deputy director of the Ministry of Health in 1958: "Our goal was to reach a satisfactory level in patient management within one to two years and the world's advanced standards in the scientific aspects of psychiatry within two to three years. In time the number of psychiatric patients in China would decrease" (quoted in Lin 1985, 11).

However, by 1957 the teaching of both sociology and psychology had been banned in universities. These branches of the social sciences were thought to be imbued with individualistic, bourgeois tendencies that should have no part to play in the new China. The effects of this on the holistic understanding of the etiology of mental illness, its treatment, and its rehabilitation have been highly detrimental and long-lasting. For most of the fifty years following Liberation there was no input from clinical psychologists, counselors, social workers, or occupational therapists into either the training of those working with mentally ill people or their treatment. Even now there is a lack of understanding about the way that the social milieu affects behavior, and scant attention has been paid to the personal psychological aspects which shape and frame each individual's experience of psychotic illness. Although there are now degree programs in social work and clinical psychology, those who graduate do not generally choose to work with mentally ill people, preferring more lucrative and less stressful positions (Lou, Pearson, and Wong 2012; Sha et al. 2012). It also needs to be remembered that during this period people were not allowed to choose where they worked or what job or profession they entered. Thus doctors and nurses were assigned to psychiatric hospitals without necessarily having any feeling or interest for the work, something which naturally affected levels of motivation and commitment. Inevitably this had an effect on the standard of service offered (Pearson 1995).

Psychiatric Resources

Two sources indicate the increase in the number of psychiatric facilities—admittedly from a very low baseline—that took place between 1949 and 1958. The first is a document that was published in 1959 called *A Collection of Theses on Achievements in Medical Science in Commemoration of the Tenth National Foundation Day of China*. It contained an essay by Wu Chengi-i on psychiatry. He says,

Sixty-two new hospitals were built throughout the 21 provinces and autonomous regions, with a total number of beds fourteen times greater than before Liberation. In 1950 the number of beds in the psychiatric wards was 1.1 percent of the total capacity and in 1957 it was 3.6 percent. There are now quite a few psychiatric sanatoriums in various areas for the chronically ill. The hospital staff increased as more hospitals and more beds became available. The number of doctors in 1958 was 16 times that in 1949. The increase in the number of nurses was twenty-fold. (Kao 1979, 110)

Unfortunately, Wu did not provide information about the numbers he was working from and there is no way to check the accuracy of his claims. But his statement does suggest that concern about the provision of psychiatric services was on the health agenda.

The second document is more specific. This is the Five-Year Plan published in 1958, known as the *Circular of the Ministry of Health Concerning the Issuance of the National Mental Illness Prevention Work Plan (1958–1962)*. It states that there were about one thousand psychiatric beds at the time of the Liberation and fifty or sixty "mental disease specialists," although the document does not say what training they had received or where they received it. It continues,

According to incomplete statistics, there are now in China 46 mental hospitals and clinics with 11,000 beds in 21 provinces and municipalities and the number of professional personnel for mental illnesses has been increased to 5,000 or more among which some 400 are doctors (including some 30 doctors of Chinese medicine). Ending in 1957, some 73,000 mentally ill persons were treated and among them some 27,000 recovered. (Kao 1979, 122)

There were very few resources available to establish and fund new facilities. The *Chinese Journal of Neurology and Psychiatry* from this period describes how one facility was set up in Nanjing by the Department of Civil Affairs. It was for long-term psychiatric patients who were originally vagrants for whom this government department, and not the Department of Health, was responsible (Zutangshan jiaoyang yuan 1958). It seems probable that it was included as a way of encouraging authorities in other areas to adopt a similar strategy. The authorities took over a temple forty miles outside the city (not in use since 1949), which had no electricity, no running water, and no transport access. As the authors say, "The hospital was established with the spirit to conquer difficulties" (Zutangshan jiaoyang yuan 1958, 259). The staff consisted of eight cadres, only two of whom were (unspecified) "medical workers." The rest of the staff were described as "caretakers" and were ex-residents of the Department of Civil Affairs facilities for the poor and sick. Not surprisingly, most of the "caretakers" were frightened and reluctant, armed for their task only with exhortations to develop "the spirit of running a hospital with hard work, economization and the spirit to serve the patients with all your heart" (Zutangshan jiaoyang yuan 1958, 260). The article is quite forthright about the difficulties they faced (e.g., fleas and incontinence). It describes the painful mistakes made on the road to the realization that inmates did very much better under a regime that provided meaningful occupation and cultural and recreational activities, and that sought and acted on inmates' opinions. Much of the increase in psychiatric facilities that China saw between 1949 and 1958 was probably organized along similar lines.

Principles and Plans

THE NANJING CONFERENCE

A landmark event in the development of policies regarding psychiatry during this era was the First National Conference of Psychiatric Specialists at Nanjing in 1959. It was organized by the Ministry of Health and was attended by over ninety people holding key positions in the field of mental health (Ho 1974). The conference was influential in setting directions for mental health policy. Most particularly it advocated a move away from Western domination of theory and practice and toward developing indigenous texts, expressed in the slogan "destroy superstition, believe in ourselves." It focused on the need for collective action to overcome the problems of mentally ill people, manifested in a willingness to move out of the urban centers and to provide services in the rural areas; and condemned "individualistic" practices. It demanded that practitioners move away from the use of restraints and explore ways of implementing dialectical materialism and thought in treatment. Above all there was to be "no more shrieking in the adult wards and no more crying in the children's wards" (Ho 1974; Chin and Chin 1969).

Not everyone agreed with the adoption of these new principles and apparently there were heated debates at the conference about the advisability of giving up the use of restraints and mechanical treatments. One has to bear in mind that at the time there was very little else, so this was akin to asking doctors to give up virtually all practices that were familiar to them, and to substitute a form of political education in which none of them had experience and for which there was no existing proof of efficacy. It was finally agreed that the use of restraints was to be abandoned and that wards were to be unlocked but there is no evidence to suggest that these policies were implemented. If they ever were, the old practices were certainly in evidence again by the early 1980s, based on my own observations. At the conference, difficulties impeding progress were discussed; these included problems in hiring suitable staff. There was a reluctance to take up mental health work because it was seen as a low-status job that carried a high risk of being physically and verbally abused by patients.

THE FIVE-YEAR PLAN, 1958–1962

The National Five-Year Plan of 1958 turned out to be the only five-year plan dealing with mental health matters for many years, and it played a major role in shaping psychiatric services for decades. Consequently it is of some importance and will be discussed in detail. It began by stating, "Mental illness is one in which the higher nervous activities of the human body are chaotic and there is a mental block. It brings not only pains and distress to the patient but also brings certain perils to industrial and agricultural production as well as social security."

The unpleasant nature of the illness for the sufferer was acknowledged but more concern was expressed about the economic consequences for the nation and the effect that people with mental illness could have on public order. This is a theme that has remained a constant in formal government policy statements about mental health. The document is notable because it did not try to gloss over the many problems that had to be faced, and it conceded that many people with mental illness received either no treatment or ineffective treatment. Neither were they well cared for by their families. The authors estimated that two hundred per hundred thousand of the population in China were suffering from a mental illness. The plan was critical of the macro level of health organizations, which concentrated too many of the few available resources on "what is new, what is big, and what is regular," which is to say Western, at the expense of looking at cheaper, more efficient and effective solutions to service provision. Authorities focused too much on hospital-based services and too little on providing outpatient facilities and early and preventive treatment.

Hospital managers were criticized for caring more about the convenience of staff than the comfort of patients. Some were said to lack professionalism, and it was claimed that there were "still some working personnel who dislike patients, discriminate against them, and despise them." The plan suggested that managers should not automatically assume that patients cannot have an opinion worth listening to and should take their wishes into account whenever possible.

The plan advocated the following:

1. Three kinds of organizational patterns: a medical base, a preventive unit, and sanatoriums for long-term care.
2. Caring for people in their homes or sending them to rural areas where there was a need for labor. The latter does not seem to have been common in practice, presumably because villagers did not want to receive unskilled, mentally ill urbanites who, in their turn, were equally reluctant to relocate.
3. Four kinds of cures: Chinese and Western medicines and physical therapy; proper labor therapy; therapy through organized sports and cultural amusements; and systematic educational therapy (in practice this tended to be political education).

With regard to treatment, the experience and expertise of Chinese medicine were to be "seriously summarized and propagated." Frontal lobotomies were categorically forbidden, as were other clinical methods that could "injure the lives and health of the patients . . . [and] binding or imprisoning of patients must be resolutely opposed." The establishment of "mental disease sanatoriums" and "mental disease convalescent villages" were also mooted. These were expected to be at least partly self-supporting through agriculture, light industry, and handicraft work but if they ever existed they were not a significant part of service provision.

Six regional centers of excellence were to be established in Beijing, Changsha, Chengdu, Guangzhou, Nanjing, and Shanghai, all places where the medical missions had been predominant. These regional centers were to be responsible for training personnel, particularly at the middle levels, to work in treatment and prevention of mental illness. They were also to train administrative cadres and to undertake research. In their work they were "to adopt the communist working style of imagination, outspokenness, and daring."

Each province was enjoined to establish a regional hospital center (colloquially known as a "leading hospital") that in addition to providing inpatient care was expected to guide preventative work and the training of relevant personnel. A joint planning structure was to be set up involving the three major government departments involved in the care of people with mental illness—Public Health, Civil Affairs, and Public Security, known as "three men leading groups"—which existed at all levels of government administration from ministerial to street and village. This continues to be the mechanism by which mental health services are coordinated in the PRC, although the China Disabled Persons' Federation has in many places now been co-opted.

Building more hospitals was not seen as a solution to problems posed by mental ill-health; resources were simply not available. Instead local authorities were encouraged to provide more outpatient services and some beds in local general hospitals, although Lin (1985) remarks on how extremely rare it was for this to happen, a fact which he, rightly, interprets as yet another manifestation of the widespread stigma that mental illness experiences, even among the medical profession.

Leaving aside the rhetoric and taking into consideration the lack of financial and human capital in the PRC in 1959, there is much in this plan that is forward-thinking and admirable. At the very least it shows that mentally ill people were part of the agenda and that there were those in positions of influence who viewed their situation with compassion and concern. What happened to these ideas as they percolated out into the real world is, of course, another matter. Unfortunately, that world was about to face the essentially man-made disasters of the Great Famine (Dikötter 2010) and the Cultural Revolution. Millions died, through starvation, chronic malnutrition, murder, and suicide. The agenda became an irrelevance.

The Cultural Revolution

Formally the Cultural Revolution lasted from 1966 to 1976, although the first four years are generally agreed to have been the worst. Professionals and intellectuals

were vilified, removed from their posts, and sent to work as agricultural labor-
ers, or put to work in various menial positions. Many hospitals closed, or maintained bare functionality. Naturally this had an effect on psychiatric services, but
it is not easy to determine exactly what this was. There are no statistics, policy
plans, or research reports to guide us, and much of what we "know" is based on
articles published by the few foreigners who were allowed to visit (Lazure 1964;
Thompson, McKenzie, and Peart 1967; Chin and Chin 1969). Cerny (1965) has
been widely quoted but may never have visited China. Once China began to open
up, more reports from visitors began to appear but these visitors tended to be
those considered "friends of China." They generally purveyed the party line, and
were uncritical (Sidel 1973; Sidel and Sidel 1973, 1982; Adams 1972; Sainsbury 1974;
Ho 1974). Furthermore, many of these articles are based on visits to the same two
hospitals, the Shanghai Number One and the Beijing Medical College Third Hospital. These were two of the best psychiatric hospitals in China, and the quality of
their medical staff and general practices cannot be considered to be typical. They
were also very close to the political heartland.

Revolutionary Approaches to Mental Illness

Sidel (1973) describes in some detail the principles of revolutionary optimism that
governed psychiatry during this period:

1. The feelings of individuals should be subordinated to the needs of the group
   of which they are members—the family, the classroom, the commune, the
   entire society.
2. Individuals are part of something larger than themselves; the revolution.
   This revolution will ultimately be victorious.
3. The participation in an ultimately victorious revolution gives meaning and
   joy to life, even if the road to revolution is paved with personal sacrifice.
4. People have an infinite capacity to learn, to modify their thinking, to understand the world around them, and to remold themselves through faith in the
   revolution and for the sake of the revolution.

This approach to the patient, as a conscious being with a capacity to learn
and change, continues an age-old approach to human beings and their essential
educability which is Confucian in origin. By being presented with correct ideas
and exemplars people could be changed for the good. The major technique to
help patients develop rational thought was the study of Mao's works, particularly "Where Do Correct Thoughts Come From?" and the ones referred to as "the
three constantly read articles": "In Memory of Norman Bethune," "To Serve the
People," and "The Foolish Old Man Who Could Move Mountains." Staff were expected to take the lessons contained in what were essentially allegorical tales and
help patients apply the lessons to their own lives. It is most unlikely that Mao's
thoughts had much part to play in the control and treatment of active psychosis

but they may have helped in what we would think of as the social rehabilitation of the patient. Furthermore there is an argument to support the view that this was part of a process of normalization: psychiatric patients were subject to the same expectations of political indoctrination as all other citizens. This could be interpreted as an act of respect, albeit ineffective in controlling and treating psychotic symptoms.

Hospitals in China since 1949 have tended to use the imagery of the army; illness and incorrect thoughts were the enemy to be defeated and, of course, social relationships were ordered in a strict hierarchy. The political climate and the imagery involved in revolution made the use of a military model almost inevitable. Wards were divided into "fighting groups," with the positions of corporal and sergeant being taken by model patients, known as Red Sentries—they were considered to be on the road to recovery and were expected to set a good example and look after newer and sicker patients (Ho 1974; Frears 1976; Lu 1978). Doubtless this also had the advantage of alleviating staff shortages and reducing the wages bill.

What Happened to Psychiatric Personnel?

This is a question that is frequently asked but which cannot be answered with any certainty. Those who survived this period are reluctant to talk about their personal experiences, and when they do it is with the understanding that their narratives are not broadcast. Medicines, food, and other necessary goods were in short supply and could not be guaranteed. "Politics taking command" meant chaos in terms of hospital administration. In some hospitals, doctors were assigned to menial positions, such as cleaners, while those with better political backgrounds but little or no medical training were moved to management or therapeutic posts. The CCP ruled, but it was not always possible to determine what that meant. Strife frequently broke out between different political factions among the staff and people did what they needed to do to survive. Some took the only means of escape open to them and killed themselves. Once it was over the survivors had to find ways of working and living together, and this has mostly been achieved by acts of collective amnesia, or at least silence. Experiences and the emotions that accompany them are boxed up and hidden in a dark place. It is a very different coping mechanism than talking, "getting it off your chest," seeking resolution, but in the Chinese context it is the preferred coping strategy.

Sidel (1973, 732), a very firm "friend of China" during this period, comments that "the psychiatric hospitals were the only segment of Chinese life that we saw in which depression rather than exhilaration was the predominant affect."

Seeking Truth from Facts

Following the advent of "ping-pong diplomacy," the PRC in the late 1970s and 1980s began its gradual process of opening up to the outside world, a process that included psychiatry. Articles on Chinese psychiatry written by psychiatrists themselves began to appear in the literature (Liu 1980; Liu 1981; Jiang 1988). The attendance of Chinese psychiatrists at international conferences became the norm and academic exchange programs began to take place, such as, for instance, the one between the University of Washington, led by Arthur Kleinman, and Hunan Medical College in Changsha, led by Young Derson (Kleinman 1986). These activities have allowed greater understanding among all parties. Some of the characteristics that had made China seem so "exotic," like the emphasis on Mao's works in treatment, rapidly faded. On this subject Young is quoted as saying, "We do not believe that you can get a disease from a wrong idea—nor will a 'correct idea' cure a patient. We try to teach the meaning of illness, based on scientific knowledge" (Achtenberg 1983, 373).

Published reports and my own experience of visiting, teaching, advising, and consulting at various psychiatric hospitals in the PRC make it clear that conditions, in most cases, might best be described as "bleak" and profoundly institutional. Wards were and are routinely locked, lacking in personal space (e.g., lockers) and devoid of anything that might remind patients of a previous life, like a photograph (Visher and Visher 1979; Wilson and Hutchison 1983; Parry-Jones 1988; Priemus-Noach 1988; Pearson 1995). Insulin shock therapy was still routinely being used in the 1980s, especially in the less prestigious hospitals. It was and still is routine practice to give ECT without anesthetic (Tousley 1985; Parry-Jones 1986; Thornicroft 1987; Pearson 1995). This seems to be partly due to different attitudes toward pain and partly for the wholly pragmatic reason that it is advisable for an anesthetist to be present, and for most hospitals this would be an impossible expense. Lobotomies were also being performed (and possibly still are) but this has rarely been recognized.

Traditional Chinese medicine (as was true of Western medicine until the 1950s) had not developed a drug that would effectively control the symptoms of active psychosis, although sedative preparations were well known. The first drug to do this was chlorpromazine (known as Largactil in the United Kingdom and Thorazine in the United States). It was approved for use in treating schizophrenia by the U.S. Food and Drug Administration in 1954. Naturally, it quickly became widely used despite the unpleasant side effects (e.g., lethargy, weight gain, and tardive dyskinesia). By the late 1970s its use was common in China and, as Chinese drug companies were able to manufacture it themselves, it was also inexpensive. Chlorpromazine has been credited with greatly speeding up the deinstitutionalization movement, enabling the closure of the large psychiatric asylums in countries like the United Kingdom and the United States. However, some say that this had more to do with the vast amounts of money that could be made by authorities selling off the sizeable grounds on which the asylums stood (Barham 1984; Scull 1985). As China had never developed an extensive network of institutional care for mentally ill people, the same effect was not witnessed there. Rather it reduced the physical restraint, isolation, and abuse that mentally ill people were subject to and allowed them and their families to live a semblance, at least in many cases, of normal life.

More intriguing is the widespread use in China of clozapine, the first of the atypical antipsychotic medications to be developed. It was first introduced in 1971 but was not licensed for use in many countries, notably the United States, because of its side effects, particularly acute agranulocytosis. It was not approved by the Food and Drug Administration until 1989, and even then only as a second- or third-line treatment for resistant schizophrenia. China saw things differently, and clozapine began to be used there as a first-line treatment for schizophrenia in the early 1980s (Pearson 1995). At that time China felt under no obligation to be bound by Western copyright laws. Without the authorization of the original drug company that developed clozapine, China made its own version. China's experience with the drug has been generally positive; psychiatrists find that it is effective and has fewer side effects than the earlier generation of psychotropic medications, such as chlorpromazine and haloperidol. Chinese psychiatrists report that clozapine is the most commonly used antipsychotic in China (Wang and Li 2012; Tang et al. 2008); reportedly between 25 and 60 percent of all patients with schizophrenia use it. Of these, it has been estimated that 0.21 percent develop acute agranulocytosis, of whom one-third die (Tang et al. 2008). These authors suggest that Chinese psychiatrists need to pay more attention to potential toxic side effects when making drug choices. Because it is manufactured in China and is relatively cheap, clozapine tends to be the medication of choice for treating schizophrenia in remote and economically deprived areas. In major cities doctors and patients prefer the newer generation of atypical antipsychotics, such as risperidone and olanzapine, which are much more expensive (and thus generate greater income for doctors and hospitals), and have a higher status because they are seen as "foreign," although they are not necessarily more efficacious. Doctors in America continue to recommend the use of clozapine only as a second-line treatment in resistant cases (Remington et al. 2013).

Psychiatric Facilities

The *1992 China Statistical Yearbook* states that there were 449 psychiatric hospitals in China, providing eighty-nine thousand psychiatric beds. An internal document on rehabilitation reported that the Ministry of Civil Affairs was responsible for thirty-five thousand beds, which constituted 33 percent of all hospital beds for those with a mental illness, and that 85 percent of those beds (at that time) were occupied by people with a chronic mental illness. A pamphlet produced by the West China University of Medical Sciences in 1990 reported that there were 473 psychiatric institutions under the Ministry of Public Health, 190 under the Ministry of Civil Affairs, 81 under the Ministry of Industry and Mining, 23 under the Ministry of Public Security, 24 under the armed forces, and 12 under local collectives. Unfortunately the pamphlet did not distinguish among hospitals, research institutes, departments of psychiatry in medical schools, psychiatric wards in general hospitals, and freestanding clinics. This was the period when private "psychiatric hospitals" began to open, made possible by changes in funding rules, but no records were kept of their numbers, size, or anything else. The 1987 document *Opinions about Strengthening Mental Health Work* (discussed further below) stated that there were six beds (for psychiatric patients) per thousand patients. It is simply not possible to be precise about what was provided and in what quantity, but it does not seem unreasonable to say that for a population of over one billion it was grossly insufficient, particularly since, as we will see later, community-based facilities provided little coverage.

Staff

To facilitate a more comprehensive grasp of the context in which patient care took place, some, albeit brief, information needs to be provided about staffing because, at least in this period, it was very different from the international norm. Occupational therapists, psychologists, and social workers were effectively non-existent, leaving only doctors and nurses. The 1931 League of Nations Health Organization's *Report on Medical Schools in China* recommended a two-level system of medical education for China: national colleges at the university level to produce "high level physicians" in a five-year program, and provincial-level medical schools to train medical practitioners in a three-year program (Lucas 1982). This two-tier system remained in place after the Cultural Revolution. Little psychiatry was taught in either program, nor was there a national system of accredited, postgraduate specialist training in psychiatry (Liu and Jia 1994), although some hospitals in major centers had initiated postgraduate training in psychiatry (Xia and Zhang 1981). Up until the 1990s doctors were not permitted to decide where they worked or in what specialty, so many of those assigned to work in psychiatric institutions had no natural affinity for it. As the system became more flexible the situation changed somewhat but it created a different problem: psychiatry was a very unpopular area, and once choice was allowed it became much harder to recruit doctors—willing or unwilling (Pearson and Phillips 1994).

Nurses were in even shorter supply than doctors. By the end of 1991 there were 3.99 million medical doctors and only 1.01 million nurses, according to a report from the State Statistical Bureau reported in the *China Business Weekly* (March 8–14, 1992). The World Bank report on health care in China (1992, 98) described nurses as "too often confined to semi-skilled and house-keeping functions." Bueber (1993b) describes psychiatric nursing as a fledgling discipline and reports that the first national psychiatric nursing association was not formed until 1990. Many nurses had no formal training and learned by watching older nurses on wards. Even those who had some training (two- or three-year pro-grams in the provincial-level medical colleges) would not have been taught about psychiatric nursing, which was not seen to be much different from general nurs-ing. In sum, nurses in psychiatric hospitals were assigned to their jobs and had little or no training in working with people with a mental illness. Because of the stigma and fear associated with this client group, nurses were also likely to be very reluctant recruits and to bring to their work all the negative stereotypes and misinformation that laypeople have about people with a mental illness. Bueber (1992) reported that it was not unusual for nurses to be so mistrustful of patients that they refused to reveal their names to their charges, and that many truly be-lieved that they could "catch" schizophrenia from their patients. The potential for the therapeutic role of nurses in the care and treatment of patients was not recognized, so nursing staff evaluations in psychiatric hospitals were based on activities like giving intravenous and intramuscular medication, inserting a uri-nary catheter, and making beds (Bueber 1993a).

The State Council Document of 1987

The Second National Meeting on mental health was held in Shanghai in 1986, jointly called by the three government ministries most involved with psychi-atric provision: Public Health, Civil Affairs, and Public Security. This meeting produced the first major assessment of the state of psychiatric care, as well as guidelines for future directions, since the Nanjing meeting in 1959. The result-ing document, entitled *Opinions about Strengthening Mental Health Work,* was approved by the State Council and published in 1987. The contents of this docu-ment have been extensively discussed in Pearson (1995), so the details will not be replicated here. In summary, it painted a dire picture of psychiatric service provision in China. Mental health work was being ignored by local cadres and its importance not recognized, despite there being an obvious increase in mental illness. Agencies doing mental health work were insufficient, as were hospital beds, funding, and manpower. Hospitals were described as run-down and their facilities as primitive and frequently located far away from the populations they were supposed to serve. Community care and rehabilitation was said to be almost nonexistent. The government was said to allocate only half the funds to psychiat-ric hospitals that it gave to general hospitals at the same grade. Particular concern was expressed about the problems that those suffering from mental illness posed to social order, and the "most pressing case" was said to be those hospitals run by the Ministry of Public Security for mentally ill people who had broken the law. Half of all patients (estimated to number ten million in total) were said to relapse and cause "serious danger" to society. Numerous examples are quoted, including that of a man who set fire to the Daqing oil refinery, causing one hundred mil-lion renminbi's worth of damage. Concern was expressed about the paucity and quality of staff, who suffered heavy workloads, high-risk work environments, low pay, and poor promotion prospects. In addition they were stigmatized and their work unvalued by others because of their close association with mental patients (the well-known contagion effect in stigma).

The analysis of difficulties was surprisingly honest, but the proposed "solutions" considerably more anodyne. These included setting up a joint committee of the three ministries at all administrative levels to guide national and local mental health work; incorporating mental health work into the "construction of a socialist spiritual civilization"; putting more effort into training personnel and carrying out scientific research; developing mental health legislation; developing community-based treatment and management programs for people with mental illness; actively pursuing public education programs to increase the general public's knowledge about mental illness and to decrease levels of stigmatization directed at mentally ill people; and actively pursuing alternative, nongovernmental sources of funding for the provision of institutional and community-based services. However well-meaning, these structures are not adequate for the provision of psychiatric services to a population of over one billion people. The suggestions constitute not much more than a wish list, with little in the way of service design, planning targets, implementation strategies, and clear operational guidelines. Most significantly, the issue of funding is glossed over, as are the huge problems of providing services for a rural population that at that time constituted 75 percent of the total (Phillips and Pearson 1994b).

The issues involved in funding health care in general and psychiatric care in particular in China have defied all solutions. The major advances in health characteristic of the early days of the rule of the CCP were achieved through tried and tested public health measures. Once the PRC passed through the health transition (see chapter 1), inadequate resource levels and irrational distribution of what resources there were proved intractable problems (Henderson 1990). Severe mental illnesses had never enjoyed that initial honeymoon period. They are often recurrent or chronic and therefore expensive to treat over the course of a lifetime. Urban dwellers prior to the Deng Xiaoping era had health insurance because they mostly worked for the government or state-owned industries and thus had access to psychiatric hospitals. But the vast majority of the population in the rural areas had little or no insurance coverage, and the cost of an average stay in a psychiatric hospital of three or more months was more than could be borne by a commune or individual family. Indeed, length of stay has been demonstrated to be more closely correlated to ability to pay rather than to severity of the condition (Phillips, Xiong, and Xiong 1993; Pearson 1995).

This situation changed through the 1980s and 1990s as the government withdrew central funding for hospitals, which were told that they had to become self-funding. At the same time, individual enterprises were allowed, people and families could set up businesses, and health insurance became less generous and less common, except for the privileged few who worked for the government. Psychiatric hospitals had two strategies to earn the money they now needed to cover operating costs and salaries/bonuses. They could operate sideline enterprises (e.g., running restaurants or factories, opening a holiday camp, renting out land and fishponds) and/or raise their fees (Pearson 1995; Phillips and Pearson 1994a). The end result was a vicious cycle of inpatient treatment becoming increasingly expensive and occupancy rates declining because families could not afford the fees (Pang and Kao 1995). As we shall see in the following section, there were other consequences when it came to developing community-based care and rehabilitation services outside the psychiatric hospitals.

Into the Community

Since the 1950s, "care in the community" has been the catchphrase that has guided the planning and provision of services for people with mental illness in countries able to afford to run large psychiatric hospitals. Ostensibly this was because of the realization that to deprive so many thousands of their chance to live a normal life was no longer tenable. Underlying this laudable motive was, first, the awareness that hospital services were expensive to run, and the hope that community provision might be cheaper; and second, the desire to realize the substantial sums that could be raised by selling to property developers the land on which they stood (Barham 1984). The various PRC documents discussed so far have made references to noninstitutional community-based care and have acknowledged its desirability, but a coordinating vision of how this could be achieved was obviously lacking.

That is not to say that there were no community-based projects in operation (Pearson 1992). Shanghai had developed its own system based mostly on guardianship networks and work station therapy (Zhang, Yang, and Phillips 1994). In theory at least, each patient had a guardianship network consisting of three people: a family member of the patient, a medical person, and a local cadre from the street organization or local residents' committee. Each was supposed to keep an eye on the patient, ensure they were properly cared for, and negotiate a return to the hospital if they presented social order issues. In reality the responsibility fell on the family but at least they should have had people to turn to if they needed help. Each street organization was supposed to provide a work station for daily activities for people with a psychiatric illness in their area, usually staffed by retired people who were volunteers and received a small stipend.

In other areas of China medical staff had set up home-based psychiatric beds and community support and visiting programs. The best known were probably those in Beijing's Haidian district—the "hospital and community integration model" (Shen 1983)—and in Yantai in Shandong Province (Wang, Gong, and Niu 1994). There was also a rural "community beds" scheme organized by the West China University of Medical Sciences in Chengdu. Some places used factories as the basis for community support via the *danwei* (workplace). In a classic example of an individual with passion making a serious difference, Wang Xishi, working in Shenyang, set up a factory that printed cinema tickets staffed by people recovering from mental illness (Wang 1994). It was an economic enterprise like any other and was independent of state financial help, but it turned a healthy profit and was self-supporting. Neither the Yantai model nor the one in the Haidian district survived the demands of the market economy that emerged in the 1990s (Ma 2012).

So it could be argued that the PRC did, indeed, have an integrated model of hospital and community care for people with mental illness (Pearson 1992). The problem was that not only was there no mechanism to spread these ideas beyond the original location and its sphere of influence, but there were severe internecine rivalries that stopped a model with proven efficacy from being adopted countrywide. Issues of both vertical and horizontal integration abounded, and they severely affected support for services that were supposed to help keep patients out of the hospital. As we saw earlier, state funding was withdrawn from hospitals throughout the 1980s and 1990s, and the simplest way of replacing this money was by raising fees. There was little motivation for hospital-based psychiatrists (and most were hospital-based), particularly outside the major centers, to try and keep patients out of their beds—it was like asking turkeys to vote for Thanksgiving, and as a funding strategy it was fundamentally flawed. A further complication was that even when patients were fortunate enough to have health insurance, it only covered inpatient care (Liu et al. 2011a).

Families had to fund anything outside of the hospital themselves. Yet it remained obvious that the way forward could not be building more hospitals, as such a policy was unaffordable and out of step with modern thinking.

The Eighth Five-Year Plan, 1991–1995

Most unusually, the Eighth Five-Year Plan contained a Work Program for Disabled Persons, initiated by the China Disabled Persons' Federation established and led by Deng Pufang, the son of Deng Xiaoping and himself a wheelchair user. The federation was set up in 1988, in affiliation with the Ministry of Civil Affairs, and rapidly began to take very significant steps to raise the profile and meet the needs of people with a disability. As mentioned earlier, this included encouraging the government to undertake the first-ever survey of the numbers and types of people with a disability in China: 51.64 million in 1987 (Tian et al. 1994).

Several very senior psychiatrists approached Deng Pufang in 1988 and persuaded him that people with psychiatric disorders should be included under the umbrella of his organization. With his agreement the Chinese Rehabilitation Research Association for the Mentally Disabled was formed in 1989 as a branch of the Chinese Rehabilitation and Research Association for Disabled Persons, which was in turn part of the China Disabled Persons' Federation. Thus it came to be that the work plan for disabled persons included in the Eighth Five-Year

Plan contained chapter 3: "a system for the prevention and treatment of psychiatric disabilities." Most psychiatrists working in China at that time considered this a most ambitious and hopeful development and one that could possibly turn back the tide of institutionalization. Extensive details of the plan are provided in Phillips and Pearson (1994a) and will not be repeated here.

Essentially the framework was that of the community-based Shanghai model (guardianship networks, work therapy, and home care) in sixty experimental sites, thirty in urban areas and thirty in rural ones. Twelve ministries were consulted and involved in formulating the plan so that the problem of horizontal integration mentioned earlier was hoped to be overcome. The plan also included mandated administrative structures and training programs to create the necessary trained personnel. One obvious problem from the beginning was that funding was supposed to be raised locally from the sixty sites, and for this purpose local governments were authorized to raise 0.05 RMB per head of population in their area (at the time about one cent). It was never likely that such limited funding would be able to provide the wide range of activities envisaged. Time showed that where similar services already existed the plan stimulated enthusiasm and motivation, at least initially. The major practical problems were insufficient funding, lack of trained personnel, and low motivation on the part of local officials. A top-down plan dependent on voluntarism and community compliance might have been feasible in the pre-reform era but was much less viable in the decentralized competitive environment of post-reform China. Seen from the position of local officials, they were, and are, given impossible targets to reach across many different areas with insufficient resources. Their careers depend on meeting such targets. It is not hard to understand why they prefer easy-to-measure one-off interventions like cataract and orthopedic operations or cleft palate repairs, which make people more or less instantly functional with no overhead expenses.

The 686 Project

This project was a serendipitous byproduct of the PRC government's response to improving the national health system following the SARS epidemic in 2003. It was the only noninfectious disease project to be developed. Known formally as the Central Government Support for the Local Management and Treatment of Severe Mental Illnesses Project, it was nicknamed the 686 Project because the government initially injected 6.86 million RMB to get it started. It was modeled on the World Health Organization's recommendations for creating integrated inpatient and community-based services for mentally ill people, with a focus on rehabilitation and recovery rather than the control of serious symptoms and the maintenance of public order. As the coordinator of the project describes it,

> The specific goals of the project were to a) establish an integrated identification and treatment system for individuals with mental illnesses who are poten-

tially violent or disruptive; b) increase treatment rates for persons with serious mental illnesses; c) increase community awareness about the characteristics and treatment options for persons with severe mental illnesses; d) increase the rates of successful recovery and rehabilitation; and e) alleviate the pain and suffering of patients and their family members. (Ma 2012, 172)

The project established sixty demonstration sites: one urban site and one rural site each in thirty provinces, independent municipalities, and autonomous regions. Each site had a minimum population of four hundred thousand individuals, and the total catchment population was forty-three million, or about one-thirtieth of the national population. The components of the intervention included patient registration and initial assessment, free medication and regular follow-up in the community, management of community emergencies, and free emergency hospitalization. The project identified and treated many patients who had previously been locked up or restrained in their homes by family members, still a frequent and widespread occurrence in China. As part of this process of implementing the project a large number of training materials for different types of personnel were developed (Ma 2012).

By 2008 the model was considered sufficiently mature to merit scaling it up to the whole country. By the end of 2010 a total of 280,000 people with serious mental illnesses had been registered in the system (Ma 2012). The project has been welcomed within and outside China (Good and Good 2012; Jenkins 2012) and it has provided the greatest cause for optimism for the development of adequate psychiatric services for the Chinese population since 1949. It is too soon to judge whether the effects of the project will be sustainable nationwide and sustainable within the constraints of available funding. So far, there seems to be little published research that has evaluated the outcomes of this new model for patients (and their families) treated within it.

First National Mental Health Legislation, 2012

Another reflection of governmental concern with mental health and its long-standing association with social order is the passage into the statute books of China's first national mental health legislation. This was adopted by the Standing Committee of the National People's Congress on October 26, 2012, and became law on May 1, 2013. Serious debate about such a law began in 1985. Since then various local pieces of mental health legislation have been passed, most notably in Shanghai. Such local statutes function as experiments with the law on a small scale to gain experience and identify good practice, and are a common practice in the Chinese legal process. But it is far too soon to say what effect this law will have on the treatment of those with mental illness and how extensively its provisions (which will require a huge increase in the number of psychiatrists and other psychiatric professionals as well as other resources) will be implemented (Chen, Phillips, and Cheng 2012).

Conclusion—Families and Community

In China the family is morally and legally responsible for controlling the behavior of its family members. In relation to people with a mental disorder this tradition dates back at least to the Yongzheng period and the enactment of the registration and confinement laws of the Qing Code implemented in 1731, 1755, and 1766 (Ng 1990). This translated into a form of house arrest, with families expected to create a secure, barred, and locked room in the home to contain and restrain the sick person. Local authorities provided ropes, chains, and shackles—certainly cheaper than providing accommodation in jails, which would have been the only alternative. As we have seen, this tradition of family responsibility has continued through the centuries and is still relevant today. We have seen, too, that a concern for containing the potential for disruption to social order that mentally ill people present permeates policies, both ancient and modern.

This is enshrined in the stated goal of the guardianship networks (a means to maintain mentally ill people outside the hospital): "to observe the patient's mental health condition and report to relevant health personnel in case of disorderly conduct or breach of the peace" (Xia, Yan, and Wang 1987, 83). In Western countries the idea of community care is construed as the provision of services outside of institutions so as to maximize conditions of normal living, increase patients' sense of self-worth and value, and increase quality of life. The concept of community care in the Chinese context is dominated by the need for surveillance and control. But on its own terms, it works. Both Qiu and Lu (1994) and Zhang, Yan, and Phillips (1994) have demonstrated that guardianship networks are successful in preventing relapse, increasing social functioning, and reducing socially disruptive behaviour. The issue is not necessarily the design of services but their paucity. Whatever is written about services, the fact remains that the majority of mentally ill people in China were and are cared for by their families (Pearson and Lam 2001; Phillips 1993), some with loving kindness, some not.

It is thus surprising that family care is not recognized by authorities and policymakers as the major resource for caring, and little effort is made to work with family members, either therapeutically or as partners in care (Phillips and Pearson 1994c). Their efforts are taken for granted and grossly undervalued. Policies need to recognize that families caring for people with schizophrenia have needs of their own—for support and to be accepted as having intimate knowledge of the patient that should be integrated into any care and treatment plan. Where family-oriented projects—for instance, psychoeducation training for families and family resource centers (Pearson 2007; Pearson and Lam 2001) or therapeutic interventions for families (Zhang et al. 1994; Yang and Pearson 2002)—have been set up, outcomes have been good. Efforts have been made to create family mutual support groups in a number of cities (e.g., Wuhan, Shashi, Guangzhou, Beijing), but these have had varying success and have not taken root as well as might have been hoped.[2] Even the recent 686 Project has little to say about family carers other than the built-in assumption that they must continue to do their duty, despite the high emotional, social, and financial costs to those involved. Nor should it be forgotten that the level of stigma experienced by people with mental illness and their families is high and pervasive (Phillips et al. 2002; Yang et al. 2012). Families carry out their obligations in a social environment that is profoundly unsupportive and in many cases actively hostile.

The experience of mental illness in China is played out against a backdrop of a turbulent and changing political and economic environment where the needs are overwhelming but the resources made available are scant. The cultural context is one that values order, stability, and conformity and construes mental illness as the antithesis of this. Within this framework, the major focus is not on the well-being of individuals and families but on maintaining conditions in which the collective is as little disturbed as possible. These basic precepts have not fundamentally altered from 1898 to the present day. What has changed is the increasing honesty with which the problems in the system are analyzed, and the sophistication of the proposed solutions (Ma 2012; Liu et al. 2011a). While the goal of accessible, affordable, and effective treatment for seriously mentally ill people has not, as yet, been achieved, at least it has not been abandoned.

Notes

1. Michael Phillips, personal communication with the author, December 24, 2013.
2. Ibid.

Part III
Adaptations and Innovations

9 Foreign Models of Medicine in Twentieth-Century China

Xi Gao
Translated by Sabine Wilms, Xi Gao,
and Bridie Andrews

Competing Models during the Republican Era: Japan, Europe, and the United States

> The people of my humble country do not know how to pay attention to health care (*weisheng*). In particular, they do not know that a country's strength and prosperity are held up entirely by a strong and vigorous citizenry and that they must therefore pay attention to healthcare. We rely completely on the enthusiastic guidance from all of you assembled here to allow researchers in healthcare to develop and advance from one day to the next. Moreover, the destitute men, women and children in China depend on your church for protection and nurturance, as well as on the instruction in culture and knowledge. This is the great benefit provided by your church to my country. . . . In particular, we hope that you will continue, upon your return to your home country, to advise and protect the people of my humble country as before, in order to transform everybody into strong, healthy and cultured citizens in the future.

This statement was made by Yuan Shikai on January 15, 1913, in front of foreign medical representatives of the China Medical Missionary Association in Beijing ("Dazongtong jiejian boyihui waiguo yishi daci" 1913, 91). Coming from the first president of the Republic of China, Yuan Shikai's speech represents a positive attitude by the Chinese government toward foreign physicians. We can tease out at least two major points he wanted to communicate. First, health care is the foundation for the health of citizens, and healthy citizens are a symbol of the culture of a nation. Second, foreign physicians are able to protect and guide Chinese people toward becoming healthy and cultured. And yet, this perspective contrasts sharply with the disdain in traditional Chinese culture for the medical profession, which is regarded as a lowly craft. According to the *Li Ji* (*Book of Rites*), the literate elite of traditional China generally looked down upon medicine in the context of "all those who hold skills to serve their superiors, such as clerks, archers, physicians, diviners, and the hundred artisans." The fact that in the present case the position of health care and of doctors had been elevated by the government to one that concerned the survival of the race and the nation's virtue and culture must certainly be looked at as peculiar. The only explanation for this oddity is that the Chinese term for health care, *weisheng,* that Yuan Shikai placed such faith in did not refer to the techniques for "safeguarding life," as in traditional language and literature, but to a system of knowledge that the Chinese people did not yet fully understand.

This system of knowledge from abroad is the subject of this chapter. In Chinese it is refered to as "new medicine" or "Western medicine." We will focus on exploring the following questions: What were the core contents of the different models of foreign medicine in twentieth-century China? What were the different ideological and historical trajectories that brought them to China? What were the key factors that ultimately determined the choice of the Chinese people? And lastly, what kind of a knowledge system was it that China constructed as a result?

Government Medicine: The Japanese Model

The earliest people to introduce foreign medicine to China were British and American missionaries. Medical schools served as important bridges of communication, Chinese-language medical textbooks and instructors were key vehicles, and missionary societies also sent Chinese students to Europe and the United States to study abroad. Missionaries with some clinical experience, a bit of background knowledge in Chinese literature, and introductory scientific knowledge in Western medicine were in agreement with the Chinese literati class and the new government officials that health care was the path to a strong nation. Elite Chinese promoted medicine with the goal of strengthening the country and protecting the Chinese race. Prior to 1900, Western medical education in China was almost completely in the hands of European and American missionary societies: among the eight schools of Western medicine, seven were run by European or American missionary societies and only one was state-run: the Tianjin Medical School (founded in 1893), whose predecessor had also been a hospital run by the London Missionary Society.

A number of changes took place in the early twentieth century. First, the dominant force in disseminating medical information changed from foreign missionaries to the Chinese people and the Chinese government. In other words, Chinese doctors (of both traditional Chinese and Western medicine), students returning from abroad, and Chinese intellectuals superseded medical missionaries as the key players in the transmission of medicine. Chinese people actively promoted and selectively adopted foreign medicine, which underwent substantial transformation in the process. Second, these role reversals caused the dissemination of medicine to move further and further away from the goal of missionary work, which was replaced with the new goal of constructing a vigorous and cultured state. The requirements of this nation-building phase created a fertile, though highly politicized, environment for the introduction of modern medicine. To be precise, the development and transformation of foreign medicine in twentieth-century China unfolded under the leadership of the government and expressed itself in the specific educational system and health care structures the government chose to imitate. The system first chosen by the Chinese government for imitation was the Japanese model.

After the defeat of the Qing dynasty troops in the Sino-Japanese War of 1894, both the Chinese court and the general public turned to their eastern neighbor and paid close attention to how Japan had succeeded in modernizing and expanding by following the example of the West. Kang Youwei put forth the strategy of "taking one's formidable foe as one's teacher" and proposed that China should carry out reforms by imitating Japan's education system. Zhang Zhidong believed that Japan would be an easy example to emulate since the political conditions and people's customs were similar. In his words, this was a case of "twice the results with half the effort" (Chang Chih-Tung 1900). Imitating Japan as a shortcut to studying the West was a view that was advocated by people like Liang Qichao and Wu Rulun and was accepted by the general consensus of China's elites. In 1896, the Qing government began sending students to Japan. Their numbers reached between ten and twenty thousand people by 1906 (Sanetō 1983). By 1907 there were at least 127 Chinese students in medical school in Japan (Yiyao xuehui 1907). In 1902, when Yuan Shikai founded the Beiyang Military Medical College in Tianjin, he selected a Japanese-style organizational system and invited Japanese medical officer Higara Seijirō (正平贺精次郎) to serve as head instructor. His hiring marked the beginning of the end of the era of European and American missionaries and doctors' monopolizing the enterprise of Western medicine in China.

According to the Memorial on Regulations for Colleges promulgated by the Qing government in 1903, there were three categories of college-level preparatory courses, with the third category being premedical preparatory courses. The regulations for premedical courses stipulated thirteen credit hours of German-language instruction and four credit hours in either English or French, thus clearly emphasizing the need to study German in order to enter medical school. In 1904, the Qing Ministry of Education promulgated regulations for universities: "Each department should, in general, be run in accordance with the regulations in force in Japanese medical schools and technical colleges" ("Yike daxue zhangcheng shangque" 1905). Academic programs in medicine were four years in length, with German as the primary foreign language and curricula that were basically identical to those of Japan's Imperial Universities.[1] Nevertheless, the fact that no courses were established in anatomy or histology was broadly condemned in China, the main argument being that if China was to truly study Japan, why not do so thoroughly ("Yike daxue zhangcheng shangque" 1905)?

The medical college at the Metropolitan University in Beijing invited Ding Fubao, who had studied medicine at Dongwen College in Shanghai (a Japanese-style college), to serve as physiology instructor there. In 1909, Ding received an order from the provincial governor of Liangjiang to travel to Japan to investigate "the various medical specialties in Japan, the stages of medical reform in the initial years of the Meiji government, the Chinese drugs in use by the Japanese people, as well as the regulations and curricula of the medical colleges and hospitals" (Ding 1949). In Japan, Ding toured the Imperial Medical Universities and Kitasato Shibasaburō's Institute for Infectious Diseases. Upon his return, he composed an article introducing the Japanese medical education system, hospital regulations, and examination system for physicians (Ding 1910). He proposed that to improve the state of medicine in China, the Chinese had to learn from the experience of Japan, and that "following the Japanese example was more convenient than the European and American model" (Ding 1949). In addition, Ding invested a huge amount of energy and effort in translating Japanese medical literature, ultimately translating and composing nearly a hundred books on medicine. These included textbooks and academic treatises, but his greatest influence stems from his writings that popularized medicine and science. His *Ding Shi Congzhu* (Master Ding's collected writings) was widely popular for a while and became a key source of information on Western medicine for the Chinese people (Niu 2004).

If the nineteenth century was when Christian missionary hospitals and clinics allowed the general population in China to experience the marvels of Western medicine for the first time, it was the great number of medical translations from the Japanese, with their emphasis on diseases, germs, physiology, and hygiene, which introduced Chinese intellectuals to the principles of Western medical science. In the words of Wu Dui, "If we want to strengthen the nation, we must strengthen the people. If we want to strengthen the people, we must strengthen their bodies. Let us please start with health care" (Wu 1907). This demonstrated how the term "health care" (*weisheng*) had become a commonplace expression in the political discourse of the Chinese intelligentsia at the beginning of the twentieth century (Zhang 2009b), to the point where even Yuan Shikai, whom we cited at the start of this chapter, clearly understood the significance of this "way of health care."

After 1900, educational reform according to the Japanese model became an important element of the New Policies, and educational experts and public opinion in Japan only added fuel to this fire. As the Japanese scholar of pedagogy Kano Jigorō 嘉纳治五郎 claimed, "Now that Japanese education experts have been traveling to China and taking responsibility for China's development, they have achieved in one or two years the same results that western missionary educators took decades to obtain" ("Jianashi de Qing guo jiaoyu tan" 1902). The Japanese *Daily News* of May 21, 1907, went even further in advocating for investments in education in China: "We should encourage Japanese universities to make special arrangements to accept Chinese students for higher education." As a result, large numbers of Japanese teachers appeared in Chinese medical colleges, to the point where there were as many as fifty Japanese professors of medicine teaching in China in 1909 (Yoshino 1910). In addition, Chinese study-abroad students returned home and threw themselves into medical education and the dissemination of medicine. A 1915 survey of China by the Rockefeller Foundation found that, with the exception of the Beiyang Medical College and the Guanghua Medical College in Guangdong, practically all private and public medical schools in China were influenced by Japan and had faculty that either were educated in Japan or were Japanese professors (China Medical Commission of the Rockefeller Foundation 1914).

Nevertheless, a statistical analysis of Western-style medical schools in China prior to 1911 shows that out of a total of thirty-one schools, twenty-two (or 70 percent) were Christian medical schools, five were Japanese-style medical schools, and four were established by the provincial or national government, or by private foundations, to teach Japanese-style medicine. Only a single medical school was established by the Japanese: the Nanman (South Manchurian) Medical College, founded by Japan's imperialist South Manchurian Railway Company in 1911 (Li 1987, 410–411). Furthermore, from the 1880s the newly reestablished China Medical Missionary Association began to consider how to develop Western medical education in China. Medical missionaries had a wealth of practical experience in medical education as well as considerable success with its local implementation in China. Moreover, there were schools with a long history, such as John Kerr's Boji Medical School in Canton. European and American schools therefore had a slight edge over Japan, in terms of sheer numbers, quality of education, and valuable experience.

The question then becomes, why did the Chinese people select the Japanese model? The answer lies in the difference in each country's intentions for establishing medical schools. Around 1901, the China Medical Missionary Association was already aware that China needed medical schools and realized that medical education offered unprecedented opportunities for development and growth. Neverthelesss, its starting point was to meet the need for Chinese assistants in missionary hospitals in order to create greater opportunities for propagating Christianity (Whitney 1901). What was concerning the Christian hospitals at that time was the fact that they had to make difficult choices in the training of their students and assistants and were deliberating such technical questions as whether instruction should be in Chinese or in English (Whitney 1901b). In this context, whether Chinese graduates could be "certified" or "qualified" were key issues, as the Medical Missionary Association deliberated medical education (Cousland 1901). However, the modern medical education that Chinese people understood was one that existed within the organizational structure of a university; they saw the creation of medical colleges as a necessary step in the context of national educational reform. The goal of missionary medical education differed fundamentally from that of the late Qing government: one was trying to establish "Western-style government" while the other was concerned with transmitting "Western skills" (Zhou 1934). The state's political goals related to the construction of a national government, and this determined the choice of the medical education system. For the missionaries, medical education stopped at the level of improving technical skills, and their ambition in medicine was limited to pursuing advancement in medical specialties and at most elaborating on the scientific nature of medicine. This contrast is perfectly illustrated by a comparison of publications in China by the two camps: between 1898 and 1911, at least twelve Chinese translations of Japan's school system and education law were published (Tan 1980), and the periodical *Jiaoyu Shijie* (World of education) published another ninety-seven articles on Japanese education law between 1901 and 1903, as important reference information for the education system being drafted by the Qing Ministry of Education. At the same time, the Medical Missionary Association published its position on education only in the English version of the *China Medical Missionary Journal,* and practically nothing in Chinese. Evidently, the association had not completed any plan for medicine as a service to the state, with the inevitable result that its model of medical education lost out in the state-building activities of the late Qing New Policies era.

There is one more important point to consider. After the government had investigated Western systems of education, it realized that "universities in Western countries place great emphasis on medicine, with Germany at the forefront of this development. And Japanese medicine is heavily indebted to Germany." It therefore required that medical preparatory courses "must include the study of German," and "must add the subject of Latin, since the technical terms in medicine and chemistry in Western languages all use Latin" (Zhu 1987). Obviously, the late Qing government possessed clear knowledge regarding their choice of a medical system, and what they chose was not the Western model but the model of German medicine—the most advanced medicine in the world. And the reason why they imitated Japan was due to nothing but the fact that it could function as a linguistic bridge and therefore offered the additional benefit of serving as a shortcut. Even though the Ministry of Education clearly adopted Japan as its model, there were some scholars who considered the education system in Japan most deficient and claimed that textbooks were far superior in Germany. Lufei Kui, for example, criticized this approach by stating that the government's decision to imitate Japan was nothing but the position of politicians (Lufei 2007). In 1911, the provincial governor of Xijiang, Zeng Yunzou, requested that upper-level medical colleges be established in the provincial capitals by imitating "the German system of medicine and specifying school courses and regulations in accordance with the established methods of all countries East and West" ("Di yi qian yi bai wu shi qi hao, zhezou lei" 2006 [1911]).

The entire situation changed, however, when the Qing government was overthrown and the Republic of China was founded in 1911. In 1912, the Republican government convened a temporary national council on education to discuss a new national education system. Among the ninety-four conference participants, 50 percent had either studied in Japan or visited Japan for observation and study (Tian and Yu 2010), while only 10 percent of attendees had studied in Europe. Numerous proposals were submitted to advocate for the Japanese model, but attendees also felt that "the Japanese state system is different from ours, and we must also choose appropriate methods from Europe and America" (Woyi 1912). Among the medical representatives at the conference were Tang Erhe, who had studied in Japan and Germany and had returned to China with a doctorate in medicine from Germany; Yu Richang, a graduate of St. John's University; and Zhang Jiguang, originally secretary-general of the Ministry of Education. While studying in Japan, Tang Erhe had joined the Revolutionary Alliance (founded by Sun Yat-sen) and had closely associated with Sun Yat-sen and Zhang Taiyan. He was also a close friend of Cai Yuanpei, the first minister of education in the Republican government, and served as examiner for the "Proposals for Education" on the State Education Committee ("Linshi jiaoyu weiyuanhui jishi" 1912). He was a key instigator of the government's decision to choose the Japanese model.

On November 22, 1912, the Ministry of Education promulgated regulations for professional schools in medicine, which differed somewhat from the educational system in the Qing period: medicine was included among the professional schools, "with the aim of cultivating skilled specialists in medicine" ("Guoli Beijing yixue zhuanmen xuexiao zhangcheng" 1920). Imitating Japanese professional schools, the length of study was set at four years, with forty-eight subjects, and German was required as the first subject of study ("Zhonghua Jiaoyujie" 1913). The appearance of these regulations was directly influenced by Tang Erhe. Ten days before the promulgation of the rules for medical schools, Tang was invited by the Ministry of Education to serve as principal of the state-run National Medical College in Beijing, which we can regard as a step by the Ministry of Education toward implementing its system of medical education. The curriculum at the National Medical College was arranged in strict accordance with the rules of the Ministry of Education, with a total of forty-three subjects.[2] There were three terms a year, with German required for all four years. One deviation from Western and Japanese medical curricula was that first-year students were required to attend classes on physics and chemistry, because China lacked a system of preparatory courses ("Guoli Beijing yixue zhuanmen xuexiao zhangcheng" 1920). Tang Erhe personally went to Japan to purchase textbooks and teaching equipment and invited Japanese professors and Chinese students who had returned after studying in Japan to assume teaching responsibilities. The state-run National Medical College thus became representative of Japanese-style medical schools.

When the Ministry of Internal Affairs in January of 1914 published the "Statutes for Dissections" that had been proposed by Tang Erhe, this marked a new departure for modern medical schools in China. Knowledge of anatomy had been introduced to China in the seventeenth century by missionaries and had first been taught in missionary hospitals, but it had suffered from restrictions imposed on it by China's traditional beliefs and the legal code. The Qing government's medical schools had not permitted courses in dissection, and the missionary schools made do with models to lecture on anatomy. So Chinese students, unlike those in Japan, had never before been able to gain anatomical knowledge through human dissection. After the promulgation of the 1914 Statutes for Dissections, missionary medical schools also profited from this development and combined to conduct the first lawful human dissection for the purpose of teaching in China (Cormack 1914). This situation demonstrates that it was the needs of the government that dictated the speed of scientific development in China.

There are two other areas where Japanese influence left obvious traces in the government's approach to medicine. The first is the system of managing public sanitation and epidemic prevention. In 1902, during the last years of the Qing, Yuan Shikai took control of the Bureau of Sanitation in the provincial yamen in the city of Tianjin and converted it to the Beiyang Bureau of Sanitation. Graduates from the Beiyang Medical School held the posts of sanitary officers (Gan 1907), and this is regarded as China's earliest Chinese-run sanitary organization (Fang 1928). Influenced by Japan, Yuan Shikai strengthened the supervisory and administrative authority of the police to manage public and environmental health and sanitation. In 1905, he established a Ministry of Police in Tianjin, which was responsible for public sanitation, and additionally created a Bureau of Sanitation and a Bureau of Official Medicine. In charge of managing public health for the entire country ("Xunjingbu nipin weisheng guwenguan" 1906), these offices were staffed predominantly by health care workers from the Japanese faction. During the late Qing and early Republican years, almost all rules and regulations that concerned the supervision of the professional practice of medicine and pharmaceutics, prevention of epidemic diseases, and punishment for violations of unclean food and sanitation regulations, were either direct translations of Japanese rules (Jin 1985) or minor adjustments of them (Iijima 2000). And yet, these regulations failed to be implemented in practice. The so-called pursuit of hygiene was still limited to cleaning streets and dispensing simple medicines (Yu 2011b).

The second aspect of Japanese influence on government medicine was the attempt to abolish traditional Chinese medicine. This was inspired entirely by the actions of the Meiji Restoration to abolish Chinese medicine in Japan, and the most extreme instigators of this effort in China were Chinese who had returned from studying in Japan. One of these, Wang Qizhang, advocated "the use of political means, to imitate contemporary Japanese measures of banning traditional Chinese medicine . . . to exterminate it." Yu Yunxiu, a member of the Central Health Care Committee who had also been a student in Japan several years earlier, committed himself wholeheartedly to advocating for medical reform and in 1929 published a "proposal to abolish the old medicine, to sweep away obstructions to medicine and hygiene." The six measures listed in this proposal, such as examinations and retraining for practitioners of traditional Chinese medicine, the prohibition of schools or dissemination of information on traditional Chinese medicine, etc., were entirely copied from Japan (Hao 2005). And the main political supporter behind these two activists was Wang Jingwei, who had received government funding to study in Japan in 1903 and was in charge of the Administrative Yuan. As his contemporaries described him, "he goes around everywhere lobbying for Japan's Meiji Restoration, the first act of which was the abolition of Chinese medicine" (Chen 2000).

Foreign Models and the Modernization of Medicine in China

If we compare Japan's system of health care administration during the Meiji years with government regulations on health care by the Shanghai Ministry of Works and the Tianjin Provisional Government (Dutong Yamen), it is not difficult to see that the centralized system of health care formulated during the late Qing and early Republican period borrowed from the experiences of many countries. It adopted content and institutions from the health care supervisory systems of England, France, and Japan. One noteworthy point concerning the structures for health care administration is that Japan, after comparing health care regulations in all the European countries, had been inclined toward the British model (Ono 1997). The earliest institutions for health care administration in China were those established by the Shanghai Ministry of Works in 1863. Placed under the responsibility of British doctors, they gradually created public health structures, setting up institutions like isolation hospitals, hospitals for venereal diseases, and preventive inoculation stations. They formulated regulations for nursing and expanded sanitary administration to include medical treatment, epidemic prevention, venereal disease control, environmental hygiene, food hygiene, and prison hygiene. China's first forerunner of a modern public health bureau was the Tianjin Provisional Government's *service de santé* (*weisheng bu,* or health service), which had been set up by Eight-Power Allied Forces in 1900 in the wake of the Boxer Rebellion and was run by French and Japanese medical officers. Its administrative responsibilities included the supervision of environmental hygiene in the cities, disease prevention and control, health care statistics, quarantines, the monitoring of water quality, physical examination of prostitutes, dietary hygiene, death statistics and burial, vaccinations and inoculations, and the construction of public cemetaries (Ren 2009). After Yuan Shikai took control in 1902, he asked the original director of the service, the French medical officer G. Mesny, to assume the role of consultant. He also retained a number of the original hygiene policies, such as a system for street cleaning, waste management measures, water quality monitoring, and a system of hygiene inspections. The bureau was likewise influenced by Japan, and after the founding of the Republic it restored certain measures that had originally existed but had then been abandoned, such as physical examinations of prostitutes and the management of graveyards (Ren 2009).

When the Republic of China was founded in 1911, Sun Yat-sen's secretary and personal friend, the physician Lin Wenqing, who had received his medical training in England, was appointed as the country's first director of the Health Department. In 1913, the Health Department was transformed into the Health Division under the Police Department in the Ministry of Internal Affairs. It consisted of four branches with distinct responsibilities: (1) managing health care–related organizational structures, handling hygiene in cities and on roads, and indigent health care; (2) hygiene and infectious diseases, epidemic prevention, and quarantines; (3) managing hospitals, physicians, midwives, and pharmacists; and (4) handling cleanliness and hygiene in medicinal substances, pharmaceutical products, and food (Fang 1928). There were clear differences from Meiji Japan's health administration in the two branches of health care and epidemic prevention (*Yizhi bainianshi* 1974a), and the restructuring of the four branches according to the Japanese system was not completed until 1921 (Kōseishō imukyoku 1974). Consequently, even though the system of health care under Yuan Shikai's government and in the first years of the Republican period was for the most part managed by Japanese-style physicians, its organizational structures and health care regulations were by no means all derived from Japan alone.

Two other details concerning the new Republican Health Department are conspicuous. The first branch also was charged with creating "a system for investigating health-related writings and reports," and the fourth branch included a "smoking prohibition." These two health regulations did not appear in either Japanese or British health care regulations. The latter was a rule formulated in an attempt to improve the state of general health in China (see chapter 4 in this volume), but the former is an example of the influence of tradition on health care in China. Control over public opinion and an emphasis on the ruler's authority were inevitable results of the autocratic culture of traditional China, and even though the imperial system had been abolished, the traditions of ideological control remained. What was different was that the politics of health care during the Republican era looked to the West in search of scientific foundations and political support. Wu Lien-teh, a prominent Malay Chinese who had trained in Britain, criticized the choice of Japanese methods which had resulted in control over health care being placed in the hands of the police instead of in a separate health care administration. For him, this meant that China's system of health care was inferior to those in Europe or the United States. Wu believed that the United States' system of health care management would be a more appropriate model for China (Wu 1934).

In 1927, Yan Fuqing, the director of the Hsiangya (Hunan Yale-in-China) Medical School responded to suggestions by John B. Grant of the Peking Union Medical College (PUMC) and proposed the creation of a separate Health Department to the Republican government. He also wrote up a blueprint for how it might be operated (Yen 1928). In the same year, Hu Tingan, a doctoral candidate in public health at Germany's Berlin University, also proposed a "program for implementing health care administration in China" to the Republican government on the basis of his practical experience at the public health office in the city of Berlin. In his opinion, consideration of the present economic and financial difficulties in China made the American-style model of a multilayered organization with many subordinate structures an inappropriate choice for China because such a system required financial strength and support. Instead he suggested that China should adapt a combination of the experiences of public health administration in countries like England, the United States, France, and Germany (Hu 1928). After comparing the mortality and birth rates of China to those of the various Western European countries, Huang Zifang, the director of the Beijing City Bureau of Public Health, believed that the reason why China so clearly lagged behind advanced countries in the world was that its pursuit of public health was not developed. He therefore suggested that China should make it a priority to preserve the health and safety of its population (Huang 1927).

Under the influence of a continuing push by China's medical elite to advance public health in the government ("Yuanqi" 1929), a health department was finally created in 1928, and Liu Ruiheng, president of the Peking Union Medical College, was elected as its vice director, based on the recommendation by John B. Grant. His appointment marks the end of the period when China turned to Japan to study European and American medicine. In November of that year, the Health Department published its administrative regulations, creating five departments: general affairs, medical administration, sanitation, epidemic prevention, and statistics. In December, it announced guidelines for a national system of sanitary administration and set up public health offices at the provincial level and bureaus of health at the city and county levels. These guidelines showed clear differences from the Japanese system in terms of the institutional structures to be established and their range of responsibilities. Imitating the American model, the Health

Department created a Central Board of Health, which was charged with overseeing the health care of the entire country. It also set up an International Advisory Council and invited the director of the League of Nations Health Organisation Ludwik J. Rajchmann (1881–1965), the Rockefeller Foundation's Victor G. Heiser, and Sir Arthur Newsholme, who had been chief medical officer of the United Kingdom, to serve as consultants ("Waijiaobu pinqing Laximan" 1929).

In July, Ludwik Rajchmann led a delegation from the League of Nations Health Organisation (LoNHO) to advise the Health Department ("Waijiaobu pinqing Laximan" 1929) and decided that LoNHO should collaborate with China's Health Department to address the problems of health care in China. This was to include restructuring China's seaport quarantine administration; creating mechanisms for training administrative staff for the Health Department; assisting with the establishment of central health care facilities and laboratories; setting up provincial hospitals; and establishing close collaboration with the Far Eastern Epidemics Intelligence Bureau in Singapore ("Weishengbu guwen laximan yijianshu zhaiyao" 1930). In addition, the Health Department set up a special Editorial Committee, which was in charge of translating books and articles to introduce British, German, French, and Russian health care and educational systems.

John B. Grant was clearly highly influential in the early stages of China's public health administration. In 1926, he collaborated with the Beijing Municipal Police in setting up the Beiping First Health Demonstration Station to run a pilot scheme for American-style public health services. This station functioned not only as a base for coordinating student training in fieldwork, but also as an arena for advanced training for the many health care administrators who received their training here (Jin 1985). Jin Baoshan can serve as a perfect example: after graduating from Japan's Chiba Medical School, he worked at the Beiping First Health Demonstration Station and during his time there was greatly influenced by Grant. On Grant's recommendation, he went to study in the United States and subsequently became inclined much more toward British and American health care systems. After his return to China, he assumed key posts in public health, and made frequent trips to the United States to explore the American model of health care. In 1928 he collaborated with Grant to formulate an "Outline for Metropolitan Health Care Administration and Provisional Criteria for Evaluation," which was published in 1936 by the Department of Public Health.

During this time, there were many different voices coming from all directions that suggested that China's health care policies should not blindly imitate European and American systems of health care, to avoid choosing something that did not match China's situation (Huang 1927). The government thus dispatched health care specialists to France, Germany, and Austria to investigate their health care systems (Tan 1929). In cooperation with LoNHO, it drew lessons from the health care administrations of other European countries, such as the hygiene institutes and rural health stations in Poland (Yao 1929a) and Greece's experience of progressive health care reforms in cooperation with LoNHO (Yao 1929b), and sent health department official Chen Fangzhi to Japan to investigate hygiene research structures (Chen 1929). The Central Field Health Station, created in 1932, was modeled on Yugoslavia's Zagreb Research Institute for Public Health. The Yugoslavian institute's director Berislav Borčić was invited by LoNHO to help plan and set up the Chinese institute, which was charged with establishing various mechanisms for health care–related experimentation and research and with training all sorts of skilled specialists in hygiene, health protection, and epidemic prevention (Jin 1985).

The shortage of medical specialists was the greatest impediment to medical modernization, which was rooted in the organizational disorder in medical education. Even though it had been decided in 1906 that the official medical education system should be modeled on the Japanese system, medical schools and hospitals in China were still each doing things in their own way. At the same time, neither missionary nor private medical schools were overseen by the government. In addition, German and French secular medical schools had also begun to enter the country: the German government created the Tongji German Medical College in Shanghai in 1908 and the German Medical School in Qingdao in 1911, and the French Catholic Zhendan Medical School was established in Shanghai in 1909. Each of these schools was run in accordance with the respective founding country's system of education. After the founding of the Republic of China in 1911, the new government continued as before to imitate the Japanese systems of education and health care administration. Additionally, governmental structures were changed with great frequency in the early years of the Republic, and funding for government-operated medical schools could not be guaranteed. Medical schools were divided into national-level, provincial-level, and privately run schools, each under different levels of supervision, and the Ministry of Education lacked basic powers of jurisdiction over them. As a result, regulations for schools existed in name only and even in state-run technical schools the Japanese model could not be implemented fully. Specialized medical schools hardly ever had affiliated hospitals, and entrance requirements varied greatly (China Medical Commission of the Rockefeller Foundation 1914).

Medical Schools in China during this time period can be divided into three categories: those established by missionary societies, those established by governments of or private organizations in foreign countries, and those established by the Chinese government or by private organizations in China. Instruction was given in Chinese, German, English, and Japanese, with Chinese being the most common language of instruction. Organization varied widely, with some programs lasting four years (Japan) and some five (British, French), and curricula also differed greatly (Yan 1914). Yan Fuqing suggested to the Ministry of Education and the Medical Missionary Association that cooperation between China and foreign countries was the most ideal path for developing medical education in China (Yan 1915). He also suggested that China should follow Japan's example of having two levels of medical education—medical colleges aimed at cultivating highly skilled individuals, and technical schools for training secondary-level practitioners (Yan 1914)—in order to solve China's shortage of physicians and instructors in medicine.

Beginning in the 1920s, the future of China's medical education became the issue of greatest concern for the medical elite. At the same time that they were attacking the current Japanese-style education system, they were actively promoting the English, German, French, and Russian systems of medical education.[3] Wu Lien-teh noted that the U.S. medical education system had been quite disorganized before World War I but had carried out the Flexner reforms after the war, creating uniform standards for educational institutions that allowed medicine to progress (Wu 1934). The educational administration system in the Republican period had been based purely on the U.S. model (Sun 1934). In 1929, the Ministry of Education accepted a suggestion by the League of Nations to invite a number of medical leaders from Beijing and Shanghai to form a National Medical Education Committee to discuss the establishment of a national system of medical education ("Jiaoyu bu pin ding yixue jiaoyu weiyuan" 1929). Members included Zhu Minyi (trained in France, chair of the National Health Congress), Lin Kesheng (trained in the United States, professor at Peking Union Medical College), Yu Yan (Japan), Yan Fuqing (United States, president of the National Zhongshan University Medical College), and Xu Songming (Japan, president of Beiping University Medical College). The members of this committee formulated a ten-year education program. In 1930, the Ministry of Education invited Knud Faber from Göttingen University to come to China and assist the committee in its work. After surveying the state of medical education in China, Faber concluded that it would not be appropriate to apply foreign standards to China's education and suggested a two-tiered system of education (Faber 1931). In addition, the National Health Congress invited leading medical figures and members of the Chinese Medical Association to discuss the development of medical education (Zhu 1932). In 1929, Lin Kesheng, representing the Chinese Medical Association, also proposed a two-tiered system ("Cheng Zhongyang zhixing weiyuanhui" 1929). China's medical circles unanimously approved this plan to change the original system of technical medical schools into a two-tiered system (Zhu 1932), namely, a six-year program of university medical colleges and a four-year program of technical schools. According to Yan Fuqing, chair of the National Medical Education Committee, the technical schools should coordinate with the Health Department to train medical personnel with a practical orientation and to use clinical medicine and social medicine (including public hygiene and preventive medicine) to solve the shortage of medical personnel in China (Yan 1935).

The leading forces for this second model of medical education were primarily the medical elites from the European and American factions. Where they differed from their predecessors was in their attempt to modify foreign perspectives to integrate them into China's economy, culture, and society. As a result, they opposed an all-out imitation of foreign models:

> Up until now, all the medical schools in China have continued their old practices as before. Among them, a great number have directly copied foreign countries, without paying any attention at all to China's society and economic environment, as well as to the particular needs of different human beings. (Yan 1935)

Foreign models had therefore to be adapted to China's national circumstances in terms of knowledge as well as professional work. In 1935, the Ministry of Education promulgated a provisional schedule of classes for university medical colleges and courses in medicine. But this curriculum was criticized by another faction of scholars, who argued that it plagiarized the course structure of the Peking Union Medical College and emphasized pragmatism over theory, replacing education in hygiene with public health and neglecting "the entire field of hygiene studies." Claiming that it was not necessary to adopt PUMC's practice of establishing tropical medicine and parasitology as independent programs ("Xijing yishi gonghui" 1935), the critics charged that "it was by no means a perfect curriculum," since American medicine was not as advanced as German medicine and many of the American textbooks had been translated from German to begin with. These critics therefore suggested that China should consult German, Austrian, Swiss, Dutch, Danish, Japanese, and other curricula before reformulating its own (Li 1935). They even went so far as to say that emulating the United States would prevent China from training and cultivating its own outstanding physicians since the emphasis on clinical instruction would result only in the creation of assistants who had to rely on supervision by foreign staff. Since this system would not be able to create leaders in medicine, it was "not suited to the modern condition of China" (Li 1935). In the end, however, the PUMC-inspired curriculum was adopted in the form of a statute after slight revisions.[4] In 1936, Yan Fuqing, the chair of the National Medical Education Committee, introduced the ordinance at a plenary meeting of the Chinese Medical Association. In his eyes, the government had taken a giant step toward the unification of the education system. At the same time, he also expressed his gratitude to the missionary schools for their active cooperation (Yan 1935), which allowed China's medical education to forge ahead toward modernization.

Medical Models and Medical Factions

Up until 1936, both the medical education system and the health care administration system had clearly emerged on the basis of lessons learned from the experi-

Table 9.1. Structure of the German-Japanese medical faction in Republican China

Language	Representative schools	Representative figures	Organizations and media
German, Japanese	Shanghai Tongde Medical School National Beiping Technical Medical School Nanman Medical University Shanghai Tongji Medical University	Tang Erhe Zhu Minyi Hu Tingan Hou Ximin Chen Fangzhi	Chinese Pharmaceutical Society Republic of China's Society of Pharmacology *Zhonghua minguo yiyaoxue huibao* (Report on pharmacology in the Republic of China) *Tongji yixue yuekan* (Tongji medical monthly) *Tongren yuekan* (Tongren monthly)

ences of foreign countries, but they also established native Chinese institutions and methods, including conducting instruction in Chinese. Nevertheless, the divergence of medical factions that had arisen due to differences in educational backgrounds continued to be present and they consistently affected or even constrained the progress of modernizing medicine in China. This situation constitutes an important special characteristic of China's path to medical modernization. Medical circles in China were directly divided into a German-Japanese current, a British-American current, and a French-Belgian current, demarcated by language and each forming its particular and distinct pedagogical methods, academic specialties, and ideas about health care administration. Each current had famous physicians to serve as its representatives, created academic organizations, and possessed academic periodicals and representative medical schools, where each produced individual lines of transmission in Western medicine.

The German-Japanese current was made up of two groups, namely, Chinese students who had studied in Japan or had graduated from Japanese-style medical schools, and students who had studied at German medical schools in China or who had gone to Germany for their studies and returned to China (see table 9.1). Japan's medicine had originated from German medicine, and China's Japanese-style medical schools also venerated German medicine and universally chose the German system of education and German-language instruction. Furthermore, some of the students who had studied in Japan went to Germany for advanced studies after graduating in Japan. The academic system followed by the German-

Table 9.2. Organization of the Anglo-American medical faction in Republican China

Language	Representative schools	Representative figures	Organizations and media
English	Shanghai St. John's Medical College Hunan Xiangya Medical College Peking Union Medical College National Shanghai Medical College	Liu Ruiheng Yan Fuqing Lin Kesheng Jin Baoshan	China Medical Association China Medical Missionary Association *Zhonghua yixue zazhi* (China medical journal)

Japanese current was therefore German medicine. National Beiping Medical University and the South Manchurian (Nanman) Medical University were two schools that were able to compete with the British-American current, and Knud Faber estimated on the basis of a survey that Nanman Medical University had attained an academic level that was on par with Japan's Imperial Universities (Faber 1931).

There are two other points worth noting. First, a highly influential periodical of Japanese-style medicine circulated in China, called *Tongren yixue* 同仁醫學, which had been created in Tokyo by the Association of Chinese Medical Students in Japan, who supplied manuscripts to introduce the newest medical research results from Japan to China. Second, Yu Yunxiu, who had studied in Japan, took it upon himself after his return to China to criticize traditional Chinese medicine. Learning from Japan's experience with its governmental policies for handling Chinese medicine there, he started a movement in China to abolish traditional Chinese medicine and to lead China's traditional medicine onto a path of "medical revolution."

In fact, though, the earliest group officially dispatched by the Chinese government to study abroad was sent to the United States. Between 1872 and 1875, four groups of youth were sent there, of whom three students ended up becoming physicians (Gao 1982). Nevertheless, the first representatives of the Anglo-American faction were trained in missionary schools in China, and it was only after the founding of the Republic that the dominant force in the British and U.S. current was made up of students who had studied in England or the United States and had returned to China (see table 9.2). In 1921, the Rockefeller Foundation invested a huge amount of money to establish the Peking Union Medical College on the model of Johns Hopkins University, which became the most magnificent medical college in China, the most advanced in terms of facilities, the most abundantly funded, and the strongest in terms of faculty qualifications. Representing the standard of American-style medicine, not a single medical college in China was able to compare with it.

Speaking strictly in terms of numbers, the number of students who studied in England and the United States was far lower than the number who went to Japan. As the statistics of the China Medical Association from 1915 demonstrate, among Chinese doctors of Western medicine, sixteen had degrees from the United States, seven had degrees from England, and four hundred had degrees from Japan (Greene 1918). Nevertheless, a closer look at the schools that the members of the two factions attended reveals that those who went to Japan mostly chose mid-level technical schools and that there were very few students who graduated from Tokyo Imperial University or Kyoto Imperial University (China Medical Commission of the Rockefeller Foundation 1914, 8). In contrast, students who returned from England or the United States all came from schools such as Yale, Harvard, or Edinburgh University. In 1925, Hu Xiansu, who had received a PhD from Harvard University and was a professor in the Department of Biology at China's National Dongnan University, estimated that those who had studied in Japan were the most active in revising laws and organizing the military, while many also focused their energy on political revolution. The greatest shortcoming for students returning from Japan was "the fact that they were not patient enough to continue studying and graduate from advanced-level schools in Japan and engage in graduate-level studies at the Imperial Universities" (Hu 1925). According to national statistics of graduating universities for physicians from 1929 to 1932, among 186 graduates from Japanese schools, 71 (about 40 percent) had come from medical technical schools, while only 10 had graduated from the departments of medicine at the Imperial Universities. Graduates from American schools, on the other hand, generally came from Harvard, Pennsylvania State University, and Johns Hopkins University, and among those who had studied in England, more than half were graduates from Cambridge (Xu 1933). The medical world in China at that time thus judged students who had studied in Japan as lacking specialized knowledge and appraised Japanese-style physicians as being less qualified ("Zhongguo de yixue jiaoyu" 1933, 205). In an analysis of the educational and study-abroad history of China, it is true that the number of students who went to Japan was far greater than those who went to Europe or the United States, but numbers are only one superficial criterion, and the quality of their studies and the level of education they received are also an important basis for evaluation.

The influence of the French and Belgian faction was the weakest, dominated by students who had studied in France and by graduates of the Shanghai Zhendan University Medical College. This group lacked an organizational structure, but Zhendan University began publishing the *Zhendan Daxue yike zazhi* (Zhendan University journal of medicine) in 1929 and produced a total of fourteen volumes plus four additional issues. The most prominent representative of this faction was Song Guobin, a graduate of Zhendan University's Department of Medicine. He served as editor-in-chief of *Yiyao pinglun* (Medical critic), an important medical periodical during the Republican period. In its pages, he introduced Louis Pasteur's scientific achievements and published constructive and influential articles concerning the establishment of medical education and health care management in Republican China. Song Guobin warned the physicians in the French and Belgian faction against getting bogged down in the struggle between the different factions, believing that "if we speak of factions in accordance with scholarship, we can receive the benefit of group discussions, but if we leave scholarship out when we speak of factions, it is nothing but a fight over privilege and power" (Song 1935).

In reality, the lines of demarcation between the scholarly factions were not clearly distinguished, especially since there were times when people could switch sides. Jin Baoshan, for example, switched from the Japanese current to the British-American current, and the Guangdong National Zhongshan University Medical College was transformed as a result of the restructuring of the school administration from a school of the British-American faction to a German-system institution (Huang 1988). Moreover, the differences among these three academic factions in terms of scientific knowledge were not that great after all. For example, in regard to education, each faction emphasized the need to learn from other educational models in the world, including the Soviet model, in order to create a unified national education system. And even though the 1935 curriculum had been created on the basis of the PUMC model, its critics focused on minor details such as the fact that parasitology should not be a separate course of study and that it was inappropriate to replace "hygiene studies" (*weisheng xue*) with "public health" (*gonggong weisheng*). Confronted with the criticism that the new curriculum was emphasizing clinical training at the expense of theoretical research, Di Ruide from PUMC composed an article emphasizing that his school had done an excellent job at integrating theory and practice (Di 1934).

At its root, the dispute among the academic factions was a struggle over political power, the explanation for which can be found in China's long and drawn-out history and tradition. The dominant scholarship in China had always been determined by the rulers in the government or chosen in accordance with the rulers' preferences. Even in the twentieth century, scholars who had received a full-fledged Westernized education still understood this truth about China, namely, that the selection and final decision regarding a model of medicine was intimately connected to the personal inclinations of political leaders. As Jin Baoshan, the director of the original Bureau of Sanitation, pointed out in his memoir, the backer of the Anglo-American faction was Chiang Kai-shek, while the backer of the German-Japanese faction was the "CC Clique," led by Chen Lifu and Chen Guofu (Jin 1985). In the initial stages of constructing the Ministry of Health, John

Grant used the resources provided by the League of Nations to help support Chiang Kai-shek. The resulting Central Field Experimentation Station and Central Hospital that he established were intended to train medical cadres and to organize local health care institutions. The personnel for both research and clinical work all came from PUMC. This situation was critized by the German-Japanese faction, which claimed that this sort of cooperation amounted to an American colonization of medicine in China (*Shidai gongbao* 1933). Especially after 1945, Chiang Kai-shek's government was completely inclined toward the United States, and the provision of staff to the Health Department was dominated by Western medicine of the pro-U.S. faction, which became one aspect of China's pro-U.S. policies (Jin 1985). The goal of the dispute among the academic factions thus was a struggle over the discourse of health care and over the country's health care–related resources. This fact was well understood by the medical circles in the Republican period. It was also the reason why every faction emphasized the need for unity and cooperation in the effort to establish the ideal unified system of medical education. But conflict among the factions persisted nonetheless, both beneath the surface and in the open.

> The source of medical factionalism in today's China, in my view, does not come from socially minded physicians but from medical functionaries in the government. I see their primary characteristics as careerist ambition rather than personal sacrifice in the interest of justice and truth. Therefore, we must unanimously and sincerely devote ourselves and quickly resolving these disputes. Our principal aims should be to eliminate factionalism and prejudice, thereby creating a harmoniously scientific nation. It is our responsibility to use our knowledge to promote the advance of medicine and pharmaceutics in China. In that case, there can be a glimmer of hope for the future of medicine, instead of this never-ending strife between different political currents. (Hu 1934)

If we examine these developments chronologically, we see that the period of innovation during the late Qing from 1904 to 1911 and of the Beiyang government from 1911 to 1927 is characterized by the dominance of the Japanese model of medicine. During the period from 1927 to 1949, by contrast, the British-American model of medicine was dominant, while the medical models from other European countries provided auxiliary input. So we can say that this was the period of pluralism in medical models. The special characteristics of these historical stages can be illustrated even more clearly by the choice of health department leaders by the Republican government (see table 9.3).

Between 1928 and 1949, most leaders of the central government's health department came from the British-American system, while mid-level administrators were for the most part people who had studied in Japan, and local healthcare offices were staffed mostly by people who had studied in Germany. For example,

Table 9.3. Training and national allegiance of government heads of medical departments during the Republic of China, 1912–1948

Period	Director of the Health Department or Ministry	Academic Faction
1912–1928	Wu Sheng (June 1912–1917)	Studied abroad in Japan
	Liu Daoren (1917–1920)	Studied abroad in Japan
	Wang Xi (1920–1924)	Not a medical professional
	Ren Huanli (1924–1926)	Not a medical professional
	Lin Yanjing (1927–1928)	Studied abroad in Japan
1928–1948	Chen Fangzhi (1928)	Studied abroad in Japan
	Xue Dubi (1928)	
	Liu Ruiheng (1928–1938)	Studied abroad in Japan
	Yan Fuqing (1938–1940)	Studied abroad in Japan
	Jin Baoshan (1940–1947)	Studied abroad in Japan
	Zhou Yichun (1947–1948)	Graduated from missionary medical school
	Lin Kesheng (1948)	Studied abroad in Japan

the director of the Nanjing health office, Hu Dingan, and the director of the Shanghai health office, Yu Yunsong, both belonged to the German faction, and the person in charge of the Shanghai Physicians' Association was Song Guobin, a representative of the French faction. This kind of pattern explains why no single foreign model was able to completely dominate. It is noteworthy that during the time when they were borrowing directly from Europe, Chinese physicians of all persuasions were agreed that they should also consult with Japan regarding its experience with European models. And during the time when American-style medicine served as the dominant model in China's medical education, both the general population and the academics in China continued to believe that German medicine was the most advanced medicine in the world and that German physicians were the most brilliant practitioners and the most admired physicians (Jin 1985).

Clearly none of the academic currents managed to establish itself as the absolute authority. The influence of each current served to balance the influence of the others, preventing any one faction from imposing a single model for the development of medicine, pharmaceutics, and health care in China. This multiplicity created a multidimensional space for China to create its own model of medicine and science.

This multifaceted prospect was destroyed by the Soviet model, expressed in the slogan "Take the Soviet Union as our teacher," after 1949. For a relatively long timespan afterward, medicine in China followed only a single model,

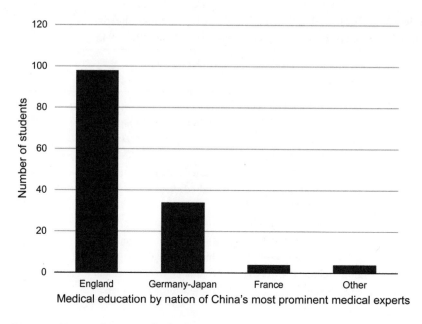

Figure 9.1. Training locations of China's most celebrated medical scientists. *Source:* Cui and Wei (1987).

namely the Soviet-style, or socialist, path of medicine. Nevertheless, the book *Zhongguo dangdai xixuejia huicui* (Biographies of contemporary China's most distinguished medical experts), published in 1987, provides information regarding the medical models from the West that socialist China ultimately approved. Compiled under the leadership of Cui Yueli, the director of China's Ministry of Health, it records the 140 people the editors believed to have made the greatest contributions to medicine in China, including medical scientists, specialists in clinical and preventive medicine, and specialists in pharmaceutics. In this list, ninety-eight are associated with the British-American system, twenty-one with the German system (also including Austria), thirteen with the Japanese system, and five with the French (including one Vietnamese). In addition, there is one person from the Soviet academic current, one who was trained after 1949, and one who was not associated with a medical college (see figure 9.1).

These famous medical figures had the following study-abroad experiences: thirty people in the United States, four in England, two in Canada, fifteen in Germany, two in Austria, six in Japan, two in France, one in Vietnam, and one in the Soviet Union. For more details, see figure 9.2.

Evidently, the Anglo-American system was still emphasized after 1949 and its graduates were given creative opportunities to serve the new state. At the same time, within the German-Japanese current, the number of students who studied

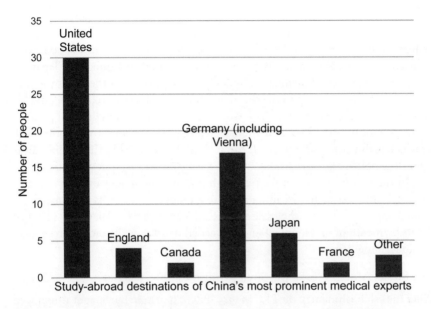

Figure 9.2. Study-abroad destinations of China's most celebrated medical scientists. *Source:* Cui and Wei (1987).

in Germany was far higher than that of students in the Japanese system, which once again proves that the quality and quantity of students who went to study in Japan was not on par with the German contingent. By examining this kind of statistical data we can see past the rhetoric and discover that in the end, the personal preferences of those in power could not defeat the basic patterns of scientific progress, and the changes in national politics could not interrupt the long process of continuous development that had been necessary for the creation of a medical system adapted to China.

Summary of the Influence of Foreign Medical Models during the Republican Era

In the twentieth century, the United States and each of the countries in Europe made significant contributions to the development of modern medicine in the areas of medical education, scientific research, and health care administration. Because the developments in medicine that the Chinese people were exposed to took place in so many different areas in the various foreign countries, it was not an easy task to choose the perfect model to adapt to the Chinese experience. In the end, numerous foreign medical models and styles coexisted in space and time, namely the Anglo-American current, the German-Japanese current, and the French-Belgian current, as well as the Soviet current from the 1950s on. Experiences from all of these models were applied at one point or another in the history of the development of contemporary medicine in China, even to the point of being used as templates. The Chinese government turned readily to standards of health and hygiene in the Western countries to allow China, like Japan, to join the ranks of world medicine as quickly as possible. Nevertheless, it was also forced to squarely face up to the social, economic, and health-related conditions in China, and therefore chose its lessons selectively. Harmonizing the political and academic benefits of each method, it created a certain compromise, the result of which is difficult to formulate. It can perhaps be described as a tendency away from "the politicization of health care" toward "the sanitization of politics."

In the first fifty years of the twentieth century, the modernization of medicine in China was begun by imitating foreign models, but in its response to repeated opposition to the wholesale application of any one model, China searched for its own path of development and succeeded in creating its own native model of modern medicine.

The Soviet Model: "Take the Soviet Union as Our Teacher"

After the establishment of the PRC in 1949, PRC Chairman Liu Shaoqi announced the slogan "Take the Soviet Union as our teacher" in October of 1949, ushering in the official state strategy of the new government. This section will explore the effects of this strategy on medical development in New China. We will consider two aspects: (1) the impact of medical technical specialists from the USSR, and (2) how the Chinese medical profession responded to the new methods and technologies introduced from the Soviet Union.

The relationship between the Soviet Union and China was not limited to the Communist Party. Even prior to 1949, China's Nationalist Party (GMD) invited a delegation of Soviet military experts to China. Between May and June of 1938, the first group of Soviet military advisors arrived in China, initially consisting of twenty-seven members but increasing in October 1939 to eighty members. These advisors were distributed throughout the entire military and related organizations and included two medical specialists, including the chief advisor of the department of military medicine. By 1942, when the Soviet Union withdrew its military personnel from China, the number of military advisors in China exceeded three hundred, in addition to two hundred technological advisors, and included medical specialists (Shen 2003, 22).

At the academic level, interest in Soviet medicine was already evident in China in the 1930s, when China's medical association introduced the Soviet model of public health ("Sulian gonggong weisheng" 1934) and Gu Yunyu (1936) published an article titled "Soviet Women's and Infants' Health." Within Chinese medical and intellectual circles, interest in the Soviet model of medicine arose on the eve of the conclusion of the Sino-Japanese War in Chongqing. Around 1944, when World War II was coming to an end, GMD health officials and the medical elite in the Chongqing area began to plan the rebuilding of China's medical system. Discussion focused on two questions: How would the government assume responsibility for providing health care for the entire population? And what were the methods by which to provide it? After studying and comparing the health care systems of Europe, the United States, and the Soviet Union, scholars concluded that the free public health care system of the Soviet Union was the ideal model and suggested that the Chinese government adopt the Soviet health care model (Zheng 1944).

The collaboration between the Chinese Communist Party and Soviet medicine started at roughly the same time as the beginning of Nationalist control. In 1941, the underground Chinese Communist Party and its Soviet comrades cooperated in Shanghai to establish the Soviet Union Times Press, which introduced Soviet literature and delivered news about the Red Army's defense of the homeland during World War II. In addition, the Times Press published the journal *Soviet Medicine,* producing ten volumes between 1945 and 1954. This journal introduced Soviet medical research, public health management and medical education, and the newest Soviet medical achievements, with an emphasis on the introduction of Pavlov's research (Min 1986).

In 1948, a book series on Soviet medicine was published that included the titles *Soviet Medical Education,* by Li Zhiyi (1948), and *Health Care of the Soviet Union* (1949) and *Workers' Health Care in the Soviet Union* (1949), both by Zhu Binsheng. Zhu was the primary author and translator of the series, and between 1949 and 1952 he translated and published a total of twenty-two Russian books on medicine. He was the key person to introduce Pavlov's theories, his study of histology, and the Pavlovian technique of "painless childbirth" to China (see chapter 3 in this volume).

Beginning in the 1930s, the American medical historian Henry Sigerist developed an interest in Soviet medicine, taught himself Russian, and researched the nation's medicine, history, society, and economy. In 1935, 1936, and 1937, he made three trips to the Soviet Union to observe medical and health care work, and subsequently published *Socialized Medicine in the Soviet Union* in 1937. In it, he described the development of Soviet medicine from a medical-history and social perspective, reporting how the Soviet Union was able to protect the health of its population and firmly establish a socialist medical system (Gong 1950). During World War II, the Soviet Red Army made an impressive show of resistance to the Germans on the Northern Front, in which the contribution of the Soviet medical corps elicited great interest from the other Allies, including the United States. This event caused a change in European and American attitudes toward Soviet medicine, and several of those nations sent medical delegations to the Soviet Union expressly to observe medical education.

As a result of this interest, Sigerist added new information to his book and republished it in 1947. This edition was translated into Chinese in 1950 by Gong

Naiquan, vice minister of the Department of Health in the East China military administration and director of the Shanghai Medical School. As Gong pointed out, "From reading this book we can learn how a leading authority in medical history from a capitalist country evaluates Soviet medicine on the basis of extensive research on medicine, both from a longitudinal and latitudinal perspective" (Gong 1950). In his book, Sigerist paid close attention to the organizational structures of Soviet medicine, the structures of public health administration, the budgetary structures of national health care, the new organization of medical education, and the administrative systems of medical centers in industrial and urban medical areas. Soviet medical circles responded quickly to this European and American interest: the head of the national Soviet medical administration, A. N. Shabanov, published a book titled *Soviet Medical Education* in 1948, which was also translated by the Times Press into Chinese.

On October 8, 1949, Liu Shaoqi issued the following statement to the China-Soviet Friendship Association: "In the past, the revolution of the Chinese People has taken Russia as its teacher. From the present on, as we build our country, we will likewise take Russia as our teacher, studying economics and education from the Soviet Union." The Eleventh Congress of the State Administrative Council decided in December 1949 to establish a People's University of China in order to respond to the needs of state building and to incrementally and strategically train cadres for the task of constructing the new state by accepting the advanced experience of the Soviet Union and inviting Soviet professors. In 1950, a People's Health Book Series was launched during the first nationwide conference on health care. In this series, specialized pamphlets were published that introduced the Soviet methods of setting up health care and Soviet health care work, such as *Thirty Years of Soviet Health Care* and *Protection of Women and Infants in the Soviet Union.*

Soviet Medical Ethics as the Basis of "Medicine in the Service of the People"

The rationale behind Minister of Health Li Dequan's 1950 promotion of the study of Soviet medical achievements was quite simple:

> Because the USSR is a socialist country, its superiority is not restricted to the fields of politics, economics, and social welfare. Additionally, its health administration and medical sciences are equally advanced. The entire Soviet health administration is designed around the needs of the people. Therefore, following the Soviet Union in health care is much better than following the medical models of capitalist countries, because it is much more appropriate to the conditions in China. (Li 1950)

In fact it was not the Soviets who introduced the idea of the primacy of "the people" in the design of medical administration; already in the 1920s, Chinese medical elites were actively debating the proper aims of a national medical system. By 1930, the consideration that 85 percent of China's population were rural peasants had led the Nationalist Health Administration to endorse state medicine in order to better serve them. Many medical professionals also supported the idea of a state medicine, because such a medical service, funded entirely by the government, would allow them to devote their energies to providing health care to China's most needy population. However, by the time of the Sino-Japanese War, this plan had only been implemented in a few rural demonstration stations (Gao 2012).

During the first meeting of the new National Health Administration in 1950, Director of the Chinese Academy of Sciences Guo Moruo explained that "the USSR already has a well-developed system of state medicine, which we have yet to realize. This is a goal that we must diligently pursue" (Guo 1950). Because of the preexisting commitment of many Nationalist physicians to state medicine, this turn toward Soviet medical policies was able to satisfy both former Nationalist and Communist medical sympathizers. "Medicine in the service of the people" became a unifying ideology. As explained in the popular magazine *Sino-Soviet Friendship* in June 1952, "The benefits of the welfare system enjoyed by Soviet workers are much better than those available to workers in capitalist countries; the Soviet welfare system is fair, perfect, and free of charge" (Ge 1952). Because the Soviet health care system emphasized the ethic of "serving the people" and provided an example for the realization of a state medical system, it was able to win the support and trust of even the former Nationalist physicians in the new People's Republic, who now actively studied it.

The new government also carried out many new measures in the name of "serving the people." Beginning in 1953, state employees received free health care. Following the precedent of the Soviet Union, by October 1957, the Chinese government had established more than six hundred specialty clinics for various epidemic diseases (such as tuberculosis, schistosomiasis, and STDs) and 1,500 epidemic prevention stations. In order to improve the health conditions of industrial workers, the government also set up a system of factory doctors similar to that found in the Soviet Union. The socialist design principles applied to the construction of new urban areas and factories also included health and sanitation planning for the workers. Additionally, the state renewed its focus on maternal and child health, succeeding in reducing infant and maternal mortality rates. In the minority areas of China, by 1954 the government claimed that it had established 350 new sanitation stations and over thirty hospitals, with two thousand health officials trained from among the minority population (Fu 1954). All of these initiatives helped the Communist government promote its image as the protector of the health and sanitation of society, and were instrumental in increasing the government's credibility among health professionals.

As we have seen, in the early years of the People's Republic the slogan "serve the people" was a way to unite health personnel from different political backgrounds around their shared aspirations. In 1953, however, the tone and meanings of the slogan changed. The 1953 Third Congress of the National Health Administration decreed that the political leadership must strengthen its ideological unity and centralization by increasing its standard of study and its implementation of Marxism and Leninism. As a result, the meaning of "serve the people" began to refer primarily to the political agenda, and became a code for separating "old" from "new" thought among health care professionals, as well as a standard by which to judge their patriotism.

In 1957, Deputy Health Minister Fu Lianzhang, in the wake of the "Hundred Flowers Movement" of 1956, felt the need to publish an article in the *People's Daily* titled "We Must Unswervingly Continue to Study Advanced Soviet Medicine." The "Advanced" in this title referred to

> a wholehearted commitment to the spirit of "serve the people." This is the starting point of our entire mission as socialist nations. Because all Soviet health care workers have this spirit, they take the people's suffering as their own suffering, the people's happiness as their own happiness, and with a spirit of self-sacrifice, they overcome all difficulties, pay attention to every detail, [and] strive to do their best to constantly promote the advancement of medicine in order to achieve the best possible preventive, clinical, educational and research medical work. (Fu 1957)

The Influence of Soviet Technical Specialists

By 1947, the Soviet Union had already begun to give formal support and aid to the Communist Party in Northeast China; between 1947 and 1949, the Soviet Red Cross and Red Crescent Societies responded to invitations from China and dispatched yearly epidemic prevention teams to the region to aid in the implementation of plague prevention and treatment. These teams, consisting of technical specialists, disinfection personnel, and nurses, carried with them large amounts of medicines, uniforms, laboratory instruments, hospital equipment, and bedding and clothing for patients. The 1949 outbreak of the bubonic plague in Chabei was swiftly extinguished with the direct assistance from the Soviet team. These Soviet teams trained large numbers of medical workers in the new scientific methods of epidemic prevention in Northeast China.

Reliable statistics concerning the numbers of Soviet technical specialists who came to work in China between 1947 and 1960 are not available. But it is undeniable that Soviet specialists had significant influence on three aspects of medicine in China: the design of Chinese health administrative systems, the organization of clinical care, and medical education.

The first Soviet health consultant was Dr. F. S. Bykov, who was invited by the Ministry of Health in January 1951. He introduced the principles of socialist medical education, the history and development of the Soviet health care system, and the organization of health services administration in the USSR, and instructed ministry officials in the design of socialist work plans (Fu 1957). In 1952, Soviet specialists assisted the ministry in running training courses in anti-tuberculosis measures in industrial settings (Wang 1952). In 1956, the Soviet technical team took part in the Chinese government's influential twelve-year planning meeting for the development of medicine, science, and technology, delivering reports on industrial health, sanitary inspection, and urban preventive networks, including detailed plans to address the endemic problems of malaria and schistosomiasis (Li 1957b; Xin 2002; also see chapter 6 in this volume).

The greatest contribution of the Soviet advisors in this period was to give the CCP officials in charge of medical education and administration the credibility as socialist leaders to win over the medical profession. At this early juncture, the many students who had been sent to the Soviet Union to study medicine had not yet returned, and the existing medical professionals had initially been reluctant to accept orders from CCP officials.

For example, in 1952, Tikhon E. Boldyrev (波尔德列夫, 1900–1984), leader of the Soviet advisory team, persuaded the party to set up a training course called "Principles of Socialist Health Administration" for high-level officials, which he also taught. He emphasized the leadership and supportive functions of health officials, thereby elevating the status of health administrators in medical decision-making processes: "For medical professionals to succeed in their work, and to solve various medical work-related issues, it is necessary . . . to have correct leadership. The duty of health leaders is to rely on the specially designed national framework proceeding from the Health Ministry though its provincial, city, county, and district offices" (Boerdeliefu 1959, 2).

For Boldyrev, "correct leadership" referred to Communist Party leadership. He designed a set of principles and methodology for party health officials to use. The most important of these principles was "collective leadership." In that era of following the "Soviet elder brother," Boldyrev's classes were influential in giving party leaders the confidence to force through the party's health care restructuring (Li 1957b).

Perhaps the most concrete manifestation of Sino-Soviet collaboration in medicine was the construction in 1952 of the Beijing Soviet Red Cross Hospital, which was designed and entirely funded by the Soviet Union as a model institution. Within five years, there were 126 Soviet doctors working in this hospital, who treated several hundred thousand Chinese patients in collaboration with Chinese doctors. But if we are objective in our evaluation of this model of "advanced scientific medicine," we must find it lacking. The main therapies in use were "laser therapy, mudbath therapy, hydrotherapy, wax therapy, and physical therapy," which were hardly the cutting-edge scientific therapies of the time

("Wei Zhongguo renmin" 1954). Even according to the Soviet ambassador to China, "The professional qualifications of medical personnel sent to China were not high, there were no doctors of professorial rank, [and] often our Chinese colleagues had higher professional qualifications" (Shen 2003, 198). Even more telling was the fact that the Beijing Soviet Red Cross Hospital only allowed access by people with special connections, by virtue of either their high rank or personal relationships. Ironically, therefore, it was precisely this hospital, touted as a model of "serve the people," that pioneered the institutionalization of privilege in medical care ("Wei Zhongguo renmin" 1954).

Soviet Medical Education to Achieve Centralized Administrative Authority

In the area of medicine, the study of the Soviet Union began with a major restructuring of colleges and academic departments. Prior to 1949, two different systems of medical education existed in China: those left behind by the Republican government and the systems of medical education in the newly liberated areas. The former consisted of both public and private, and Christian and non-Christian, medical schools. Because the Republican government had lacked the ability for systematic and forceful supervision, existing medical schools followed a large variety of models of education, including American and English, German and Japanese, and French. They had neither unified textbooks nor curricula, and their training programs varied in length. In the 1930s, the China Medical Association and the Ministry of Education cooperated in an attempt to establish standards of education for medical schools, which ultimately failed to succeed. The wartime conditions in the liberated areas, on the other hand, caused medical schools there to emphasize the training of medical and health care workers needed for combat and therefore did not give rise to any systematic educational schemes.

For the new government, "taking Russia as our teacher" was a sound strategy when considering how to manage and standardize the disorganized and chaotic medical schools that varied so widely across China. As Republican health care officials and medical educators had already learned, medical treatment and education in the Soviet Union differed substantially from practices in Europe and the United States. Soviet universities were state owned (Zheng 1944), and the higher education system was characterized by a strict division into specialties, each of which was under the dual control of its respective department and the Ministry of Education. Beginning in the 1930s, independent medical colleges and departments had been established, under the authority of the People's Health Care Association, and unified curriculum plans and teaching programs had been implemented all over the Soviet Union. The new Communist government in China wished to implement a similarly comprehensive overhaul of the education system that would replace the European and U.S. models with the Soviet model and construct a new Communist education system.

The Soviet medical specialist F. S. Bykov, who arrived in China in January 1951, was of tremendous service to Chinese health care officials in establishing a system of medical education and introducing the new medical institutions, educational structures, and methods of instruction from the Soviet Union. With his assistance, the National Ministry of Health organized medical schools into nine departments (internal medicine, external medicine, pediatrics, gynecology and obstetrics, public health, dentistry, ophthalmology, dermatology, and ENT) and established unified instructional programs for medical schools, nursing schools, and midwifery schools (Min 1952). In 1952, the PRC government implemented a restructuring of forty-four medical colleges by taking them out of the comprehensive university system and turning them into independent colleges under the dual authority of the Ministries of Health and Education, creating a genuine structure of centralized authority in medical education.

The first national conference on medical education in 1954 determined that medical education should adopt the key policies of the Soviet Union and carry out reforms in the areas of educational institutions, content, methods, and structures. The length of professional training was shortened and medical specialization was restructured into four major areas (medical therapy, health care, pediatrics, and dentistry) to be mastered in five-year programs, while pharmaceutics became a four-year program with the addition of two years of specialized training. In 1953, the Ministry of Health issued a notification calling for the use of Soviet teaching materials. As a result, a total of fifty-two Soviet texts were published in translation in 1954–1955, which were used mainly in medical colleges in Manchuria and North China. After the texts were in use for two or three years, it was realized that these Soviet-based learning materials, while extensive in quantity, were inadequate in terms of content to meet China's specific needs and also suffered from low-quality translations that caused a number of difficulties in their application. In 1956, Chinese scholars began to publish their own teaching materials in the various specialties and instituted unified curricula for each specialty. At that time, eighty-four subjects were established for advanced medical education and forty-nine subjects for secondary education (Zhu and Zhang 1990, 14). To improve the study of the Soviet experience, the vast majority of schools dropped English-language courses and established Russian as a required course. Nationally, thirty-four upper-level medical schools set up accelerated educational programs for specialized reading in Russian.

The Third Congress of the National Health Administration explicitly proposed educational reform based on the Soviet model by calling on each medical college and school to reorganize medical education on the basis of teaching and research teams. In so doing, the Congress decided that "overly departmentalized colleges should study the Soviet experience with departmentalization in medical education and carry out progressive reforms in accordance with their particular circumstances" ("Di san jie quanguo" 1954). The newly instituted plan for education comprehensively implemented the following four principles of Soviet education: integration of technical training and education in political ideology, the integration of theory and practice, the integration of basic knowledge and specialized training, and the integration of guidance by teachers and self-study by students. In regard to educational methodology, it advocated the study of the text *Pedagogy*, by the Soviet writer I. A. Kairov (1893–1978), to emphasize the transmission of knowledge, improve the outcome of classroom instruction, and stress the role of teachers as guides. Valuing the transmission of knowledge at the expense of intellectual capability, this approach was based on the maxim of "application molds expertise" as the focus of specialization. In addition to higher education, "special training courses" were established, and practical training was extended in length while the duration of formal schooling was changed to three years. Students were recruited as on-the-job health care cadres to be trained as doctors in internal medicine, external medicine, pediatrics, and gynecology and obstetrics. In terms of scholarship, the study of Pavlov's teachings was emphasized, with his medical ideas used as guidelines and his theories applied to transform contemporary medicine.

The system of higher education in the Soviet Union was marked by the fact that it had established a curriculum in politics, assembling and disseminating a system of courses in ideology that consisted of a combination of required and elective courses. In China, college-level literature and law schools in the northern region stipulated from 1949 on that students in literature, law, and education programs had to attend required courses in "dialectical materialism" and "historical materialism." This requirement was progressively extended to cover the range of colleges and universities all over the country. On October 7, 1952, the Ministry of Education issued the "Directive for Courses on Marxism-Leninism and Mao Zedong Thought," which stipulated, "Beginning in 1952, all general studies universities as well as colleges for economics and finance and for fine arts must set up a three-year sequence of three courses with a total of a hundred study hours for each year in the 'Theory of New Democracy.'" In 1953, the Ministry of Higher Education again issued a mandate that all schools of higher education without exception begin offering a course called "The Foundations of Marxism and Leninism," with a total of 136 study hours. Up to this point, the initial establishment of a system of courses in ideological and political education in Chinese universities basically followed the Soviet model of a top-down, centralized, unified, and integrated curriculum.

Following the Soviet model in medical education specifically entailed four important special characteristics. The first was the strengthening of political and ideological work. For faculty and administrative cadres, this involved advancing the study of political theory and policies; for students, it meant the inclusion of the fundamentals of Marxism and Leninism as a subject for examination. The second characteristic was an emphasis on practical application in the disciplines to mold human resources, increasing the proportion of specialized courses, and making the number of applied study hours more than half of the total number of academic study hours. The third was the systematic study of Pavlovian theory, to improve the quality of education and explain Pavlovian theory as the standard of all scholarship in the classroom. And fourth was an emphasis on education and research in preventive medicine.

Studying the Advancements in Soviet Medicine:
A Focus on Pavlovian Theory

In the initial years after the founding of the People's Republic of China, the new government's promotion of the Soviet model required not just political might but also a rational explanation. To encourage the medical elite that had remained on the mainland to accept this approach, the assistant director of the Ministry of Health, Fu Lianzhang, published an article in 1952 titled "Studying the Advances in Soviet Medicine." In this article, he put forward that "Soviet medicine is the most advanced medical science in the world" (Fu 1952), and further pointed out that it utilized the scientific method of dialectical materialism and had been developed in integration with the needs of the people. The advancements in Soviet medicine had been first manifested in the theories of Ivan Pavlov, the prominent representative of this advanced Soviet medicine whose brilliant theory of neural activity had proven pathbreaking in the field of medicine (Fu 1952).

In 1943, the Chongqing China-Soviet Friendship Association published *A Commemorative Collection of Pavlov's Works*. In 1948, the biography *Pavlov* was published in Shanghai, translated by Zhu Binsheng. The Times Press published *Pavlov's Centenary* in 1949. By 1953, it was commonplace within medical circles all over the country to study Pavlov's theories, and every medical journal and publisher was introducing and publishing numerous Soviet medical writings. According to statistics gathered by the library of Fudan University, for example, it received in total more than 90 related books in the period from 1949 to 1962, while the Shanghai library estimates that it collected 89 titles authored by Pavlov during the same period. The collection at the National Library included more than 160 titles related to Pavlov between 1950 and 1965. Medical periodicals all created special columns on Pavlov, and the Ministry of Health established a special committee to study Pavlov's theories. As Pavlov was the most prominent representative of Soviet medicine, his theories not only included academic knowledge on the nervous system but also touched on physiology, psychology, medical studies, and pedagogy, which were deemed to express the Marxist-Leninist "Theory of Reflection" on the theoretical level (Wu 1955). In 1950s China, Pavlov's teachings were identified with the doctrines of materialism and Marxism-Leninism, and were taken as the universal standard for biomedical theory. They became the concrete manifestation within China's medical circles of "taking Russia as our teacher." Pavlovian theory could furthermore be extended to "a number of issues in pedagogy" (Karpanovski 1953), and his two systematic theories could be used to analyze Marxist and Leninist epistemology and elucidate the standpoints of materialism and atheism (Pipunyrov 1956; Petrushevskii 1953).

At the same time that Pavlov's writings were turned into authoritative dogma and theory, their applicability was also expanded indefinitely, including to the area of gynecology and obstetrics. The Russian physicians Vilvovskii and Porotitsev, in cooperation with Shu Gaomu, invented a method of "painless delivery" on the basis of Pavlov's ideas, with the intention of conditioning pregnant women to avoid the suffering associated with childbirth. In 1947, Zhu Binsheng published an article in the journal *Soviet Medicine* that introduced "The Physiological Dynamics in Nikolaiev's Painless Method of Delivery" (Zhu 1947). To promote information concerning the method of painless delivery, the Ministry of Health in the National People's Government demanded in 1952 that all health institutions at the level of the six administrative regions, provinces, and cities organize their medical personnel, especially gynecologists and obstetricians, to study models for combining Pavlov's theories with clinical application, and specifically methods of painless delivery, and to widely disseminate and study theoretical and clinical reports. The Department of Gynecology and Obstetrics at the medical college of the Shanghai University of Military Medicine took the lead in implementing the method of painless delivery by psychological prevention. According to local (albeit incomplete) statistics from all over the country, the method was used on 5,934 women from June 17, 1952, when the National Ministry of Health had issued its notification to promote the method of painless delivery, to the end of September, with the result that it claimed success in 5,507 cases, or a rate of 92.8 percent. The city of Beijing, where the method was carried out not only in hospitals but also in home births, even claimed a success rate of 93.6 percent. This "painless delivery method" was even implemented in far distant Xinjiang (Fu 1952), and promoted for application by midwives in home deliveries in cities from Beijing to Shanghai, Dalian, and Tianjin (Shen 2003, 123). In 1953, Lin Qiaozhi toured the Soviet Union and subsequently published an article titled "A Simple Introduction to a Few Key Characteristics in Medicine and Science Observed on a Tour of the Soviet Union."

The first Soviet medical therapy officially promoted by the Chinese government was "histotherapy," a treatment advocated by the researcher Feratov from the Soviet Academy of Medicine and Pharmacology in 1931. Beginning in 1948, it was first tested at the China Medical University in the Northeast and from there spread to be applied in research at Harbin, Shenyang, Beijing, Tianjin, Shanghai, and Xi'an. The National Government's Ministry of Health issued the "Directive to Organize the Implementation of Histotherapy" in March 1951, regarding the therapy as one of the great discoveries in contemporary medicine ("Zhongyang renmin zhengfu" 1951). Its advocates believed that it offered an effective treatment method for several dozen chronic diseases that physicians in the past had been able to treat either only with difficulty or not at all. Besides restoring eyesight to numerous patients who had lost their vision, it had efficacy rates of more than 77.4 percent for bronchial asthma, more than 76.28 percent for peptic ulcers, and more than 75.28 percent for scar contracture. According to statistics from the above-mentioned symposium, the therapy was applied to more than twenty-eight thousand patients nationwide, with positive results in 60–70 percent of all cases (Fu 1952).

The directive from the Ministry of Health included the following four points. First, all levels of health administration institutions in large and mid-sized cities all over the country should convene symposia on histotherapy to promote the discussion and popularization of this treatment method. Second, the National Health Research Institutes, all medical schools in the country, and the research centers in teaching hospitals had the responsibility, in terms of theoretical study, technology training, and material supply of tissue, to guide the widespread application of the therapy in hospitals. Third, professional associations for medical services at all levels, associations for traditional Chinese medicine, etc., must organize meetings for academic reports; and fourth, medical journals and publications must emphasize the publication of theoretical writings and clinical reports on histotherapy. "To earnestly organize and implement histotherapy is to be regarded as the beginning of our study of Soviet medicine," the Department of Public Health declared ("Zhongyang renmin zhengfu" 1951). According to statistics, incomplete as they may be, on a national level fifty-two thousand patients had received histotherapy by February 1952, of whom thirty-six thousand were cured.

In terms of medical technology and hospital management, the Soviet Union provided its Chinese comrades with lots of assistance and new information. The establishment of the Beijing Soviet Red Cross Hospital, for example, was a concrete manifestation of its aid and cooperation in the realms of health care and medicine. It not only helped resolve many vexing questions in the medical treatment of disease, but at the same time also served as an excellent model in the areas of hospital management, medical systems, and treatment procedures.

To demonstrate the advanced nature of Soviet medicine, Fu Lianzhang again stressed the abundant experience of the Soviet Union in the realm of scientific treatment methods (such as electrotherapy, hydrotherapy, mud therapy, application of wax, cupping, massage, etc.). These forms of therapy were simple and inexpensive but certainly achieved a high level of success with a number of diseases. In addition, therapies including sleep therapy and physical exercise therapy had been proven with concrete evidence to show obvious results with numerous diseases. In Fu's opinion, this sort of advanced medical thinking and clinical experience was well worth studying with care (Fu 1952). Shi Zengrong, professor of ophthalmology at the Harbin University of Medical Science, applied a method that had been invented by the Soviet physician Vladimir Filatov called "corneal grafting," and thereby managed to restore the eyesight of a number of previously blind patients. The so-called "Novocaine Block Therapy" introduced by the specialist Grantin was used by institutions like the Harbin University of Medical Science, the China University of Medical Science, and the Changchun Hospital for Railroad Employees, and did indeed achieve initial successes (Shen 2003, 123).

In spite of this, however, Chinese medical circles continued to express doubt about the advanced nature of Soviet medicine and considered it inferior to European and American medicine. To cite just one example, even the Beijing Soviet Red Cross Hospital that had been praised by Fu Lianzhang was plagued by a number of problems. As an attaché at the Soviet Chinese embassy attested, "The level of specialized skills by the staff assigned to work in the hospital is low, and the hospital does not have a single physician at the professor level. Very commonly, the specialized skills of the Chinese physicians exceeds that of our own physicians" (Shen 2003, 198). This even reached the point where a number of doctors with insufficient specialized skills were dispatched to China. This issue was bound to cause resentment in Chinese medical circles. In his 1957 article "We Must Unswervingly Continue to Study Advanced Soviet Medicine," Fu Lianzhang emphasized that

> the advanced nature of Soviet medicine is made apparent first and foremost in the fact that it is genuinely intended for the benefit of the people. Because of the inspiration from such a lofty goal, Soviet medical workers are able to give free rein to a high degree of enthusiasm and creativity and can implement the scientific worldview of dialectical materialism to explore the profound mysteries in the world of medicine and achieve outstanding successes. In fact, it is proven that Soviet medicine is not only advanced in the areas of guiding ideology and institutional organization, but is also unsurpassed by British and American medicine in regard to a large number of academic and technological problems, such as the study of hygiene and health preservation, physiology and pathology of the nervous system, atomic medicine, etc. (Fu 1957)

Fu was reaffirming that Soviet medicine was the most advanced medicine in the world.

Reflecting on Reflecting

The experience of Chinese medical circles in studying and learning from the experience of the Soviet model of medicine in the 1950s can be summarized by the following special characteristics:

1. Centralization of medicine. Prior to 1949, the system of medical education in China was in a state of disarray, lacking proper standards or procedures and suffering from a profusion of unqualified, substandard, and irregular fly-by-night schools. All over the country, teaching materials, syllabi, and educational institutions were unified, and a national unified medical education system was firmly established. In the administration of colleges and universities, "taking Russia as our teacher" was adopted as the foremost administrative model for managing cadres. The European and American model of universities that integrated research, education, and clinical services was abandoned.

2. Nationalization of the system of medical treatment. Free public medical care was established, along with a system of health care that matched the requirements of socialism. Free medical care was implemented in the cities, medical care and labor insurance were implemented in factories, and cooperative health care measures were carried out in rural areas, all with an emphasis on the health and safety of workers and the common people.

3. Dominance of political ideology in medicine. Medicine was first praised as an example of the actualization of "serving the people," and was subsequently used for developing education in new Communist value systems, which proceeded through the ideological remolding of medical workers, the study of Marxism-Leninism, and the mastery of the scientific methods of dialectical materialism, particularly through the work of Pavlov.

4. Specialization in clinical treatment with an emphasis on practical and small-scale application. After the formation of training teams and specialization teams, the Soviet model emphasized training for clinical work as quickly as possible, especially in the fields of internal medicine, external medicine, and gynecology.

5. Emphasis on preventive medicine. In the areas of health care and epidemic prevention, the 1950s witnessed the establishment of over six hundred specialized prevention and treatment stations and over 1,500 epidemic prevention stations, teams, and units on the basis of the Soviet experience, to prevent various infectious diseases. These measures yielded significant results (Fu 1957). The ideology of protecting health and hygiene, which was of primary importance in Soviet preventive medicine, affected China's industrial health care, urban health care, rural health care, and women's and children's health care.

In the area of industrial health care, factories and mines served as the basic organizational units of health care. With the goal of promoting workers' health, improving labor productivity and safety, and protecting the construction and smooth advance of the national economy, construction site safety systems and mobile clinics were launched, organizations of on-site physicians were set up, and workers received education in common hygiene. Environmental hygiene in factories and mines and workers' sanitary conditions were improved. In the cities, zoned medical services were implemented.

Ultimately, it is impossible to find accurate information on the exact number of Russian medical specialists who were present in China from 1949, when Soviet Red Cross workers first arrived in Manchuria to assist in extinguishing the plague, until around 1960, when Soviet experts pulled out of China. According to scholars' estimates on the basis of statistics from Soviet work records, the total number was 9,313 between 1952 and 1960. In reality, though, there must have been quite a few more, including specialists in the fields of science and culture (Shen 2003, 196). While this ten-year period of studying and imitating, based on the principle of "taking Russia as our teacher," came to an end when the Soviet specialists left China in 1960, the Soviet model did not simply vanish as a consequence.

Beginning in the 1980s, Chinese scientists and scholars in medicine and education have begun to reflect on the Soviet model. Even though theoretical and historical writings generally have a negative view of the 1950s period of studying the Soviet model (Zhu and Zhang 1990; Mei 1993), in reality the Soviet model of medicine continues to influence the educational system and organization of medicine in China. Since the 1990s, medical journals have provided reference material on the reform of China's medical education and the public health care system by reprinting articles on Soviet medicine and the reform of health care economics. Since the turn of the twenty-first century, research on the Soviet model has concentrated on the realm of education (Zhang, Sun, and Zeng 2004; Huang 2007; Hu 2009). Studies by contemporary scholars in Taiwan and Hong Kong, on the other hand, have focused more on researching topics like the historical stages, educational policies, and the wholesale Sovietization of education in the 1950s. As a result, some of these scholars believe that mainland education in the 1950s and '60s was characterized by the transplantation of the Soviet model and by an emphasis on economic and governmental functions (Wang 2010).

But the lessons learned by the Chinese medical world from the experiences of the Soviets were not only, or even primarily, in the realm of medical education. When investigating this situation, recent studies fail to take into consideration the particular circumstances of the medical environment during the initial stages of nation-building in China.

Conclusions

This chapter has clearly explained that the influence of the Soviet Union on medical development in China went far beyond medical education, or even medicine. The ideology of "serve the people" emerged from the Soviet Union and became evident in every aspect of Chinese political life, including medicine. Importantly, the Soviet Union provided essential tutelage to the Chinese Communist Party in how to govern the medical profession, and professions in general. Within medical education, even though the government was advocating wholesale copying of the Soviet Union, problems with teaching materials had already led Chinese medical schools to rewrite their textbooks according to local conditions. This shows that it was not possible for the Soviet model to be reproduced wholesale, even though its influence was profound and may still be felt today, after more than fifty years. Within clinical medicine, this influence remains most pronounced in the ideology of dialectical materialism that continues to influence the teaching of diagnostics, both in modern medicine and in Chinese medicine.

Notes

1. The Chinese curriculum contained twenty-nine courses while the curriculum at Japan's Imperial Universities was set up with thirty-two courses. China omitted anatomy, dentistry, and pathologic anatomy; consolidated external medicine and pharmaceutical manufacturing; and added the courses of traditional Chinese medicine, embryology, and mycology, which did not exist in Japan. See "Memorial on Regulations for Colleges; Regulations for Universities and Research Institutes" (Zhu 1932, 1987).

2. The curriculum of the National Medical College was set up with two years of foundational courses, German, physics and chemistry, and anatomy and physiology, with the second two years consisting of clinical courses. A few courses were combined into single subjects: for example, physiology was combined with theory and experimentation in medical chemistry; theory and practice of forensic medicine were combined; and clinical lectures on obstetrics and gynecology were combined with practical application in obstetrics. The curriculum therefore contained fewer subjects than were stipulated in the rules of the Ministry of Education.

3. The journal *Yiyao Pinglun* (Discussion of medicine and pharmaceutics), which was extremely influential in China's medical circles, continuously debated the issue of China's medical education from 1929 to 1930. The journal *Zhonghua Yixue Zazhi* (Journal of medicine in China) reported frequently on each country's medical education in 1932.

4. No substantial revisions were enacted. For example, in response to the criticism that the curriculum lacked a "department of anatomy," the revised outline merely substituted "in the category of anatomy."

10 John B. Grant

Public Health and State Medicine

Liping Bu

JOHN B. GRANT (1890–1962) was the "spirit of public health" for modern China, said Franklin Ho (1895–1975) when he was interviewed by Mary Bullock on July 22, 1970 (Bullock 1980, 134n2). Ho, former director of the Nankai Institute of Economics, shared with Grant an interest in analyzing statistics and economics of public health.[1] Ho's view was further supported by those who worked with Grant at the Peking Union Medical College (PUMC). Marion Yang (1891–1983) recalled in her memoirs that Grant would talk to anybody and everybody about public health when few paid attention to it during his early days in China (Yan 1990, 143–153). For almost twenty years (1921–1939), Grant worked tirelessly with his Chinese colleagues in training a cadre of public health professionals and in creating a modern public health administrative system under the Nationalist government. His enormous work had a profound impact on China's modern health system. Recent publications on Grant indicate that his ideas on public health have valuable relevance to the current debate on the efficient delivery of health care (Litsios 2011; Bu 2012a).

This study focuses on three interrelated aspects of Grant's work that had long-term implications for China's public health profession and health care: first, the development of a department of public health at PUMC to train public health professionals; second, the creation of health stations in rural and urban settings as experiments of pilot projects to study local health conditions and deliver health services; and third, assisting the Chinese government in establishing a modern national health administration of state medicine. Each of the three aspects seemed a necessary step in the building of a national health edifice, but this neat historical hindsight should not be taken to indicate that Grant started with a blueprint in hand, for an examination of Grant's work reveals an evolving process where persistence and tactical persuasion were mixed with shrewd observation and sensitive negotiation in a tumultuous time of highly nationalist aspirations. Nonetheless, the Rockefeller Foundation's original plan for Grant's mission in China undoubtedly set the path for the development.

Grant's Mission in China and His Reviews on Public Health

In August 1921, Grant came to China as both a professor at PUMC and the representative of the International Health Board (IHB, later changed to the International Health Division) of the Rockefeller Foundation.[2] He carried three major responsibilities assigned by the foundation: (1) to develop a curriculum of hygiene and preventive medicine for teaching purposes, (2) to establish an intramural "College Health Service" for the PUMC staff, which hopefully was to serve as a model for schools and colleges in China, and (3) most important of all, to "ascertain . . . the possibility of initiating public health activities in the country, which would be of a permanent and progressive character, aiding the quicker establishment of a national public health movement" (CMB 1921).

In its 1915 report, the China Medical Commission recommended not setting up a department of hygiene and public health for reason of "impracticability" in a medical school (CMB 1921). But by 1921 this point of view had changed because of the internal need to handle the hygiene problems of students and staff at PUMC and external demands to help Chinese society with "famine relief, plague in Manchuria, and . . . preparing for a possible typhus epidemic" (RAC 1921b). PUMC did not want to weaken its prestige by not having professionals to assist China in times of public calamity. But who was going to do the public health job? Out of several candidates recommended by key medical professionals associated with the Rockefeller Foundation and PUMC, foundation leaders chose John B. Grant as the most suitable person. Why Grant? First, Grant was a recent graduate of the Johns Hopkins School of Public Health, with a medical degree from the University of Michigan. He also had experience working in China during 1917–1919 on the foundation's hookworm control program in the Pingxiang mines in Hunan Province. Second, Grant was good at administrative affairs, full of self-assurance and energy. Moreover, Grant was born and raised in China: his parents were Canadian missionaries stationed in Ningpo, Zhejiang Province. Grant spoke Chinese and understood Chinese culture. All of these contributed to the Rockefeller Foundation's decision. It should be noted that Grant was a man of independent thinking, though a tactful and persistent foundation official. As he wore two hats—professor at PUMC and the Rockefeller Foundation's IHB representative/envoy in China—he took the opportunity offered by his vested privileges and responsibilities to envision a public health system in China that reflected his own views of public health.

Grant believed that public health was an integral part of the socioeconomic development of a society and that health care could be most efficiently achieved through an integration of preventive and curative medicine in a community health service. This kind of view was not typical among the medical and health professionals in the United States, but more in line with British health reformers who advocated social medicine and state responsibility for public health. Grant received his medical education at the University of Michigan (from which he graduated in 1917) when Victor C. Vaughan reigned as dean of the medical school from 1891 to 1920. A leading figure in American medical science and public health, Vaughan was a reformer of medical education who "developed one of the first systematic courses on bacteriology and germ theory for medical students" and carried out reforms of medical education years before the landmark 1910 Flexner Report (Markel 2000; Davenport 1996; Vaughan 1926; Duffy 1992). Grant continued his public health studies at Johns Hopkins University (1920–1921), where he met and studied with the British public health reformer Arthur Newsholme. Instrumental in the public health movement that led to the establishment of the Ministry of Health in Britain in 1919, Newsholme emphasized state responsibility for public health (Eyler 1997). Grant was also influenced by the British public health physician George Newman, who published widely on the social problems of public health and emphasized the importance of preventive medicine (Seipp 1963, xiii–xiv).

Grant cited Newsholme and Newman frequently to support his idea of a combined preventive and curative medicine when he presented his proposal for a department of public health to the China Medical Board of the Rockefeller Foundation in 1923. Grant's belief in social medicine and state responsibility for public health may have very well been reinforced by his early working experiences in rural North Carolina and in Chinese coal mines in Hunan, where he observed firsthand the social causation of epidemic diseases (Bullock 1980, 135–138; RAC n.d.a). If the North Carolina fieldwork taught him the frustration and ineffectiveness of disease control when preventive and curative medicine were carried out separately, the China fieldwork in the coal mines made him realize the crippling prospect of public health work when industrial leaders and government officials paid no attention to health issues of workers. These and later experiences in China convinced Grant of the necessity of the state's responsibility to take care of the health of the people. In designing a Department of Hygiene and Public Health, Grant drew lessons from his fieldwork and adopted an innovative approach to public health education in which the integration of preventive and curative medicine was emphasized.[3] Grant would later apply his experiences in China to public health programs in other places such as India, Europe, and Puerto Rico.

Creating the Department of Public Health and Training Public Health Professionals

In October 1923, Grant sent the China Medical Board in New York an eighty-page proposal for a Department of Hygiene with a demonstration health station.

In the proposal, Grant was critical of the separation of curative and preventive medicine and was determined to avoid it in his creation of a curriculum of public health at PUMC. Grant believed that "any artificial separation of curative and preventive medicine is detrimental to the efficiency of both" and that the "medicine of the future" required the "establishment of this combined curative and preventive medicine in a community in . . . a real 'health station'" (CMB 1923, 42). By the same token, the training of public health professionals should be deeply rooted in a community where preventive and curative medicines were integrated in practice. Grant envisioned that the future of medicine lay in the general medical practitioner as nucleus working with hygiene specialists in a community (CMB 1923, 26).[4] There was, however, no available example of such an integrated model of curative and preventive medical education or practice. Grant therefore had to experiment with his own vision of a health station that would include medical services, disease prevention, and vital statistics collection. In so doing, he moved away from the primarily "laboratory-based" model of public health education that W. H. Welch (known as the "dean of American medicine") created at Johns Hopkins University, and instead he designed a "community-based" model of public health education where students directly engaged in studying public health problems in a daily routine in the real world.[5] Grant, however, did not abandon the emphasis on scientific research, a signature feature of the "Johns Hopkins Model" in his new approach to public health education.

This bold departure from the exalted Johns Hopkins model was a manifestation of Grant's independent orientation rooted in the belief of medical efficiency. Grant conducted broad research on the different models of public health education in dozens of countries in Europe and around the world. Moreover, he gathered information on the experimental health stations being built at the time by the international health officers of the Rockefeller Foundation in different parts of the world (Farley 2004). To create such a health station in Beijing, however, would require the approval and collaboration of local authorities. Understanding the way to conduct business in China, Grant made friends with Chinese leaders in the medical and governmental circles through personal ties, professional affiliations, leadership of medical associations, and mingling with persons of importance.

Instead of imposing his ideas on Chinese officials, Grant chose to work behind the scenes with Chinese medical leaders who were keen on promoting public health, and encouraged them to take the ideas to government authorities. In the early 1920s, China had no central health administration, but two government-run public health institutions—the Manchurian Plague Prevention Service (established in 1912) and the Central Epidemic Prevention Bureau (established in 1919, renamed the National Epidemic Prevention Bureau in 1925 but retaining the same Chinese name, Zhongyang fangyi chu 中央防疫处). These two pioneering government institutions of public health engaged in scientific research for the prevention and treatment of epidemic diseases such as plague, smallpox, cholera, rabies, and scarlet fever (NHACFHS 1934; Flohr 1996). Many of the medical scientists at these two institutions actively promoted popular public health education and worked with such civic organizations as the YMCA and the Council on Health Education when the latter launched health campaigns in major cities in the 1910s–1920s (Bu 2009a; Bu 2011; Bu 2009b).

The absence of a centralized health administration and the medical scientists' interest in public health presented opportunities to shape the future of the Chinese health system. Grant thought that PUMC and its Department of Hygiene and Public Health should play a pivotal role in the development of a public health administration in China by training public health specialists who would become leaders. The political chaos and instability of China, however, complicated the scheme. The nationwide anti-imperialist movement that aimed to achieve national sovereignty and unity since the 1919 May Fourth Movement set the background that required Rockefeller Foundation officials to behave cautiously in dealing with Chinese nationalist sentiment. Grant wrote to the New York headquarters that "at the present stage of the history of this country direct administration [by PUMC] of such a demonstration [station] is in my opinion a rather bad thing to do. . . . Such work should ostensibly be carried out under Chinese supervision" (RAC 1922). He encouraged his Chinese colleagues to take initiatives public in the matter of establishing a health demonstration station. In the meantime, Grant strategically took a seat on the International Board of Finance of the Central Epidemic Prevention Bureau to maintain important contacts and secure the support of key members of the central government in Beijing (CMB 1924).[6] These strategies characterized Grant's working style in China throughout the years.

Back in December 1921, just three months after his arrival in Beijing, Grant shared with Dr. Quan Shaoqing, director of the Army Medical College in Beijing and a leading figure in promoting public health in China, an outline of an experimental public health unit in Beijing. Grant pointed out that the experimental area should represent average Beijing city conditions with a population of ten thousand, and the ward of Dengshikou appealed to him because it was close to PUMC and social workers there could help advance some services of public health (RAC 1921a). Quan became the director of the Central Epidemic Prevention Bureau in 1922–1923 and was in a better position to advocate the cause, but it was his successor, Fang Qing, who in May 1925 submitted a petition to the chief of the Beijing Metropolitan Police, Zhu Shen, for "the establishment of a Station in the Second-inside-left District [of Dengshikou] in Peking for the experimentation of public health measures in co-operation with the district police authorities" (NHACFHS 1934, 107–108). Zhu Shen favored the petition and appointed Fang Qing as director of the station, with full responsibility for selecting and appointing officers and devising means to secure necessary equipment and facilities (NHACFHS 1934, 109).

The station was established in 1925 with four divisions, each (except one) headed by the leading men of the Central Epidemic Prevention Bureau: T. F. Huang (Huang Zifang 黄子方) was chief of the Sanitation Division; H. K. Hu (Hu Hongji 胡鸿基, not of CEPB) was chief of Vital Statistics; P. Z. King (Jin Baoshan 金宝善) was chief of Medical Services; and C. L. Wang (Wang Changling 王長齡) was chief of the Communicable Diseases Division. Grant took no official title but served as the superior advisor (CMB 1925c). As the work of the Division of Vital Statistics involved the investigation of causes of death and communicable diseases, it was later merged with the Communicable Diseases Division. Two more divisions were added to the station in 1930: a public health visiting division and a general administration division. The Sanitation Division investigated the sanitation of water, foods, latrines/flies, home hygiene such as delousing and general cleanliness, street cleanliness, and public health education. The Division of Vital Statistics and Communicable Diseases collected statistics of births and deaths, population, causes of death, and communicable diseases. The Division of Medical Services covered school health, industrial health, public health nursing, maternity health, infant health, and medical clinic services. The Division of Public Health Visiting made health visits to schools, factories, homes, maternity cases, and so on. The Division of General Administration was responsible for correspondence, the library, business and accounting, health publications (including monthly, quarterly, and annual reports), health education (including distribution of health literature and posters and giving health talks and lectures), cooperation with other agencies, and all other administrative matters (RAC 1930b, 7; CMB 1925d).

The station, named the Public Health Experimental Station of the Metropolitan Police Department of Beijing, was in reality a collaborative endeavor of the Peking Union Medical College, the Central Epidemic Prevention Bureau, and the Beijing Metropolitan Police.[7] The station constituted "the *practice, investigation* and most of the *teaching* fields for the work of Hygiene" (RAC 1928a). In 1928, all medical students at PUMC were required to take a three-week internship at the station in their fourth year. In the 1930–1931 academic year, a total of sixty-four medical students received public health training at the station, ranging from three months to a year in duration (RAC 1931).

Spreading Health Stations and Building National Health Administration

The work of the Beijing health station not only inspired Chinese doctors like Yan Fuqing (1882–1970) but also boosted Grant's confidence in expanding the experiment to other urban and rural areas. In July 1928, Yan and his colleagues at Shanghai Medical College (SMC) created the Wusong health station, which was clearly modeled after the Beijing health station, as a demonstration area for public health teaching.[8] Several prominent doctors who were strong advocates of public health sat on the SMC faculty, including Hu Xuanming, Huang Zifang, and Zhang Wei. Hu Xuanming was in charge of the demonstration station, where all SMC medical students were required to intern for a month. Their internship included conducting public health education and clinical treatment that was combined with disease prevention, sanitation, maternal health, and dental hygiene. In 1929 the Health Bureau of Greater Shanghai joined the college as partner to operate the Wusong station. But the station was totally destroyed by the Japanese bombing in January 1932 (Zhang 2006a, 183–184).

Although Wusong was the first rural health demonstration station in China, it was rarely recognized as such but was categorized as one of the first three rural health stations established in 1929, the other two being Dingxian, near Beijing, and Gaoqiao, of Shanghai (Li 1934a). The Dingxian health station, which was integrated into the Mass Education Movement led by James Y. C Yen (Yan Yangchu, 1890–1990), was initiated by Grant but operated and led by C. C. Chen (1903–2000). Its inception demonstrated the shift of Grant's view of rural health demonstration in China. Back in 1923, Grant thought rural public health in China "entirely impracticable" to handle (CMB 1923, 30). But by 1927 he had changed his mind and was seriously working to extend health stations to rural and urban locations as pilot experiments to achieve two major goals: the study of local health conditions and the delivery of health care services to local people. Since the extraordinary achievements of Dingxian have been well studied (Gamble 1968; Hayford 1990; Bullock 1980; Chen 1989), I will not repeat that story here. The Gaoqiao station, which has not been a focus of scholarly investigation, deserves serious attention and will facilitate a better understanding of the health station movement in the 1930s.

The Gaoqiao health station started as a collaborative project between the Rockefeller Foundation (International Health Division demonstrations) and the Health Bureau of Greater Shanghai, with budgets shared by both sides (RAC n.d.c; RAC 1928b). Gaoqiao was a better-than-average Chinese rural area, with a variety of small businesses and merchants and a 40 percent literacy rate (the national average literacy rate was around 10 percent at the time). Sitting on the east bank of the Huangpu River and the south bank of the Yangzi River, twelve miles from the city center, the area was about two hundred square li (one li equals half a kilometer) and contained about two hundred villages and a town with a population of 33,959 (RAC 1929b, 1–3). Medical services were the main activities of Gaoqiao station, though it followed the model of the Beijing First Health Station in conducting vital statistics collection, prevention of communicable diseases, and popular health education. The first quarterly report indicated lack of interest among the locals in Western medical services and health demonstration. Out of a population of 34,000, a total of 1,281 patients were treated at the station in the first three months (RAC 1929b, 19). Prevalent diseases in Gaoqiao included gastrointestinal diseases, malaria, rabies, tuberculosis, syphilis, smallpox, leprosy, puerperal sepsis, and infections of the newborn (RAC 1929b, 7). As Gaoqiao was relatively large and travel was not easy, the station developed a "traveling clinic" to give smallpox vaccinations to those villagers in the district who for various reasons were not able to come to the health station clinic. This was probably the first mobile clinic in China. It consisted of two wheelbarrows, carrying a staff of three—a doctor, a public health nurse, and a sanitary policeman—and was equipped with "a bag containing vaccines, knives, antiseptics, other necessary medical supplies and health pamphlets" (RAC n.d.e). In 1929 the traveling clinic made fourteen trips and vaccinated 634 individuals. The sixth report showed little progress in winning over the populace to Western medicine and health demonstration, as the number of patients who sought medical services remained small (RAC 1930a).[9]

The Gaoqiao experience indicated that the work of health stations was ineffective in delivering medical services and collecting data when no comprehensive rural reform was carried out to get local people involved in improving their socioeconomic and educational conditions. In contrast, Dingxian proved successful because serious endeavors were made to integrate health programs with a general reform movement for rural improvement. More importantly, C. C. Chen, director of Dingxian health programs, sufficiently trained locals to be health workers to serve their fellow villagers. This extraordinary progressive method made Dingxian unique and successful in contrast to other health stations (Bu 2012b). The Nationalist government, together with the efforts of private organizations such as the Rockefeller Foundation and local municipal governments, established more than seventeen health stations in cities and towns. Their work and limitations were evaluated by two 1934 survey studies on rural and urban practices, respectively (Li 1934a; Grant and Peng 1934). The survey reports summarized that the work of rural health stations was limited and that municipal health bureaus took inadequate measures to control communicable diseases. Local authorities claimed that poverty was the reason for inadequate health measures, but the authors of the report on urban health argued, instead, that the "chief requirement for the establishment of modern health administration appears to be competent technical personnel rather than finance" (Grant and Peng 1934, 1078).

Grant considered that the major problem was a lack of competently trained experts in public health. In order to increase the number of public health professionals and to enhance their technical knowledge, he suggested that lower-level training programs be created and taught in Chinese, and advanced programs be created and taught in English (RAC 1929a). His correspondence also indicated that he sought every opportunity to recruit quality men and able persons for public health work. In addition to sending Chinese students and medical doctors to the United States for advanced training in public health, he inquired among Chinese students who were studying at American medical schools—especially those who were studying at the medical schools of Harvard, the University of Chicago, the University of Michigan, and Johns Hopkins—to find out who might be interested in public health work (RAC 1925).

The creation of health demonstration stations was carried out simultaneously with the scheme of building a central Ministry of Health in China. Early in 1923, Grant requested that the New York office send him material regarding the organization of ministries of health in different countries for possible use in the establishment of such a ministry in China. The Rockefeller Foundation's information director sent Grant "a list of the laws and other material" regarding the organization of health ministries and laws of countries such as Czechoslovakia, Cuba, Poland, Yugoslavia, Nicaragua, Brazil, and France (RAC 1923). In Grant's view, the major obstacle in China was essentially officials' "lack of any conception of what Governmental Public Health is" (RAC 1925g). Grant and his associates, therefore, prepared a pamphlet in Chinese on public health to educate the officials in Beijing.[10] He emphasized the importance of public health for a nation's progress. Using the world power Britain as an example, Grant persuaded Chinese officials: "Gladstone, the great English statesman, is responsible for the statement that 'the first duty of government is a safeguarding of the health of its citizens.' A study of the present important position of public health in any efficient government of the leading nations of the world shows an appreciation of this statement" (CMB 1925e).[11] Grant mentioned four major divisions of a governmental public health administration—municipal, rural, provincial, and national—and emphasized the obvious importance of rural public health to a large agricultural country like China. Looking at what was being done in other large agricultural countries such as Russia and India, Grant felt the urgent need for China to pay considerable attention to this aspect (CMB 1925f). Grant sent a pamphlet on rural public health to the governor of the Beijing Metropolitan area, Hsueh Tu-pi (Xue Dupi), when he showed interest (CMB 1925b).[12]

To gain possible funding, Grant worked with his British associates in an effort to persuade the British government to allow a significant portion of the British Boxer Indemnity to pay for public health in China (after all, the British started the opium epidemic in China), but the effort did not materialize in the end (CMB 1926; CMB 1927a; Teow 1999, 130–132). Rockefeller Foundation officials such as Grant and Roger S. Greene had regular conversations with the medical officer of the British Legation, Dr. G. Douglas Gray, regarding the creation of a Ministry of Health in China. Gray thought it not worth working on and suggested focusing on the intensive training of good men for public health (CMB 1927b). He told Huang Zifang, "In my opinion the best way to go about it is to consolidate P H work round a central focus either at Peking or Shanghai, preferably the former, making a model station from which graduate students would learn the proper way of working and then return to their various cities and establish Municipal

Public Health. Then when China becomes purged of its present misrule and has a National Government you could link up these municipal schemes and weld them into a National service comprising not only municipal schemes but also a maritime quarantine service" (RAC 1927). That seemed to be exactly what Grant and his associates were working on, especially in their efforts to develop a modern health service in major cities like Beijing, Tianjin, and Shanghai.

Political stability seemed to have arrived when Chiang Kai-shek established a national government in Nanjing of a nominally united China after the Northern Expedition.[13] But misrule was not purged entirely with the Nanjing government, as different political forces vied for dominance. The creation of a Ministry of Health of the Nationalist government on October 28, 1928, revealed intense competition among and lobbying by different political and professional factions for control. (Ka-che Yip [1995, 45–47] and Xi Gao [2012, 145–148] have provided a glimpse of the intriguing story of political struggle in their respective studies.) Candidates for the position of health minister included prominent medical leaders of different factions, such Liu Ruiheng and Yan Fuqing (American-trained), Wu Lien-teh (British-trained), Hu Dingan (German-trained) and Tang Erhe (Japanese-trained).[14] Political forces of different warlords (Yan Xishan and Feng Yuxiang, for instance) and the Nationalists also juggled the position as a reward for their protégés. International organizations such as the Rockefeller Foundation/PUMC and the League of Nations Health Organization (LoNHO), with offers of international help, quietly worked behind the scenes to make sure the position was to be held and sustained by professional experts to neutralize factional infighting politically and professionally. Liu Ruiheng was eventually appointed as vice minister, the technical leader of the health administration, ensuring the professional dominance of American influence, as he was trained at Harvard University and was director of PUMC.

From Public Health to State Medicine: National Health Policy

According to Grant, China faced two immediate medical needs: "First, to control the causes of an excess mortality resulting in not less than 4 million unnecessary deaths a year. Second, to offer palliative medical facilities for a sum total of daily illnesses which probably aggregate some sixteen million cases a day and [are] now inadequately met by one-fortieth the requisite number of physicians and one-sixtieth the number of beds set as a standard for communities with only half the morbidity of China" (Grant 1928, 75).[15] How was China to take care of the health of its large population under a national health administration? What kind of health system should China have in order to effectively protect its entire population?

Given China's particular conditions, such as large population, low-level socioeconomic development, and limited medical personnel and facilities, Grant believed that the logical policy for China was state medicine (Grant 1928, 65–80). He explained that there were two types of medical systems in the world: private-run and government-run. The reason why China should adopt state medicine was that under private medicine there would be "a haphazard and inefficient distribution of curative facilities" with two outstanding deficiencies: rural areas would be insufficiently served, and in urban cities some districts would have an unjustified concentration of hospitals with duplication of expensive equipment, causing the disadvantage of other districts' being inadequately served. Further-more, under a private medical system, there would be "an unequal availability to each class of population of medical science. The rich will command the best of medical service, the poor will have it made available through charity clinics and the large middle class will be unable to afford either." In light of this analysis, Grant thought that state medicine—the entirely governmental responsibility for medical service for all people—was suitable for China, because state medicine "would make certain outstanding benefits compulsory" and "ensure an adequate position for Hygiene in General Education" (Grant 1928, 76–78).

How to implement state medicine? In Grant's opinion, the first step was to secure efficient personnel. "Such personnel," he wrote, "should equal in training and administrative ability the best medical men in the world." It was impera-tive that "political leaders appreciate that medical affairs are non-partisan and scientific in nature." Second, "the most important would be the establishment of a centralized medical authority with power to execute the adopted policy on a nation-wide scale" (Grant 1928, 79). Grant made the argument for state medi-cine on January 27, 1928, at the annual conference of the Chinese National Medi-cal Association, and he published his speech a month later in the association's medical journal. His call for state medicine set in motion an extensive debate in China over the next two decades. Chinese medical leaders supported state medicine but they seemed to understand the concept differently. Some focused on health service for all—rich or poor, rural or urban—while others emphasized the importance of a centralized health system. Xi Gao's examination of the state medicine movement indicates that the connotations of state medicine shifted from the original "health service for all" to a bureaucratic sense of a "central-ized medical system," which Chinese health professionals hoped would protect them from competition from unlicensed practitioners (Gao 2012, 144–160). The original meanings of state medicine in Grant's definition actually contained both service-for-all and the establishment of a national health administrative system as two sides of the same coin.

The promotion of state responsibility for public health was an international trend in the 1920s–1940s, spearheaded by the League of Nations Health Orga-nization. Grant had extensive working relations with LoNHO leaders such as Ludwik Rajchman, Berislav Borčić, and Andrija Štampar, who came to work in

China to help build a national health system (Borowy 2009a; Lucas 1980). LoN-HO helped health reforms in many countries, of which China was one. In fact, one of the most important functions of LoNHO, as Iris Borowy points out, was to help set up a national health system when requested by a particular country (Borowy 2009b, 361–420).

Long-Term Implications: State Medicine and Disease Prevention

Many of Grant's colleagues and students, such as Li Dequan (1896–1972), C. C. Chen, Yan Fuqing, P. Z. King, and Marion Yang, worked in socialist China and held key positions in medical institutions as technical experts. Li Dequan, for instance, served as the first health minister of the People's Republic of China (1949–1965). These people were strong advocates of state medicine and public health. They were also influenced by Grant, as most of them had worked with him and received advanced training in the United States upon his recommendation (see chapter 14). When the government promoted socialist state medicine after 1949, the ideas of state responsibility for public health and preventive medicine that Grant first introduced to his Chinese colleagues in the 1920s found an encouraging environment, where they gained new vitality and were transformed into new practices under the guidance of a distinct socialist ideology.

In the early 1950s, the Chinese government defined its national health policy by these four key principles: prevention as first priority, a combination of Chinese and Western medicine, serving the people, and combining health and mass movements. In the Cold War environment of international relations, John B. Grant could not possibly have any influence in the development of a state medical system in socialist China. Nonetheless, his ideas of state medicine and preventive medicine were embedded in the PRC's national health policy. Moreover, the influence from the Soviet Union in the 1950s further shaped China's medical landscape, particularly in terms of medical education—curricula and textbooks, the establishment of anti-epidemic disease stations, and maternal and child health stations across the nation. By the end of 1965, "all 29 provinces had anti-epidemic disease stations with analogous structures for the railway, mining industry, and large enterprises" (Bangdiwala et al. 2011, 208–209). Public health education emphasized the biomedical model of "epidemiology, school hygiene, occupational hygiene, food hygiene, environmental hygiene and radiation hygiene" (Bangdiwala et al. 2011, 209).

Although the PRC government inherited the national health system from the Nationalist government, it extensively pushed modern health into village China, setting up health centers and clinics to benefit the other 80 percent of the Chinese people.[16] The barefoot doctors, who came into being in the mid-1960s, reminded people of the rural health workers of Dingxian (see chapter 13). The Chinese government "adapted the ideas developed at Dingxian to great advantage in building a nationwide rural health care system after 1958," wrote C. C. Chen (1989, 36). The barefoot doctors, like the rural health workers three decades before them, came from the village and served their fellow villagers. They not only used herbs for treatment but also popularized the use of Western medicine in village China (Fang 2012). After a short training program, they became the paramedics of rural China, providing basic medical services and health education, and mediating between the state medicine system and rural health care.[17]

In his twenty years in China, Grant collaborated with his Chinese colleagues, making significant accomplishments in the training of public health professionals. When the Nationalist government established a Ministry of Health in 1928, a small cadre of public health specialists, many of whom were Grant's associates as former students or colleagues, formed the backbone of the public health administration. Through health stations, Grant tested his vision of a combined practice of curative and preventive medicine in a community as the best and most efficient means to deliver health care. He also achieved his ultimate ambition in China, that is, to help create a national health administration, not by dogmatically imitating the existing systems of other nations but by creatively and intelligently creating a new system to avoid the mistakes and detours that others had made and endured (Grant 1928, 65–66). Grant was sensitive to Chinese sentiment in his dealings with Chinese professionals and officials during those politically tumultuous years. His confidence in the ability of the Chinese people to carry out medical and health tasks proved to be vitally important to his many successes. C. C. Chen commented that Grant "believed that no one was better suited to solve China's grievous problems than the Chinese themselves" (Chen 1989, 38).

A fundamental belief underlying Grant's concept of medical efficiency was the technical expertise of public health professionals.[18] But in the early 1930s he began to realize the limits of technical expertise in solving public health problems. The exceptional accomplishments of Dingxian demonstrated that the public health program had to be integrated into a broader socioeconomic reform movement in order to succeed. Consequently, he worked with Selskar Gunn on a new approach to public health where comprehensive rural reform was imperative (Litsios 2005). Grant's major contribution to the formation of a public health profession in China was not just the concrete programs he created or helped create, such as the public health department at PUMC, the health education curriculum, rural and urban health stations, and the national administrative structure of a health system. More importantly, the ideas of state medicine, social medicine, and preventive medicine that he conveyed to his Chinese colleagues have left a long-term legacy. These ideas and methods of practice exerted profound influence in China under different political environments through professional continuity.

Notes

1. Franklin Ho was a Yale graduate with a PhD in economics. He created and directed the Nankai Institute of Economics during 1927–1947, making it a prominent academic institution in China. He was known for promoting and engaging in the research of "compiling statistics bearing upon social, economic, and industrial problems in China" (Chiang 2001, 78–102).

2. Grant was appointed associate professor of pathology in 1921 when he arrived in China and then professor and head of the Department of Hygiene and Public Health in 1924 when he created the department at PUMC (CMB 1925a).

3. The name of the department was changed to the Department of Public Health and Preventive Medicine, and then to the Department of Public Health.

4. It was an irony that preventive and curative medicine completely diverged in the West, while in China the government integrated prevention as the first priority of medical policy in the 1950s–1980s.

5. The public health education program at Johns Hopkins University later incorporated community field work.

6. The staff at CEPB included Chinese leaders in the field of medical science and public health, such as Fang Qing, Robert Lim, S. H. Chuan, and Huang Zifang.

7. The health station was originally called the Public Health Experimental Station, Metropolitan Police Department, Peking. After it showed some satisfactory results, the word "experimental" was dropped in 1926 and the station was called the Public Health Station, Metropolitan Police Department, Peking. Then in 1928 as the city's name was changed to Beiping with the reorganization of city districts, the station's name was changed to the Health Station of the First Health Area, Special Municipality of Beiping. In 1930, in order to reduce municipal expenditures, the Municipal Department of Public Health was merged with the Police Department and the station became the Health Station, First Health Area, Department of Public Safety, Beiping (RAC 1930b).

8. Shanghai Medical College was founded in 1927 and began classes in October of that year. Yan Fuqing was president of the college and also served as chair of the Department of Public Health.

9. The Gaoqiao station was destroyed by the Japanese when they started their full-scale aggression in China in 1937.

10. The English version of the pamphlet consisted of six single-spaced pages and was titled *Public Health in Peking*. It gave a brief history and described the organizational divisions of public health, and defined public health as "that branch of government undertaking the prevention of disease in the community. . . . The business of health protection is being undertaken" (CMB 1925e).

11. Chinese medical scientists (e.g., P. Z. King and T. F. Huang) frequently cited this alleged Gladstone statement in their advocacy of state responsibility for public health.

12. The context was that Grant was contemplating a rural health station near Beijing, but he had to walk a delicate line so as not to upset Chinese nationalist sentiment; so he made sure the appeal for assistance with public health came from the local county, San Ho Hsien (Sanhe Xian). Grant wrote, "Although, as a private organization, we are not desirous of undertaking anything in the Public Health line, we feel it incumbent upon us to answer the appeal for help from San Ho Hsien." The project of San Ho Hsien did not work in the end, which led Grant to seek an opportunity to start the health program in Dingxian in partnership with James Yen.

13. China had been ravaged by wars between regional warlords since the end of the Qing dynasty. In 1924, a revolutionary government of the United Front between the Guomindang (the Nationalists) and the Chinese Communist Party was established in Guangzhou under the

leadership of Sun Yat-sen to challenge the warlord-controlled central government in Beijing. The revolutionaries launched the Northern Expedition against the warlords in 1926–1927, with much popular support. As the United Front's military campaigns triumphed, Chiang Kai-shek, the military leader of the Northern Expedition, turned the guns against the Communists and purged them just before the new national government was established in Nanjing.

14. At one point when Grant heard that Tang Erhe was about to be offered the position of the minister of health, he asked Yan Fuqing to look into it (CMB 1927b).

15. Grant did not take into account Chinese medicine as a solution to Chinese medical needs.

16. AnElissa Lucas called this "organizational continuity" (Lucas 1980).

17. The training time for barefoot doctors varied from region to region, but mostly ranged from three to six months, and sometimes from a few weeks up to a year according to local arrangements. The doctors' retraining throughout the years to update their knowledge and skills was part of the program.

18. C. C. Chen thought that Grant emphasized academic research but did not pay enough attention to the value of clinical training of public health specialists, which limited their capability in dealing with diseases in real life (Chen 1989, 39).

11 The Influence of War on China's Modern Health Systems

Nicole Elizabeth Barnes and John R. Watt

When the nationalist government established China's first Ministry of Health in 1928, high rates of infectious disease, maternal and child mortality, and malnutrition still plagued the Chinese people, particularly in rural areas. The political and scientific reforms that swept Japan into the modern era had barely begun to take root even in China's larger cities, and the high rates of sickness and death alarmed reformers who longed to improve people's lives and raise China's standing in the international medical and political communities. Achieving this aim required the adoption of scientific biomedicine and its application to the needs of 350 million people living in considerable poverty in the countryside. Drawing on reforms initiated in Eastern Europe and the Soviet Union after World War I, reformers and statesmen came up with a low-cost strategy of improving health through public preventive care.

This chapter discusses how the Nationalist government pursued this strategy and with what results, discussing both the general situation in the country and the specific situation of Chongqing, its capital during the War of Resistance against Japan (1937–1945). In the 1930s and '40s, public health care on a scientific biomedical model was a novel idea in China. Although the outbreak of war in 1937 disrupted much of what had been accomplished in the 1930s, by then China had developed a small but growing cadre of physicians, nurses, modern midwives, and sanitary engineers capable of working within the Nationalist state's biomedical agenda to improve living conditions in China. Many of them moved to the unoccupied southwestern and northwestern provinces during the war, as did several important health agencies. These included the National Institute of Health, the National Central Hospital, and the Central Epidemic Prevention Bureau, all of which retained branches in western China after the war (Fu and

Deng 1989; ABMAC 1946). The National Guiyang Medical College (now Guiyang Medical University) remained in Guiyang, Guizhou, and new agencies were established during the war, including the Chongqing Bureau of Public Health and the Sichuan Provincial Health Administration. Rather than curtail the development of health administration and state medicine, the war moved it west.

The National Health Administration and Rural Health Care

Dr. Liu Ruiheng (劉瑞恆, who published in English as J. Heng Liu), director of the Peking Union Medical College (PUMC) and a graduate of Harvard Medical School, served as the first technical vice minister in the first Ministry of Health in 1928. Liu was one of a small handful of China's medical leaders who had been educated abroad and had returned with the aim of improving health care in China. He had worked well with Dr. John B. Grant (Lan Ansheng 兰安生), PUMC's public health director, who had grown up in China, and he knew Grant's views, and those of his students, on the relevance of state medicine to urban and rural health.

Grant had published his views earlier in 1928. In an article in the *National Medical Journal of China* (the premier medical journal for Chinese biomedical physicians), he pointed out that China suffered at least four million excess deaths per year (Grant 1928). Grant argued that this problem could only be addressed through a public health care strategy emphasizing preventive medicine, sanitation, early diagnosis, and adequate nutrition. Although no delivery system existed in 1928, Liu persuaded the ministry to study state medicine and conferred with the Ministry of Education on school health. But the Ministry of Health soon suffered three major setbacks: it tried but failed to delegitimize Chinese medicine; the minister had to resign due to a falling out between Chiang Kai-shek and the northern warlords; and the political status of the ministry was downgraded to a department within the Interior Ministry and a third of its staff were let go (Zhu 1988, 95; Lamson 1935, 463).

Prospects for implementing a rural health care strategy did not look good, but Liu and his close associate Dr. Jin Baoshan (trained like Grant in public health at Johns Hopkins University) organized a Central Field Health Station (CFHS, *Zhongyang weisheng sheshi shiyansuo*) to lead rural public health work (Wong and Wu 1936, 733–737). Politics interfered with the smooth operation of an initial model rural health service in Xiaozhuang, but two other government-sponsored county-level programs, at Tangshan and Jiangning, took its place (see figure 11.1).

By 1934, 187 health care professionals worked in seventeen rural health services. The National Health Administration adopted a plan to have a health center in each county nationwide, with a hospital and diagnostic laboratories at the county level and first aid and sanitary and preventive care in villages (League of Nations Health Organization 1937). The plan would require thousands of health

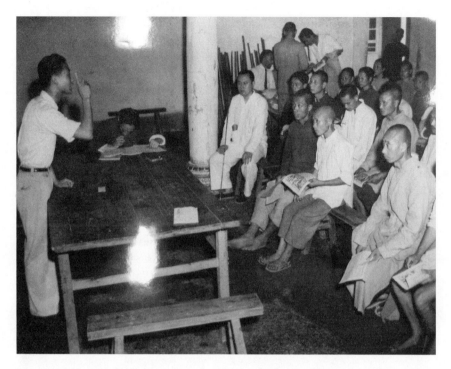

Figure 11.1. A hygiene lecture in a county health center in Jiangning county near Nanjing. *Source:* ABMAC Archives.

care workers to carry it out, so in 1935 the Rockefeller Foundation funded a Public Health Personnel Training Institute (*Gonggong weisheng renyuan xunlian suo*) to produce them.

The most important intervention by the Central Field Health Station occurred in Jiangxi Province. In 1933 a League of Nations team wrote a critical report about the marginal public health situation in that province. As a result, the National Economic Council made a grant to set up a provincial health agency and a rural health service consisting of ten centers intended for work in areas formerly managed by the Jiangxi soviet. In 1936 the Yugoslav rural health expert Dr. Andrija Štampar sharply criticized the work of these centers for failing to reach out into rural communities (ABCFM 1930–1939). But two independent county-level health programs—at Dingxian in Hebei and Zouping in Shandong—achieved more noteworthy results. The Dingxian health program bore the imprint of the Peking Union Medical College's Department of Health, for which it served as a rural health field station, and the health program director Dr. Chen Zhiqian (C. C. Chen), a PUMC graduate, became a national leader in developing the case for public health care. Unfortunately the Japanese invasion in 1937 shut down both of these remarkable innovations.

By the time the war against Japan broke out, the reformers had had nine years in which to find out what the National Health Administration (NHA, successor to the Ministry of Health) could accomplish through public health care. To a considerable extent their work depended on promoting rural reconstruction and basic literacy, and that raised major political problems for conservative powerbrokers in the Nationalist regime. Thus it is not surprising that the NHA focused attention on the two areas of special interest to the government leaders, namely, Jiangning county in the suburbs of Nanjing and Jiangxi Province, from which the main Red Army exited in October 1934 leaving only a small guerrilla force behind. But a top-down health strategy did not work well in Jiangxi. Town- and city-based health units remained in towns and cities, leaving rural health care largely in the hands of traditional midwives and disease deities. The fact that it was Nationalist Army medical men who dispensed "free medicine" and smallpox vaccine as part of an anti-Communist campaign in late 1934 indicated the lack of civilian outreach ("Health Work in Kiangsi" 1934). A modern public health care program could not easily develop in such a context.

Chongqing: Nationalist Public Health Administration in the Wartime Capital

The War of Resistance impressed upon everyone the importance of saving the country from the Japanese Army. After Wuhan, the first provisional capital, fell to the Japanese in October 1938, the Nationalist government retreated once again to Chongqing, where it founded the Chongqing Bureau of Public Health (CBPH) (*Chongqingshi weishengju*). CBPH records framed everything from anti-opium campaigns to staving off disease in the language of "strengthening the race and building the nation" (*qiangzu jianguo*) and "increasing the power of the War of Resistance and nation-building" (*zengqiang kangjian liliang*) (CMA 1940b).

The CBPH began its monumental work of cleansing the new capital in November 1938, three months after the Nationalist government settled into its wartime home. The bureau started nearly from scratch in a city where most of the residents drank water pulled straight from the river by shoulder-pole carriers; no municipal trash collection occurred; Japanese planes regularly dropped bombs on residences, schools, and hospitals; no quarantine service monitored the voluminous river traffic; and seasonal epidemics of cholera and smallpox hit twice a year. Faced with such challenges, CBPH staff set their jaws firm and their sights low, writing in the very first work report that "the greatest aim in public health is to decrease the rates of death and illness" (CMA 1938a, 181, 188; AH 1946, 1; Yip 1995, 116–118).

As other chapters in this volume illustrate, virtually everything that the Nationalist health authorities did in Chongqing had been done in China before, and almost always on the same or a similar model (MacPherson 1987; Rogaski 2004; Stapleton 2000). Yet although the Chongqing Bureau of Public Health used old methods and approaches, it did so as a central government entity in China's previously autonomous southwest, and with a new intensity of language that framed its work around resisting the Japanese. Moreover, the war years marked the apogee of the process, begun in the late nineteenth century, of imprinting individual bodies with national concerns. With an enemy army on their own soil, Chinese reformers' clarion call for strong bodies was no longer just ideological propaganda, but a response to an immediate and tangible threat. Thus, public health practices in the Nationalist state's wartime capital form a natural focal point for investigating how the war affected civilian life.

This new bureau, and the central government that directed it, changed Chongqing in three fundamental ways. First, many Chongqing residents felt the presence of the central government in their city most consistently and forcefully through the activities of the CBPH. Working to clean up the city and prevent the spread of contagious diseases, the CBPH directed and regulated the most quotidian practices of the wartime capital's residents, such as where they relieved their bladders and placed their garbage and what kinds of food and drink they could buy on the street. Its rules entered parts of life previously subject to social convention only—when to bury loved ones after their passing, when to gather in large crowds at public theaters, and where women should give birth. Second, the new municipal government, staffed with Chiang Kai-shek's chosen men, reorganized local hospitals and charitable relief organizations, placing trusted elites— many of them recent immigrants like the central government staff—in top positions, thereby changing the local power structure. The Nationalists brought new resources to the city, chiefly financial assistance and highly trained personnel, but access to these resources came with a cost, as local leaders lost their autonomy. Third, through its directives to the municipal government and the Bureau of Public Health, the central government also pushed the city's health practices in the direction of scientific biomedicine, posing a significant challenge to physicians of Chinese medicine.

The central government's move inland attracted the most elite public health personnel to Chongqing and other parts of Sichuan. Mei Yilin (梅貽林, 1896–1955), director of the Chongqing Bureau of Public Health from its inception in November 1938 through his resignation in December 1942, was one such man. The eighth child of a prosperous scholar-gentry family and the younger brother of the president of Qinghua University, Mei Yiqi (梅貽琦, 1889–1962), Mei Yilin was born in Tianjin in 1896 and belonged to the first generation of Chinese gentry to be educated at top-tier, modernized, and Western schools.[1]

When the central government's health officials arrived in Chongqing, the city boasted 313 physicians of Chinese medicine, 122 physicians of scientific biomedicine, 58 midwives, 12 druggists, and 8 pharmacy apprentices (SPA 1939).

Over one-third of the new capital's biomedical physicians migrated into the city between October 1937 (exactly one year prior to the fall of the first provisional capital, Wuhan, to the Japanese) and December 1938, peaking in the four months around the fall, September through December 1938. Popular anticipation of the central government's retreat to Chongqing unleashed a flood of new-style medical professionals into the city, tipping the balance away from the once-dominant local medicine to biomedicine.

At the same time, the war offered new opportunities for practitioners of Chinese medicine to make a place for themselves in state medicine, an important process that is more fully described in the next chapter of this volume. For example, whereas opponents of Chinese medicine had wished to make it impossible for Chinese medicine doctors to obtain state medical licenses, the Nationalist state awarded many licenses during the war. Anticipating the health needs of a population under siege, from early 1940 through October 1942 the NHA registered 513 Chinese medicine practitioners to meet "war exigencies," and allowed local health bureaus to grant them licenses. Health officials in Chongqing awarded licenses to Chinese medicine physicians and pharmacists more frequently than to biomedical practitioners, and funded the local Chinese medicine hospital (Barnes 2012b, 309–365; ABMAC n.d.e). Facing the same constraints of war, the Communists also supported Chinese medicine more than they might have had ideology alone been their guide.

Yet the primary task of the Chongqing Bureau of Public Health had little to do with medicine of any sort; sanitary engineering and basic hygiene constituted the bulk of its work. In its first month of operation, December 1938, the CBPH formed the Chongqing Municipal Rescue Team (*Chongqingshi jiuhu dui*) for air raid relief; conducted a factory health survey at all factories in the city, many of them newly arrived; surveyed the city's public toilets and planned to build ninety-eight new ones; surveyed the condition of residents' drinking water; made plans for trash incineration and night-soil processing; and requested six hundred vials of cowpox from the NHA and planned the first mass smallpox inoculation (CMA 1938a, 181–189). The new bureau got to work very quickly and was able to mobilize new projects with great efficiency because it enjoyed open communication channels up the chain of command all the way to the Executive Yuan. This, no doubt, was owing to the stature of Director Mei Yilin, who had been appointed by Minister of Health F. C. Yen (Yan Fuqing) and had his trust (CMA 1938b).

The Executive Yuan provided the new bureau with generous seed money for its first annual budget, pledging a total of four hundred thousand yuan to projects planned for 1939. These included financial assistance to the already established Municipal Hospital and operating costs for all branch organizations, as well as funds to found a Sanitation Team, a Lead Cleanliness Team, two health offices, four Maternal and Child Health clinics, an Infectious Disease Hospital, an Opium Addicts' Treatment Hospital, and a health laboratory (CMA 1938a, 182–183). The Nationalist government exhibited interest in the well-being of Chongqing residents—be it genuine, heartfelt empathy or concern for the economic and political viability of the country—by providing ample funding and detailed plans for work that systematically attacked the greatest public health scourges of the day: poor sanitation, infectious disease (with a two-pronged approach of environmental hygiene and medical care), opium addiction, and nonsterile childbirth.

Chongqing public health officials also built new hospitals and medical clinics and refurbished existing ones around the city. A survey of hospital facilities completed in May 1939 by order of Mayor Jiang Zhicheng (蔣志澄) listed only eight hospitals with a minimum capacity of ten patients and equipment up to the standard of the Bureau of Public Health. This gave the city a total of 940 hospital beds, for a population of nearly half a million, or 1.9 sickbeds per thousand population (CMA 1939b). Six months later, through a combination of increased capacity at current hospitals and the establishment of links with new ones, the bureau had nearly doubled its sickbed count, up to 1,824. This gave the wartime capital 4.1 sickbeds per thousand population, precisely double the rate of 2009, when the city proper had 2.1 sickbeds per thousand people (CMA 1939d; Chongqing shi tongji ju 2010, 5, 504). Although the latter number probably suffices for peacetime in an era when most contagious diseases have been nearly eradicated, such data confirms one of the central arguments of this chapter: Nationalist health officials worked effectively and hastily during the war, manifesting a tremendous amount of dedication. Although health conditions remained far from perfect, the relatively smooth function of public health services demonstrates their actual and rhetorical significance to a nation at war.

The Bureau of Public Health also entirely restructured the Chongqing Municipal Hospital (*Chongqing shimin yiyuan*). Bureau director Mei Yilin replaced hospital director Luo Furong (骆付榮), established a new branch location in the Nan'an district, increased its staff, and decreased its sickbeds by over half (so as to move them to other hospitals) (CMA 1939b; CMA 1939c).[2] The hospital's own board of directors had hastened these changes when they asked for a loan of ten thousand yuan from the NHA and the Central Hospital. The NHA did in fact provide this money and also funded its own handpicked staff for the hospital, including the new superintendent.[3] Accepting central government money required accepting its rules.

A look into the Municipal Hospital's records show what pushed the board of directors to ask for this assistance. A handful of merchant-gentry had started the hospital in 1934, but it did not get much business at first, because "most sick people were exceedingly suspicious of the hospital and did not dare to take interest in it." But once the war started and both the central government and thousands of refugees arrived in Chongqing, "the Municipal Hospital began to feel that we could not respond to the need" (CMA n.d.b, 1–2). In other words, the Nationalist government's retreat to Chongqing and the flood of refugees that it unleashed both caused the problem—an overload of patients—and provided its solution in the form of financial assistance and highly trained personnel.

Qi Qingxin (齊清心), the newly appointed superintendent of the Municipal Hospital, belonged to the class of Chinese who fully embraced scientific biomedicine. A forty-five-year-old man from Hebei (born in 1894), Qi was just the sort of man who would never have worked in distant Chongqing in peacetime. He had graduated from Zhili Normal University and Jefferson Medical College in Philadelphia. After a two-and-a-half-year medical internship at Jefferson Hospital in Philadelphia, Qi had served on the faculty of the Peking Union Medical College, as director of the Department of Medicine at Hebei University, and as superintendent of the Hebei Provincial Hospital (CMA n.d.c, 38). He had also written a book on tuberculosis published by the PUMC Hospital in 1925. Eminently qualified and highly paid, Qi brought new expertise and a cosmopolitan perspective on public health administration to the wartime capital's largest state-run hospital.

Other personnel sent from the NHA most likely had similar training; at the very least they had experience in the Central Field Health Station or another NHA affiliate. This meant three things: first, they had professional expertise and, given proper equipment and supplies, the ability to respond to a wide variety of patients' needs; second, they had far more training in scientific biomedicine than in Chinese medicine and would have responded to those needs from a biomedical perspective, shifting the balance of power away from indigenous medicine; and third, as non-locals from other provinces who had often received extensive training overseas, this new group of medical personnel displaced local leaders and instituted a new power structure.

This represented a dramatic shift in medical care in Chongqing. As the late 1938 survey of the capital's medical professionals showed, 39 percent of the biomedical physicians (46 people) and fully 76 percent of the Chinese medicine physicians (237 people) were Sichuan locals (SPA 1939b). Prior to the war era, the vast majority of medical professionals in Chongqing practiced local medicine. Although they certainly could have, and probably did, incorporate practices and knowledge from other medical traditions, Chinese medicine shaped their primary outlook on sickness and healing, and the arrival of physicians, midwives, nurses, and pharmacists with biomedical training changed medical practice in the wartime capital.

The arrival of the Nationalists in Chongqing changed the Municipal Hospital as well: its personnel, administrative structure, and financial situation all experienced an about-face, and the medicine practiced within its walls took a turn toward scientific biomedicine. But the arrival of new personnel from "down-river"—such as Superintendent Qi from Hebei—accorded with the institution's history; the hospital's founders and early funders all came from outside Sichuan, hailing from the Jiangnan region and the provinces of Shaanxi, Guangdong, Zhe-jiang, Fujian, Hubei, and Hunan (CMA n.d.b, 3). They were the prewar downriver sojourners whose native place associations and teahouses gave wartime refugees a home away from home. Between the late Qing years (principally from its estab-lishment as China's westernmost treaty port in 1891) and the early Republic, the majority of skilled workers who had entered new factories built in Chongqing all came from outside the province, hailing from the industrial cities of Tianjin, Shanghai, Ningbo, Changsha, and even Tokyo. The war did not change but rather capitalized on this dynamic, bringing even more out-of-towners into Chongqing who fit into the prewar hierarchy of non-native skilled workers directing local unskilled workers (McIsaac 1994, 18–19).

In addition to giving the Municipal Hospital enough money to continue and even expand its operations, by late 1940 the Chongqing Bureau of Public Health had opened the Anti-Opium Hospital, Trauma Hospital, Infectious Dis-eases Hospital, and Hongji Hospital (*Zhongguo hongji yiyuan*), as well as eight Maternal and Child Health clinics (CMA 1938a, 182; CMA 1940c; CMA 1940f; CMA 1940–1941). The Chinese Red Cross Headquarters had also opened its main Red Cross Hospital in the city, and the Chongqing branch of the Chinese Red Cross opened a branch hospital (CMA 1940f). The city also boasted multiple private hospitals and clinics, as well as three missionary hospitals (CMA 1940f; SPA 1939b). Two other municipal hospitals came much later: in August 1943 the CBPH opened a Tuberculosis Sanatorium, and in May 1944 opened the Maternity Hospital (*Chanfuke yiyuan*), each with thirty sickbeds (CMA 1943a; CMA 1944a, 17, 66). In that same month—May 1944—the NHA opened the Wartime Capital Chinese Medicine Hospital (*Peidu zhongyiyuan*), with thirty staff and an out-patient clinic and inpatient hospital, both of which treated hundreds of patients each month (CMA 1944–1945).

Lack of funding constrained all of the municipally run hospitals, and the financial situation only worsened as the war dragged on and inflation increased.[4] In October 1942, the Bureau of Public Health reported to the municipal govern-ment on the conditions of the Infectious Disease Hospital. Bureau director Mei deftly juggled his resources to accommodate building expansions and seasonal fluctuations despite the inflation that gnawed away at his budget.[5] This type of juggling happened with such frequency that, given incomplete documentation, it is virtually impossible to track Chongqing's hospitals throughout the war period. In the span of a few months, everything about a hospital might change, including its location, its superintendent and other staffing, and how many patients it could accommodate. This happened not only due to financial constraints, as in the case outlined above, but also because of the regular dispersal of the capital's population into the outlying areas to get people out of the line of enemy fire during the air raid season. When Chongqing people moved into the suburbs, the bureau still considered them its charges, and sent mobile medical teams, health clinics, and even entire hospitals out to the "dispersed region" (*shusan qu*) to provide for their medical needs. In August 1940, there were no fewer than six health clinics, six hospitals (including three trauma hospitals, one maternity hospital, one infectious disease hospital, and one missionary hospital), two mobile medical teams, and one sanatorium in this region (CMA 1940a). During the biannual vaccination campaigns conducted every spring and autumn, the bureau also sent roving teams of doctors and nurses into these outlying areas to administer shots to the dispersed population.

Vaccination Campaigns in Chongqing

Very few threats to public health worried state health officials as much as infectious diseases. In 1930, the Ministry of Health identified nine legally notifiable contagious diseases: typhoid, typhus, dysentery, smallpox, plague, cholera, diphtheria, cerebral meningitis, and scarlet fever. A National Health Administration pamphlet published in the very month of the war's outbreak stated that infectious disease caused forty-two of every one hundred deaths each year (Weishengshu 1937, 1–2). During the war years, no effective treatment or vaccine existed for three of the nine notifiable diseases: typhus, plague, and scarlet fever. Health officials repeatedly urged people to get vaccines or preventive shots when they did exist, for typhoid, smallpox, cholera, cerebral meningitis, and diphtheria. As for dysentery, prevention and treatment methods existed but conditions often precluded their effective use. In Chongqing, the Bureau of Public Health conducted mass vaccination campaigns every spring and autumn for both smallpox and cholera/typhoid (the latter diseases were often prevented through the administration of a combined vaccine). As early as December 1938, the bureau made plans for the Municipal Hospital, Bureau of Police, and Household Registration Police (*kouji jing*) to provide free inoculations (CMA 1938a, 189).

Cholera absorbed far more of the local health officials' attention, however, and they made it the top priority for 1939, a year in which the disease appeared in May—arriving on the heels of the city's horrendous May air raids—and had already claimed nearly twenty lives before the bureau could enact the plan it had drawn up for summertime cholera prevention. Once the bureau confirmed that the cholera vibrio had caused these deaths, however, it worked closely with several other organizations to put together a rapid response. The Chongqing Garrison Headquarters decided to implement compulsory vaccinations (*qiangpo zhushe*) across the board; the Bureaus of Public Health and Police organized teams of vaccinators who went door to door giving shots to all residents (almost certainly also done on a mandatory basis); the NHA, along with the CBPH, its treatment clinics, and its Industrial Health Committee, put together a total of forty vaccination teams that gave shots at wharfs, bus stations, teahouses, refugee asylums, and densely inhabited neighborhoods; the CBPH delivered free vaccines to all public and private hospitals, medical clinics, and social organizations throughout the city (bureau personnel went to the latter sites to administer the shots); the Army Medical Administration vaccinated all troops stationed within the city; police inspected all food, drink, and fruit stands throughout the city to ensure that they installed fly screens by June 1 and did not serve any cold foods or drinks or cut-open melons; the CBPH worked closely with the Bureau of Social Affairs, the Central and Municipal Party Bureaus, the Three People's Principles Youth Corps, and the New Life Movement Promotion Committee to produce and disseminate cholera prevention information to the public via leaflets, posters, radio and newspaper announcements, public speeches, and lantern shows; and the municipal government hastily set up a Cholera Hospital that opened its doors on May 25 at a local beggar asylum (CMA 1939a; SPA 1939a).

Unfortunately, other records from 1939 are no longer extant and we cannot ascertain how many people the bureau managed to vaccinate against or otherwise treat for cholera. But the 1939 epidemic convinced health authorities that cholera could come well before summer; the following year, the CBPH had vaccinated over 10,000 people by the end of May, and over 150,000 by the end of September. This method proved effective; in fact, in 1940 both the Chongqing Bureau of Public Health and the National Health Administration reported victory in controlling cholera, with not a single case during the entire year (CMA 1940d; CMA 1940e; King 1941).[6] This is a remarkable success for cash-strapped government offices working out of a new home in the midst of a war.

In 1941, the city once again vaccinated over 150,000 people against cholera, and reported only seven cases of the disease (*Chongqingshi tongji tiyao* 1942, tables 43, 46).[7] In 1943, the next year for which records exist, the CBPH vaccinated over 200,000 residents against cholera and reported no epidemic (CMA 1943b). By the late war years, cholera crept back as inflation soared to new heights and the nation's population remained highly mobile. In 1944 the bureau had planned to administer cholera vaccines to 600,000 people, but early in the year realized its limitations and decreased the plan to half as many (CMA n.d.d; CMA 1944b). In the end, the CBPH inoculated a grand total of 125,753 people, less than half as many again as the decreased plan (CMA 1944a, 15, 25, 50).[8]

Still, these vaccinations averted disaster. In July 1944, the CBPH received word that cholera was spreading in Henan Province as well as in one of Sichuan's neighboring provinces, Yunnan. In mid-August, the CBPH heard rumors that cholera had appeared in yet another neighbor, Guizhou Province, and sent a telegram asking for confirmation. This confirmation did come, and by early October a total of fifty-six cases had been reported in Guiyang, Guizhou's provincial capital. People in Chongqing grew alarmed, and a story spread that two bank employees had contracted cholera and died, but the CBPH investigation proved it to be a false rumor (CMA 1944c). Eventually cholera did appear in Chongqing, killing one Trauma Hospital patient in early November, and several people in the Jiangbei district in mid-November, at which point the CBPH sent personnel out to disinfect the area and force nearby residents to receive vaccines (CMA 1944d). No total annual death toll was reported for cholera, but this handful of cases and the bureau's response suggest that they managed to keep it to a minimum. Not so in 1945. That year, the Bureau of Public Health reported nearly three thousand cases of cholera in the wartime capital, and the dreaded disease returned the following year as well (AH 1946; CMA n.d.a).

Cholera's return to ravage Chongqing in the late and immediate postwar period does not overshadow the outstanding response of local health and relief authorities to the 1939 cholera epidemic, or their success in extinguishing cholera entirely in 1940. The Bureau of Public Health, under the directorship of a man whom his superiors knew and trusted, quickly mobilized people along both vertical and horizontal axes of power, cooperating with the National Health Administration, the local New Life Movement Promotion Committee, local doctors and nurses, and everyone in between. Although central government authorities had dismantled the local power structure upon their arrival, they put in its place a highly effective group of people who worked well together in dire circumstances. Circumstances in rural China differed drastically from those in the wartime capital, and posed many problems for health officials.

Developing Rural Health Care in West China

In the crisis surrounding the Nationalist government's exodus from Nanjing in late 1937, half of the National Health Administration's employees were sent home and never returned to government duty. The main offices were relocated to Chongqing, but several key agencies, including the Central Field Health Station and the Central Hospital, retreated to Guiyang, 330 kilometers away.

By late 1938 the Japanese military had taken control of most major cities in central and southern China. The National Health Administration responded to this situation by dividing the country into three sections. In the occupied battleground areas it aimed to provide immediate medical relief and anti-epidemic work. Within unoccupied China, in the southwestern provinces of Sichuan, Guizhou, and Yunnan, and in the northwestern provinces, the NHA planned to cooperate with provincial governments to develop local health services (ABMAC n.d.b).

The NHA also developed an epidemic prevention corps and a network of highway health stations in the battleground and rear areas. The persistence of smallpox, malaria, typhoid, and dysentery, as well as cholera outbreaks in 1939,

1940, and 1942 and other outbreaks of plague, diphtheria, typhus, and relapsing fever, made an epidemic corps a top priority. The movement of thousands of refugees who sought safety behind enemy lines triggered and exacerbated disease outbreaks. Between 1939 and 1940 the NHA established sixteen highway health stations, each of which approximated a permanent county health center. They had hospitals with thirty-bed wards, outpatient departments, and small diagnostic laboratories. By 1941 this system included forty stations and a staff of eight hundred (ABMAC n.d.c; ABMAC 1941).

The county health system, formally legislated in June 1940, formed the centerpiece of the National Health Administration's wartime work. Each county was to have a health center with a twenty-five- to fifty-bed hospital, an outpatient clinic, a diagnostic laboratory, and programs in maternal and child health, school health, communicable disease control, general sanitation, and vital statistics. Subcenters would cover a population of fifty thousand to one hundred thousand, while village health stations would serve one thousand to five thousand people. Village aides would handle smallpox vaccinations and first aid, report births and deaths, supervise general cleanliness, and carry out propaganda work (ABMAC n.d.a). At the time fourteen provinces boasted a grand total of 691 county health centers, where the NHA carried out sanitary engineering projects, and to which it supplied forty-two senior medical officers and financial subsidies (ABMAC 1941; ABMAC n.d.d).

The county health centers were divided into three grades, and most were third grade, with only one qualified nurse on staff. For example, Guizhou Province had ten first-grade, ten second-grade, and fifty-eight third-grade health centers. Only three of the 78 centers had health aides on their staffs (ABMAC 1942d). Two problems underlay this shortage of personnel: first, since its establishment in 1935 the Public Health Personnel Training Institute had managed to train 1,971 personnel by 1942 for a service that was by then conceived as requiring at least 25,000 trained staff for 780 health centers;[9] second, the centers had insufficient funding to attract and keep qualified personnel, particularly as wartime inflation worsened.

Nevertheless the NHA leaders remained determined to build the system "as a demonstration of organized medical service with the promotion and protection of the health of the mass of people as its ultimate objective" (ABMAC 1942b). Highly trained professionals staffed the wartime NHA, and the Japanese invasion aroused their patriotism. In medical and public health competence they were the equals of the foreign consultants with whom they dealt. They worked long hours in marginal offices while subjected to Japanese bombing raids and malarial infestation.

High-end agencies that the NHA developed during the war included the Epidemic Prevention Bureaus in Kunming and Lanzhou, where scientists developed vaccines and medications that constituted a key component of the preventive

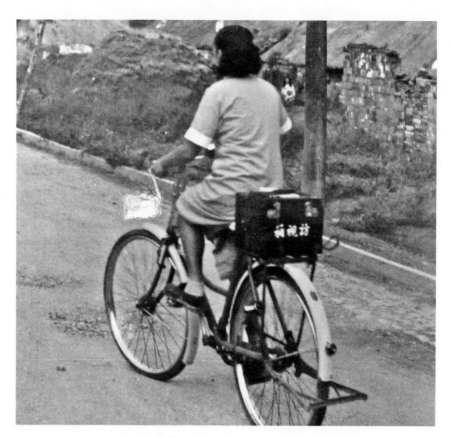

Figure 11.2. Public health nurses such as this one made thousands of home visits by foot, bicycle, rickshaw, and wheelbarrow. *Source:* ABMAC Archives.

health strategy. In August 1943 Jin Baoshan reported that the two bureaus could meet a large part of China's needs provided that materials needed for biological production could be procured in large quantities. By autumn 1944 the bureaus produced most vaccines and sera needed for epidemic prevention—a remarkable development in the midst of Operation Ichigo, the blistering Japanese military campaign that drove down through central into southwestern China (ABMAC 1944a; ABMAC 1944b).

The National Institute of Health promoted the public health care agenda at the national level. Formed around 1941 in Chongqing to consolidate the work of the Central Field Health Station, the Public Health Personnel Training Institute, and the management of model county health services, the National Institute of Health presents a picture of the ups and downs that the National Health Administration encountered during the Japanese war. Its research departments aimed to demonstrate that certain public health services were essential to national reconstruction (ABMAC 1942a). A study of vital statistical data in the Dingjia rural district in Bishan county, Sichuan, found that 41 percent of the admittedly small sample (227 cases) died before the age of six, and that the mean age of death was a little over twenty-nine years. These results reflected the discovery that 234 out of 266 births (88 percent) were unattended by any midwife—old-style or new (RAC 1945b).[10] This finding provided a corrective to the assumption that the unsanitary practices of old-style midwives were solely responsible for the serious maternal and child health problems in China.

The troubles that the National Institute of Health endured resulted in large part from circumstances beyond the control of its staff. In a 1945 report on problems with the Bishan Health Demonstration Center, the NIH noted paltry results because in five years the county magistrate had changed five times. With such turnover, the county would never assume fiscal responsibility for the NIH subsidy. But in Shapingba, a demonstration district near Chongqing, where the NIH registered over twelve thousand home visits in 1945, all types of home services reportedly showed a marked improvement in quality and quantity as compared with 1944 (RAC 1945a) (see figure 11.2).

Provincial Initiatives in West China

Provincial health administrations, such as those of Sichuan and Guizhou Provinces featured here, supervised public health care at the county level. An account by the Guizhou health commissioner Dr. Yao Kefang (姚克方), compiled in 1942, indicates that before 1937, two trained sanitary inspectors working for the Civil Affairs Bureau ran all health administration in Guizhou. The Provincial Health Committee, established in April 1938, built health stations in nearly every county throughout the province by late 1940. Guizhou suffered from approximately eight hundred thousand malaria cases and eighty thousand malaria deaths each year, so the Provincial Health Committee established an antimalaria corps in 1938. This grew into a full anti-epidemic institute in 1941, with one experimental and six field stations, and six mobile anti-epidemic units. Cholera epidemics in 1938, 1939, and 1942 kept these units busy. The province completed a water system for Guiyang in 1940, and it operated ten delousing stations (ABMAC 1942d). Guizhou's public health care system vigorously addressed the epidemic problems facing the province, and began developing a cadre of trained nurses and midwives and a modern municipal sanitary system.

A 1943 report for Guizhu county, just south of the provincial capital of Guiyang, shows insight into the challenges of introducing public health care in rural southwest China. This community of 166,819 possessed a university college, two middle schools, and an anti-aircraft training school, but still had a low literacy rate of only 15 percent, and locals believed in folklore and witchcraft. Popular fears made it difficult to administer vaccines; only 9 percent of the people were vaccinated against smallpox and 10 percent against cholera. Many maternal deaths occurred during childbirth because the women were "too illiterate or shy" to come to health stations for attention. The hilly terrain made it difficult to move out beyond ten kilometers from substations except in the instance of an epidemic or difficult delivery. Large numbers of schoolchildren suffered from trachoma. However, as a field training center for the medical colleges in Guiyang, the county offered rich opportunities for teaching the principles of public health care. The director, a physician from Hong Kong with advanced degrees in public health, was highly qualified to direct this task (ABMAC 1943).[11] Since both medical colleges in Guiyang were committed to improving public health care, their students graduated with significant knowledge in this field of medicine.

Sichuan organized the most ambitious campaign to promote public health care during the War of Resistance. This was not surprising since the health commissioner, Chen Zhiqian (C. C. Chen), had been an advocate of public health care since his student days at the Peking Union Medical College. In a summary of his work written in 1945, Chen pointed out that as long as transportation was so backward and ignorance so common, one could not hope for spectacular progress in public health, particularly since the Nationalists regarded it a matter of "theoretical and remote importance" (RAC n.d.c).[12] In other words, the top Nationalist leadership did not understand or care about the importance of public health to national strength and security. Nevertheless, by the end of the war 131 out of 137 counties in Sichuan had a rudimentary health organization, and the county services employed 122 fully qualified doctors, nurses, midwives, engineers, and laboratory technicians (RAC n.d.c). These centers collected enough data to emphasize the importance of sanitary engineering for public health, which Chen believed to be more important than advanced medical knowledge.

Maternal and child health also progressed significantly. The infant mortality rate in Sichuan, at about 126.5 per thousand, compared favorably with rates in Beijing and Nanjing. But MCH stations could reduce the infant death rate to about 73, and Chen increased the number of stations from one in 1939 to forty-four in 1945 (RAC n.d.c). In times of inflation public health training suffered by comparison with clinical training, which led to more prosperous careers. This, more than anything else, bothered Chen, who bemoaned the fact that because of inflation "all normal thinking stopped"; civilization of a higher order crumbled under the pressure of everyday needs and the craving for money.

Chen serves as an example of how health care survived and even thrived in the war period thanks to the dedication of individuals like him: idealists determined to strengthen their country through public health care. Earlier accounts have implied that health care reformers did not accomplish much in the tumultuous war years, but close examination of the documents reveals a different interpretation. Chinese medicine reformers demonstrated their importance to the state at a time when their country needed them the most, laying the groundwork for the incorporation of Chinese medicine in the Communist period. Health reformers also began the process of getting communicable diseases under control and tackling the terrible mortality in the realm of maternal and child health. It would take decades to educate enough nurses and midwives to handle this problem, but the groundwork was laid at this extraordinary time when war was shaking China to its foundations.

Notes

1. Mei attended Nankai Middle School in Tianjin, Qinghua University in Beijing, Rush Medical College in Chicago, and Johns Hopkins University in Baltimore.

2. In June 1938, minister of health F. C. Yen (Yan Fuqing) ordered the Chongqing municipal government to make many of these changes (CMA 1938c).

3. In 1939, the Bureau of Public Health transferred thirty thousand yuan in financial assistance to the Municipal Hospital from the Executive Yuan (CMA 1938a, 182–183).

4. For example, in 1944 the Trauma Hospitals exceeded their budget by over seventy-six thousand yuan (CMA 1945).

5. For an example, see CMA (1942).

6. King reported that the NHA had inoculated two and a half million people against cholera between the beginning of the war in July 1937 and May 1941 (King 1941, 2). For an analysis of the gender implications of this vaccination campaign, see Barnes (2012a).

7. The gender differential in these vaccinations is huge: 113,513 men and 37,356 women were vaccinated.

8. The bureau inoculated 46,165 people between January and March; 55,722 between July and September; and 23,866 between October and December. No numbers were reported for April–June, the high vaccination season. The bureau also reported its own grand total, from October 1943 through late November 1944, of 146,904 cholera vaccine recipients and 9,817 mixed cholera-typhoid vaccine recipients (CMA 1944a, 79).

9. Number trained is from ABMAC (1942c); number of trainees desired is from ABMAC (1942a).

10. The child mortality rate did not differ greatly from the 45 percent death rate of children by the age of five reported by the NHA at an international conference in 1937. But the 1937 report was based on conjecture, whereas the Bishan finding was based on actual data.

11. The author of the report was Dr. Sze Tsung-sing (Shi Zhengxin 施正信), director of the county health station and chair of the Department of Public Health at National Guiyang Medical College ("Tsung Sing TZE" 1997).

12. Chen's annual reports, available in the Rockefeller Archive, provide a detailed picture of his work as Sichuan commissioner of health during the War of Resistance against Japan, and of his philosophical commitment to public health work.

12 The Institutionalization of Chinese Medicine

Volker Scheid and Sean Hsiang-lin Lei

THE COMMUNIST VICTORY in the Civil War of 1945–1949 and the proclamation of the People's Republic in October 1949 did not augur well for the future of Chinese medicine as an independent medical tradition. Under the slogan "co-operation of Chinese and Western medicine" (*zhongxiyi hezuo*), the Communist Party (CCP) in Yan'an had utilized Chinese medicine to gain the support of the rural population and to meet health care needs in settings where Western drugs and technological resources were scarce. Ideologically, however, the party's leadership was committed to establishing a health care system modeled on the West, particularly Russia, in which there was little room for a medicine considered to be a remnant of feudal society and its irrational superstitions. In Nationalist-controlled areas, meanwhile, the Chinese-medical infrastructure created during the 1920s and '30s had been all but dismantled (Deng 1999, 176–191). And yet, less than ten years later a large-scale effort was underway to rebuild Chinese medicine as a modern tradition that would make a unique contribution to the health care of China and even the world. On October 11, 1958, Mao Zedong famously declared Chinese medicine to be "a great treasure-house" and demanded that its resources be forcefully developed. Another quarter of a century later, in 1982, the principle of "paying equal attention to Chinese and Western medicine" was enshrined in the PRC Constitution. Ever since, the country has enjoyed the fruits and problems of an officially plural health care system. (For foundational accounts of Chinese medicine in contemporary China, see Cai, Li, and Zhang 1999; Meng 1999; Taylor 2004; Wang and Cai 1999; Zhang 1994; Zhen and Fu 1991.)

The process that led to the creation of this system was neither linear nor the outcome of a well thought-out master plan. Rather, it was "the product of an undetermined and piecemeal process" (Taylor 2004, 151). The emergence of plural health care in contemporary China thus might be said to mirror the tortuous, painful, and frequently contradictory path the country itself has taken into the present. For this reason alone, narrating the history of Chinese medicine in contemporary China is best accomplished by linking it to that of the wider body politic of the country.

This narrative can be divided into six periods, although no fixed boundaries exist between them: (1) the period from 1911 to 1948, during which practitioners of Chinese medicine organized the National Medicine Movement to resist the oppressive regulation attempted by the state and strove to assimilate Chinese medicine into the emerging national system of health care and education, (2) the period from 1949 to 1953, which was characterized by attempts to subsume Chinese medicine into a biomedically dominated health care system; (3) the period from 1954 to 1965, during which the CCP, under the direction of Mao Zedong, switched to a policy of supporting the development of Chinese medicine and its institutional infrastructure; (4) the period from 1966 to 1976, which includes the Cultural Revolution, when activity in the field of Chinese medicine contracted under the guidance of ideological simplification; (5) the immediate post-Maoist era, which lasted from to Mao Zedong's death on September 9, 1976, to the Tiananmen Massacre in 1989, spanning the feverish decade of the 1980s, when not only the field of Chinese medicine exploded once more into a myriad of options and possibilities; and (6) the period from 1989 to the present, during which Chinese medicine has been guided toward integration into the technoscientific networks of a global health care system.

Viewed against the development of Chinese medicine over a longer period, the most noteworthy feature on which to focus in narrating Chinese medicine's development in contemporary China is not its ongoing encounter with the West, but rather the fact that, for the first time since the Song dynasty, the state now assumed direct and deliberate responsibility for regulating the field of medicine. In doing so, it fundamentally transformed the alignment of all other agents in this field, as well as curtailed the degree of movement available to them.

1911–1949

It is a great irony that the turning point in the modern history of Chinese medicine was an event that was meant to put an end to it. In 1928, amidst civil war, social unrest, and foreign occupation, the Nationalist Party (Guomindang) finally terminated the political chaos of the Warlord period (1916–1928) and formed a new government for China. Even though the Nationalist Party controlled only certain regions of the country, the regime nevertheless dedicated itself to the project of state building and to an agenda of radical modernization. As health care came to be accepted as an important part of the government's modernizing ambitions, the Nationalist Party established the Ministry of Health in the new capital of Nanjing. With the exception of the Song dynasty (960–1279) (Goldschmidt 2009), this was the first time that China had a national administrative center to take charge of all issues related to health care. In the next year, the First National Health Conference, which was dominated by practitioners of Western medicine, unanimously passed a proposal to abolish the practice of Chinese medicine. To the great surprise of almost everyone concerned, this resolution mobilized the previously unorganized practitioners of Chinese medicine into a massive National Medicine Movement (*guoyi yundong*), formally instigating a decade-long collective struggle between the two factions of medical practitioners (Lei 1999).

Largely drafted by Yu Yan (1879–1954, also known as Yu Yunxiu), the proposal passed at this conference required traditional practitioners to register with the government and to attend government-sponsored supplementary education courses in order to continue practicing medicine. Registration would end on the last day of 1930, and the supplementary classes would be offered for only five years. Traditional practitioners were not allowed to organize schools, advertise in the papers, or spread propaganda through traditional medical associations for the promotion of traditional medicine. Since traditional doctors would run out of legitimate ways to train the next generation within five years, the ultimate goal of the proposal clearly was the abolition of Chinese medicine.

Ironically, Yu's proposal provoked practitioners of Chinese medicine into organizing themselves into a national association, thereby turning traditional Chinese medicine into a national entity. In order to mobilize a mass protest against Yu's proposal, practitioners of Chinese medicine in Shanghai organized a national assembly starting on March 17, 1929. The protest was first organized by the All-China Medical and Pharmaceutical Associations (*Shenzhou yiyao zonghui*), which had organized the earlier campaign aimed at assimilating schools of traditional medicine into the educational system in 1913. Facing the threat of abolition, 262 delegates representing 131 organizations attended a three-day convention at the General Chamber of Commerce in Shanghai. More than two thousand practitioners of Chinese medicine closed their clinics for half a day to support this demonstration. More than anything else, what exhilarated the participants in this conference was the simple fact that they were gathering under one roof and serving as representatives of a national assembly. To consolidate this alliance, a new organization was created, the National Federation of Medical and Pharmaceutical Associations (NFMPA). Under the federation, branches were established at the provincial, county, and district levels. Within three years, the number of member associations increased from 242 to 518, including affiliates in Hong Kong, the Philippines, and Singapore. Thanks to Yu's proposal, an international network of Chinese medical practitioners was constructed.

To emphasize the point that their objective was not to preserve Chinese medicine as a "cultural essence" of traditional China, representatives of this assembly voted to change the official name of their profession from "Chinese medicine" (*zhongyi*) to "National medicine" (*guoyi*). Symbolically, the first day of the demonstration in support of traditional medicine, March 17, was designated as *guoyijie* (National Medicine Day) and was observed by supporters of Chinese medicine every year until the Communists took over China. Oppressed as a group by the state, traditional doctors in response strove to organize themselves into a national group. The name "National Medicine Day" testified that the modern history of Chinese medicine began on March 17, 1929, when traditional practitioners as a group encountered the first modern Chinese state.

When the Nationalist Government established the semiofficial Institute of National Medicine on March 17, 1931, it at once symbolized and embodied the vision of "national medicine" that had been developed since the 1929 confrontation. First of all, the Institute of National Medicine reinforced the vision that the objective of this movement was to make Chinese medicine thrive alongside the modern state, rather than preserve it as an authentic cultural essence of traditional China. Moreover, as traditional practitioners struggled to turn the Institute of National Medicine into an administrative branch of the state in charge of regulating the affairs of Chinese medicine, they strove to make Chinese medicine a part of the educational and health care system of modern China. On the other hand, the Nationalist government had identified the central objective of the Institute of National Medicine as "to use scientific methods to put into order Chinese medicine and to improve therapeutics and the manufacture of pharmaceuticals." Generally referred to as the "scientization of Chinese medicine" (*Zhongyi kexuehua*), the institute's official objective forcefully imposed upon Chinese medicine the dominant ideology of scientism and thereby shaped the development of Chinese medicine in the twentieth century.

While practitioners of Western medicine demanded a wholesale abolition of Chinese medicine, they enthusiastically supported conducting scientific research on Chinese herbs, which were perceived to be the raw materials of nature. This interest in Chinese drugs was partially influenced by the Japanese tradition of pharmacological research on Chinese *materia medica*, but more directly it was inspired by the world-famous discovery at the Peking Union Medical College of the drug ephedrine for asthma relief, from the Chinese herb mahuang. K. K. Chen and Carl F. Schmidt co-authored their original paper on ephedrine in 1924; within five years, research on mahuang had grown into a small industry, resulting in the publication of five hundred research papers on ephedrine all over the world. To summarize this enormous amount of research, Chen and Schmidt then co-authored a 117-page review article, titled "Ephedrine and Related Substances," in the 1930 issue of the *American Journal of Medicine* (Chen and Schmidt 1930). Thanks to the ephedrine discovery, the investigation of Chinese drugs became a nationally recognized research priority, a development that paved the way for what the American Association for the Advancement of Science characterized in 1960 as "the exalted position of pharmacology" in Communist China (Way 1961, 364). Moreover, in 2011 a study of Chinese drugs won the most prestigious medical research award ever bestowed on Chinese scientists: the Lasker Award, nicknamed "America's Nobel Prize," was granted for the discovery of artemisinin, for the treatment of malaria, from the Chinese drug qinghao.

The National Medicine Movement was neither a passive movement of resistance nor a conservative movement aimed at preserving a fragile tradition. While it is conventionally remembered as a response of resistance against the governmental threat of "abolishing Chinese medicine"—and the government indeed kept proposing other hostile regulations after the confrontation in March 1929—nevertheless, for proponents of this movement the core of their struggle was not resistance toward the state but the pursuit of new professional interests that had been created and sanctioned by the modern state. It is beyond doubt that state intervention did pose a serious challenge to Chinese medicine; nevertheless, the newborn Nationalist state opened a whole new horizon of possibilities which were never accessible to traditional practitioners before the Republican period. As the Chinese counterpart of the privileged Western medical profession, practitioners of Chinese medicine strove for the following from the state: (1) an official state organ run by themselves, (2) a state-sanctioned license system, and (3) the incorporation of Chinese medicine into the national school system. The Nationalist Party Congress passed a resolution demanding "equal treatment for Chinese and Western medicine" in 1935; the following year, the government promulgated the Regulations for Chinese Medicine. In addition, the Ministry of Education promulgated the Temporary Outline for the Curriculum of Schools of Chinese Medicine in 1939. Practitioners of Chinese medicine, at least on paper, had achieved an "equal" legal status to that of practitioners of Western medicine, although none of these regulations had been put into practice when the Sino-Japanese War broke out in 1937. Paradoxically, the alliance between the state and Western medicine, which caused the most severe challenge to Chinese medicine, also enabled Chinese medicine to transform itself into a prestigious modern profession contributing to the official knowledge of the state. In this sense, it is ironic that biomedical doctors not only posed the most serious threat to Chinese medicine, but they also introduced the unprecedented possibility of collective upward mobility to practitioners of Chinese medicine. The new status of Nanjing as the state capital, and the associated potential for collective social mobility, are essential for understanding the modern history of Chinese medicine.

1949–1953

When Mao Zedong proclaimed the establishment of the People's Republic on October 1, 1949, he did so as a figurehead of a movement able to project its will and its dreams onto the entire country. From this position of strength the CCP set out to deliberately shape both the overall structure of the health care system and the role and relations of its individual components. In practice, these efforts were oriented by "four great guiding principles" formulated during the First and Second National Health Conferences in 1950 and 1951: (1) medicine had to serve the working people, (2) preventive medicine programs were to be given priority over curative ones, (3) Chinese medicine was to be united with Western medicine, and (4) health programs were to be integrated with mass movements (Cai, Li, and Zhang 1999, 6). How these principles were to be translated into practice was not specified, however. As a consequence, concrete policies were shaped by complex power struggles among political factions in the CCP and the Ministry of Health over such translations. Broadly speaking, while the Ministry of Health was dominated by biomedical physicians who favored modernization along Western—and specifically Soviet—models of professional health care, the CCP under the leadership of Mao Zedong favored prevention, mass campaigns, and the subordination of professional knowledge to revolutionary ideals (Lampton 1977; Taylor 2004).

The new slogan "unify Chinese and Western medicine" (*zhongxiyi tuanjie*)—coined by Mao Zedong, but flexible enough to accommodate different interpretations—thus governed health care policy involving Chinese medicine in the early 1950s. Pragmatically, it allowed the sizable manpower of the Chinese medicine sector—estimated at around three hundred thousand physicians in 1949—to be recruited into the official health care system, specifically to the mass action programs favored by Mao Zedong. For this purpose, Chinese medicine physicians were taught to administer vaccinations and provide other basic medical care. In return, they were granted the right to practice, provided they could demonstrate some basic proficiency in biomedical knowledge. There was no intention, however, of extending this right indefinitely, or of creating a separate space for Chinese medicine within the overall health care system. Rather, it was to be assimilated into a "new medicine" (*xinyi*) that would once and for all remove existing divisions in the field of medicine (Wang and Cai 1999, 5–10).

Utopian visions of a "new medicine" to arise from the fusion of East and West, science and tradition, had constituted a recurring theme in the writings of a wide spectrum of reformist physicians from the late 1920s onward (Lei 1999). At the conservative end, scholar physicians like Qin Bowei (1929) or Ding Zhongying (1936) thought of "scientization" as systematization. For them, making Chinese medicine more "scientific" meant uniting the many competing currents within Chinese medicine into one medical system while, at the same time, effectively enhancing the value of its core doctrines. More radical modernizers like Lu Yuanlei (1934) and Zhang Cigong (Zhu 2000), on the other hand, were critical of what they viewed as the unscientific and mystical nature of Chinese medical learning. For them, the real value of Chinese medicine lay in the experience (*jingyan*) of generations of physicians embodied in classical formulas, diagnostic techniques, and styles of medical practice, all of which might be analyzed by and integrated with scientific (that is, Western) medicine (Lei 2002; Lai 2003).

In the political climate of the early 1950s, it was this latter position that resonated most closely with the thinking of leading Ministry of Health bureaucrats at the time—including then–vice minister He Cheng (1901–1992) (Yu and Zu 2006), a government department in which Chinese medicine lacked any official representation at the time. If the ministry had to bend to the official party line regarding the union of Chinese and biomedicine, a line that many of its members implicitly and sometimes explicitly opposed, it sought, at the very least, to ensure that Chinese medicine was thoroughly reformed and scientized (Lampton 1977; Taylor 2004). This is apparent in the focus on acupuncture and Chinese medicinals that dominates medical research during this period. Acupuncture was perceived as being both uniquely Chinese *and* explainable by Pavlovian neuropathology—a Soviet and therefore politically correct way to do science. Chinese medicinals, on the other hand, could be framed in nationalistic terms as constituting the concrete embodiment of the Chinese people's experience in their struggle against disease. Furthermore, strategies for translating such experience into biomedical practice and thereby separating it from traditional doctrines had been developed since the 1930s.

Working outward from such concrete research efforts, it was decided to apply the same strategies of scientization to Chinese medicine as a whole. The First National Health Conference proposed that Chinese medical research centers be established throughout the country, although it took until 1955 for this policy to be actually implemented (Lampton 1977). Leading strategists within the Ministry of Health also deemed it "not too late to train large numbers of new physicians possessing both adequate levels of scientific training and experience as replacements" for traditionally educated physicians once they had outlived their pragmatic usefulness (Cui 1997, 218). Between August 1950 and December 1951, the new government thus passed a series of laws that redefined the entitlement to practice Chinese medicine. Licenses were granted only to those physicians who had graduated from a college in Republican China, or who had passed one of the national licensing examinations that had been sporadically carried out during this period. The new laws thereby prevented all self-trained physicians, as well as those educated within traditional master/disciple relationships, from continuing to practice.

In 1952, a new licensing examination was introduced. Because it tested mainly Western medical knowledge, the failure rate was so high that it excluded the majority of Chinese medicine practitioners (Wang and Cai 1999, 8). In many cases physicians were able to exploit legislative loopholes and carry on as before. But a significant number did give up their practices. As a consequence, in a city like

Shanghai, which still had the most vigorous Chinese medical infrastructure, the number of Chinese medicine physicians decreased by around 11 percent between 1949 and 1953 (Wang 1998, 68; Zhang and Shao 1998, 137).

At the same time, the government began to organize the large-scale reeducation of practicing Chinese medicine physicians through so-called "Chinese Medicine Improvement Schools" (*Zhongyi jinxiu xuexiao*). The purpose of these schools, which continued to function until the end of the decade, was to raise the level of biomedical knowledge and political awareness among Chinese medicine physicians. They succeeded in familiarizing physicians who previously had no understanding of Western medicine with its main concepts and ideas, and thereby paved the way for the integration of Chinese and biomedicines at the institutional level during subsequent decades. In addition, a number of young but already established physicians were selected on the basis of competitive examinations to study Western medicine for five years (Cai, Li, and Zhang 1999, 87; Taylor 1999; Wang and Cai 1999, 86–87).

The intended unification of Chinese and Western medicine had clear political functions, too, inasmuch as Western medicine was perceived to be a tool with which to remedy the ideological shortcomings of traditional physicians. Mao Zedong, for instance, stated during a meeting of the CCP Central Committee in 1953 that, in the course of uniting the two medicines, "Western medicine definitely must smash the sectarianism [of Chinese medicine]" (Cui 1997, 155). As with so much else, in opposing the real diversity of Chinese medicine with the imagined unity of biomedicine Mao and the CCP enacted well-established perceptions of tradition, science, and the modern, even as they were bending them toward new ends. The existence of diverse currents of practice in Chinese medicine was widely recognized at least since the Jin-Yuan dynasties and was seen as a necessary condition of clinical effectiveness. At the same time, the implicit challenge of such diversity to the unity of orthodox tradition made it forever suspicious to large sections of the elite. In the early twentieth century, such established tropes were readily employed by modernizers such as Liang Shuming (1893–1988) in his juxtaposition of Western and Chinese medicine:

> What is referred to as medicine in China is in fact [nothing but] craft. Prescribing in Western medicine proceeds on the basis of matching specific diseases with specific prescriptions [so that there is] little variation [among individual physicians' treatment]. The highest-caliber Chinese physicians however rely on context and individual ability in writing out their formulas. Ten different physicians will thus write out ten different formulas that can, moreover, be extremely different [from each other]. (Liang 2002 [1921]

In that sense, reeducating Chinese physicians was not merely an effort at helping them to become modern but the continuation of an age-old preoccupation with containing the dangers of heterodoxy. Economically, too, the state began to undermine the independence of the Chinese medicine sector and to assimilate its physicians into state-controlled institutions. Chinese medicine was initially excluded from the country's new national insurance scheme, although the government established a number of Chinese medicine clinics for party cadres. The government also encouraged physicians to give up their private practices and join into larger cooperative clinics (*lianhe zhensuo*). While private practice was fully abolished only in 1966, the number of physicians in private practice in Shanghai, for instance, had already declined from 3,308 in 1948 to about 1,000 in 1965 (Wang 1998, 68–70; Zhang and Shao 1998, 140). Yet, as the following example demonstrates, these transformations at the level of the institutional infrastructure were facilitated by other types of continuities, extending back to the early Republican period and beyond, that demonstrate both the support of Chinese physicians, specifically those in urban centers, for early Maoist reforms and their ability to flexibly adjust to changing socioeconomic and political realities.

One of the first Chinese Medicine Improvement Schools (*Zhongyi jinxiu xuexiao*) in the entire country was established in Shanghai, following a meeting on January 19, 1951, attended by over one hundred physicians. The meeting was chaired by Ding Jimin (1912–1979), grandson of the famous Ding Ganren (1860–1926), who in 1916 had founded the Shanghai Technical College of Chinese Medicine (*Shanghai Zhongyi zhuanye xuexiao*), the most influential Chinese medical school in Republican China, and Lu Yuanlei (1894–1955), one of the most outspoken modernizers of that period. In 1952, the same group of physicians also assumed a leading role in establishing the Chinese Medicine Outpatient Clinic directly subordinated to the Shanghai Municipal Bureau of Health (*Shanghaishi weishengju zhenshu zhongyi menzhensuo*). Organized to serve the health care needs of party cadres, the clinic merged the private practices of leading Shanghai physicians into one single institution. The clinic had six departments—internal medicine, gynecology, external medicine, pediatrics, acumoxa, and traumatology—and functioned until September 1955 when it moved to new premises and changed its name to Shanghai City Public Health Care Outpatient Clinic No. 5 (*Shanghaishi gongfei yiliao diwu menzhenbu*). By that time, Lu Yuanlei had died while Ding Jimin had been promoted to the position of deputy director of the No. 11 People's Hospital (*dishiyi renmin yiyuan*). The hospital was controlled by the same party unit as the No. 5 clinic, and had been established in 1954 as the first Chinese medicine hospital in Communist Shanghai. It had 150 beds, and its physicians, many of whom were Ding Ganren's most influential disciples, treated over a thousand outpatients a day.

1954–1965

Contemporary Chinese histories of the period claim that the CCP has always taken a principled stance to protect and promote the development of Chinese medicine. In fact, this position only emerged in the years between 1954 and 1956. Furthermore, it did not reflect a conscious policy shift; rather, it was the outcome of a series of events that led to and fed off each other in ways that were not planned but which eventually provided Chinese medicine with an institutional infrastructure and framework of clinical practice that endures to this day. The origins of these developments can be traced to shifts in the balance of power between "reds" and "experts" within the health care sector.

As previously explained, the Ministry of Health in the early 1950s was largely run by biomedical physicians whose policies were guided by professional rather than ideological agendas and who resisted political control by the center. Beginning in the mid-1950s, the CCP leadership became increasingly unwilling to tolerate such autonomy but emphasized the importance of adhering to party policies. In the ensuing political struggles, attitudes favoring Chinese medicine initially appear to have been nothing more than a convenient stick with which to beat the biomedical professionals dominating the Ministry of Health. Beginning in 1953, the ministry was accused of a lack of leadership, and this escalated in July 1954 into an outright attack by Mao Zedong himself on the ministry's policies vis-à-vis Chinese medicine. Mao went as far as threatening the abolishment of any department that would fail to successfully implement policies regarding the unification of Chinese and biomedicines (Lampton 1977). By September 1954 Liu Shaoqi pronounced that "despising Chinese medicine is servile and subservient bourgeois thinking" (Cai, Li, and Zhang 1999). In 1955, First Vice Minister He Cheng himself was dismissed, following a public confession in the *People's Daily* in which he admitted to having opposed Chinese medicine because he "was divorced from Party leadership" (Lampton 1977).

As a consequence, Chinese medicine was increasingly accorded value in its own right. It was accepted into the national insurance scheme, and in October 1954 the Culture Department of the CCP Central Committee made recommendations regarding the improvement and strengthening of Chinese medicine that included the establishment of an Academy of Chinese Medicine (*Zhongyi yanjiuyuan*), the integration of Chinese medicine into the larger hospitals, and a general expansion of the scope of Chinese medical work.

Overall, however, the larger goal of creating a new society and a new medicine still guided this reevaluation of Chinese medicine. Mao Zedong noted that the experience of the preceding years demonstrated the mistaken assumptions underlying current policies. He then changed course and reversed the roles of student and teacher. From then on, emphasis was to be placed on Western medicine physicians studying Chinese medicine. Those physicians who, through their studies and commitment, would "abolish the boundaries between Chinese and Western medicine" would thenceforth form the spearhead of the new medicine (Cui 1997, 155). Mao Zedong's goal at this stage most definitely was not to ensure the survival of Chinese medicine as an independent tradition. Rather, he was trying to subordinate Western medicine to Chinese medicine in an attempt to ensure adherence to the party line throughout the health care sector, not only within the Ministry of Health but also at lower-level institutions. To this end, to force doctors from the two traditions to work together in order to create, eventually, a medicine of China capable of serving as a world medicine was a convenient test of where physicians' loyalties lay (Taylor 2000, 112).

At Mao's specific behest, young doctors of Western medicine from all over the country were summoned to Beijing in 1955 to be reeducated in the first experimental class of Western medicine doctors studying Chinese medicine (*diyijie xiyi xuexi zhongyi yanjiu ban*). Many of these young physicians, who shared with other intellectuals a perception of Chinese medicine as old and backward, were none too pleased about this invitation (Ma 1993, 583–584). Later, however, the considerable status associated with this class allowed many of its graduates to advance into influential positions within the Chinese medical sector. Eminent Chinese medicine physicians from all over China, particularly from Sichuan and Jiangsu, were likewise called to Beijing as teachers and advisors to the Ministry of Health. The resulting concentration of senior practitioners in Beijing not only facilitated the establishment there of the Academy of Chinese Medicine in 1955, but also located these physicians much closer to China's new political center of power (Zhongguo kexue jishu xiehui 1991).

Following Beijing's lead, classes of various duration and quality were soon established throughout the whole of China for Western medicine doctors studying Chinese medicine. These Chinese medicine courses were integrated into the curriculum of Western medicine universities, colleges, and schools. By 1960, thirty-seven full-time courses had trained more than 2,300 physicians, while an additional 36,000 Western medical doctors had received training in Chinese medicine even as they continued to carry out their medical duties (Cai, Li, and Zhang 1999, 14). Physicians of Chinese medicine were also admitted to existing Western medicine hospitals and clinics, and new hospitals of Chinese medicine were established. This strengthening of Chinese medicine's role within the health care sector was reflected in a new alignment between Western and Chinese medicine, and was expressed in the slogan, "Chinese medicine must become scientific, Western medicine must become Chinese" (*zhongyi yao kexuehua, xiyi yao zhongguohua*) (Ma 1993, 575).

The "integration of Chinese and Western medicine" (*zhongxiyi jiehe*)—a concept initially developed by Mao Zedong in 1956 to describe the second attempt at creating a new medicine in China—thus guided CCP policy from the mid-1950s onward. Unification of both medicines remained the ultimate goal, but it was accepted that this would take longer than previously estimated. Chinese medicine physicians and their supporters, sensing that the political mood had changed, seized the moment in order to lobby for the establishment of an independent Chinese medicine sector. Their campaign received a major boost in 1956 with the founding of four Chinese Medicine colleges (*zhongyi xueyuan*) in Chengdu, Beijing, Guangzhou, and Shanghai. Resources were made available for developing an administrative infrastructure charged with supervising the research, education, and practice of Chinese medicine at both the national and provincial levels. By 1961, tertiary colleges, research institutes, and teaching hospitals could be found throughout the country (Liu and Cui 1990; Zhu and Zhang 1990).

This sudden and vigorous expansion of the Chinese medicine sector caused new problems for policymakers. The most urgent involved manpower. Relying only on physicians graduated from the new colleges would have meant scaling back the ambitious scope of the program. The government therefore decided to revitalize the traditional apprenticeship system, despite its associations with feudal ideology and society. Beginning in 1957, selected students were assigned to established physicians of Chinese medicine, and special classes were set up in order to supplement such apprenticeship training with lessons in theory, Western medicine, and politics. As a result, the number of physicians of Chinese medicine increased rapidly in both rural and urban areas. In Shanghai, for instance, it almost doubled in the course of less than ten years, though this number still lagged behind the even more rapid growth of the Western medicine sector (Wang and Cai 1999, 86–95).

If it was the state that had engineered this expansion, it was also the state that decided the direction it would take. Through a series of loosely connected initiatives that have continued to define the identity of Chinese medicine up to the present, the development of Chinese medicine was thereby integrated into the CCP's more comprehensive project of nation building and socialist modernization. Though these initiatives differed in their aim and scope, their common denominator was the simplification, regularization, and systematization of traditional modes of practice. New national textbooks and teaching materials compiled under the direct supervision of the Ministry of Health attempted to condense the often contradictory information contained in classical texts into a more coherent system, while translating their content into modern Chinese. The goal was to detach learning from the idiosyncratic interpretations, experiences, and habits of individual teachers, and provide all students with equal access to the resources of tradition. As a consequence, even as they claimed to represent the accumulated knowledge of the past, these textbooks delineated Chinese medicine in an entirely new fashion.

Some commentators view this reorganization as so radical that they speak of a paradigm shift separating today's "traditional Chinese medicine" (TCM) from the scholarly medical tradition of old. Others, including the majority of Chinese medicine physicians, emphasize continuity and view modern reorganizations of learning and practice as merely another stage in the ongoing development of tradition. Both sides agree, however, that the model that organizes and, by implication, epitomizes contemporary Chinese medical practice is *bianzheng lunzhi*, or "pattern differentiation and treatment determination."

Bianzheng lunzhi describes an idealized clinical encounter as constituted by two separate yet tightly integrated processes of translation. In the course of the first step—"pattern differentiation"—the symptoms and signs elicited by way of the four examinations are organized into distinctive clinical patterns, descriptions of which can be found in the classical literature. These patterns are similar to syndromes in biomedicine. However, their primary purpose is not to define disease, but rather to grasp the moment-by-moment unfolding of pathological processes. In the language of Chinese medicine, patterns of this kind describe pathologies of qi transformation (*qi hua*). In a second step, one responds to these disorders with appropriate treatment strategies designed to balance or control the disordered process. If the physician's subjective understanding of the patient's body is expressed through these patterns, a reverse process happens in treatment strategies, which translate this subjective understanding back into materially manifest herbal medicines or acupuncture point prescriptions (Farquhar 1994b).

Although physicians had practiced medicine in just this manner for centuries, the definition of *bianzheng lunzhi* as representing Chinese medical practice per se is the definitive product of its institutionalization in Maoist China. *Bianzheng lunzhi* initially occupied this position because it was able to reconcile most effectively the multiple forces involved in this process of institutionalization. It has held the position because it has proved itself sufficiently sturdy and flexible to accommodate the changing contexts of practice since then. It played on ideological, linguistic, and conceptual similarities between older notions of pattern diagnosis in Chinese medicine and modern Marxist dialectics. It also brought together the Maoist emphasis on practice and the definition of Chinese medicine as constituted by "experience" that had been worked out in the 1930s. Physicians during the 1950s reconceptualized pattern diagnosis as being concerned with recognizing and overcoming the contradictions thrown up by the encounter between human beings and their environment. Focusing on patterns rather than disease, furthermore, provided a useful boundary marker that differentiated Chinese from Western medicine. At the same time, it allowed Chinese medicine physicians to integrate their practices into a biomedically dominated health care system and thereby fulfill their obligation to modernize (Karchmer 2002).

1966–1976

Mao Zedong's Great Proletarian Cultural Revolution, which destabilized Chinese society throughout the "lost decade" from 1966 to 1977, can be understood at least in part as a radical attempt to solve contradictions that by then had become visible, and not only in the domain of medicine. Frustrated with the manner in which old social practices and habits continued to undermine China's movement toward socialism, Mao unleashed the power of youth in a struggle against the "four olds": old ideas, old culture, old customs, and old habits. Meanwhile, individuals and groups at all levels of society used these campaigns to settle private scores against coworkers, neighbors, family members, and others for their own selfish purposes and simple acts of revenge (Thurston 1987).

Much of Chinese medicine's infrastructure—ancient texts as well as modern institutions—was destroyed in a short-lived frenzy of violence. For ideological reasons, medical doctrine was simplified to the greatest possible extent, and practice rather than book study became the proper guide of action. The integration of Chinese and Western medicine became the only legitimate way to practice, and the Chinese medicine sector rapidly contracted even below its pre-1949 levels. A survey commissioned by the Ministry of Health in 1978 established that between 1959 and 1977 the number of people employed in the Chinese medical sector declined by a third, from 361,000 to 240,000 people, while in the Western medical sector it almost quadrupled, from 234,000 to 738,000 (Meng 1999, 744).

The repercussions of the Cultural Revolution for individual lives were frequently devastating. Renowned physicians, who only recently had guided the development of the new Chinese medical orthodoxy under the direct supervision of the party, were now branded "forces of evil," subjected to torture and abuse, and prevented from carrying out scholarly work or engaging in medical practice. Some were killed; others committed suicide or died as a result of physical and emotional trauma. Most others were sent down to the countryside or employed in factories in order to attend to the health care needs of workers and peasants rather than those of the party elite.

Finally, if the 1950s had witnessed a concentration of resources in the cities—exemplified by Chinese medical hospitals and colleges, most particularly in Beijing—the period of the Cultural Revolution shifted at least some of these resources to the countryside. Due to the relatively small number of Western medicine physicians in rural areas, the population there still relied on a mixture of self-help, Chinese medicine, shamanism, religious healing, and folk practitioners for most of their health care needs. The establishment of the three-tier health care network (*sanji weisheng baojian wang*), with its emphasis on the delivery of basic health care needs at the village level through barefoot doctors (*chijiao yisheng*), dramatically changed this balance.

Sometimes condescendingly referred to as "half peasants half physicians" (*bannong banyi*) by their college-trained peers, barefoot doctors received basic training in both Western and Chinese medicine, and then worked under or together with college-trained senior doctors. When not engaged in health care, they would continue to participate in agricultural tasks. Their therapeutic repertoire included the use of biomedical pharmaceuticals where available, acupuncture for toothaches and other painful conditions, and Chinese herbal formulas prescribed symptomatically rather than on the basis of the more complex pattern differentiation. Barefoot doctors were responsible for immunization, disease prevention and family planning services, midwifery, and other basic medical care, as well as health education. Problems that exceeded their skill were referred up the network to county- or provincial-level clinics or hospitals, where more specialized care was available (Chen 1989; Jia 1997; White 1998).

Barefoot doctors, and the three-tier health care network into which they were integrated, constituted an efficient use of resources much admired by foreign experts at the time. The barefoot doctors fundamentally changed patterns of morbidity by greatly reducing the impact of infectious and parasitic diseases, still the main causes of death in rural areas prior to the 1960s. Hence, while images of barefoot doctors administering acupuncture helped to popularize Chinese medicine in the West (Fogarty 1990), their impact on patient behavior in China itself was rather different. They provided access to effective biomedical care on a large scale to a population that had never before been able to afford such luxury. Injections, drips, and those who delivered them became the first port of call for anyone seeking help outside of the home or family (Lora-Wainwright 2006).

1976–1989

The most violent phase of the Cultural Revolution lasted only until 1968, but it was not until Mao Zedong's death on September 9, 1976, that the revolution's force was finally spent. Two years later, the CCP officially acknowledged its failures. It embarked on an ambitious program of reform and development under the slogan of "the Four Modernizations" in agriculture, industry, science and technology, and national defense. Creating "socialism with Chinese characteristics" implied that Chinese classical culture could once more be valorized—though this time in the service of a transition modeled on Western market economics (Baum 1982; Ong 1995). The contours of post-1979 reforms in the health sector reflect these ideological reevaluations and tensions. They can be summarized by four new maxims: (1) to emphasize hospital-based services rather than primary or community care, reversing the priorities of previous policies; (2) to move toward reprofessionalizing medicine (implying that specialist knowledge was to be valued above that of political cadres); (3) to depend on technology, including the transfer of technologies such as tools and personnel from developed countries; and (4) to establish a plural health care system (Henderson 1989).

The contours of this plural health care system emerged incrementally through a series of Ministry of Health meetings and conferences during the late 1970s and early '80s. In 1976, Chinese medicine colleges resumed teaching degree courses, while the new chairman of the CCP, Deng Xiaoping, personally initiated a program aimed at revitalizing the Chinese medicine sector. In 1980, the Ministry of Health committed itself to the so-called "three paths" policy, which stated, "Chinese Medicine, Western Medicine and Integrated Chinese and Western Medicine constitute three great powers which all need to be developed and which will coexist for a long time." Two years later, in 1982, the phrase "to develop modern medicine and our nation's traditional medicines" (i.e., not only Chinese medicine but also the medicine of China's non-Han minorities) was formally written into the new Constitution of the People's Republic of China. The number of Chinese-medicine physicians reached a historic high in 1985, while in conjunction with its policy of reform and opening up, the Chinese government began to take more decisive steps toward promoting the globalization of Chinese medicine (Wang and Cai 1999, 17–21).

In the long run, therefore, the Cultural Revolution merely interrupted the process of expansion and modernization that had been set in motion during the previous decade. And yet, inasmuch as it also constituted the endpoint of the Maoist project, it marked a break whose long-term consequences for the field of Chinese medicine are only gradually becoming apparent. As the predominance of the center was shattered, regionalism and particularistic social relations once more became potent forces in Chinese political and social life. Integrated Chinese and Western medicine—so powerfully promoted during the Cultural Revolution—emerged as a potent third force within China's health care system that continuously threatens to disrupt the stability of its parent. As China marches toward a neoliberal market economy that is socialist only in name, Chinese medicine, too, is subject to reconstruction by economic forces that appear to be far more powerful and corrosive than those unleashed by successive waves of Maoist revolution.

During the 1980s—a period that may yet come to be seen as the final flowering of Chinese medicine as an independent medical tradition—such developments were as yet only barely visible on the horizon. It was a decade of ferment and, at least initially, fervent optimism. Economic reforms promised undreamt-of prosperity, and China's intellectuals were dizzy with the new modernity opening up before them. A range of "fevers" swept the country: "new methodology fever" explored the possibilities of rational science; "root-searching fever" tried to understand the present through the possibilities of the past; and "*qi gong* fever" tried to cure everything by getting in touch with specifically Chinese energies. Meanwhile, "Chinese medicine fever" (*zhongyi re*) had erupted in the West and offered physicians in China new forms of legitimization, new students, and new possibilities of escape (Chen 2003; Jing 1996).

Inevitably, the Chinese medicine sector, too, became infected. But its inherent traditionalism—and perhaps its constant engagement with the materiality of the body—ensured that the fever never reached the levels it did in other cultural arenas. Yet, for a while at least, the strategies and tactics by which Chinese medicine should be inherited and developed (*jicheng fazhan*) appeared to be up for genuine discussion. Some physicians turned with renewed vigor toward the integration of Chinese and Western medicine, hoping to move forward more easily now that they were no longer constrained by Maoist ideology and the material deprivations of revolution. Others went beyond reductionist biomedicine, in an effort to align their ancient tradition with the dynamic sciences of the late twentieth century: systems theory, cybernetics, and quantum mechanics (Dong, Hou, and Zhang 1990).

These terms imply that the development of Chinese medicine during this period of opening up became ever more enmeshed with practices, ideas, and cultures stemming from places other than China itself. Our vignette on the globalization of the Chinese medicine treatment of menopausal symptoms, presented in the textbox at the end of this chapter, seeks to capture the complex dynamics of this process by way of a practical case study. The anthropologist Mei Zhan (2009) speaks of the "worlding" of Chinese medicine to point out that the diffusion of Chinese medicine around the globe, just like its ability to assimilate the non-Chinese in China, is not a process of moving a discrete entity from past to present, East to West. Instead, it involves ongoing "syntheses" (Scheid 2002) or "articulations" (Langwick 2011), bringing bodies, diseases, technologies, selves, and whatever else may be necessary to solve the problems at hand into ever-new conjunctions with each other—conjunctions that may be stable for varying periods of time but that equally threaten to fall apart at any moment and therefore require ongoing efforts to keep them in place.

1989–Present

In 1989 the Chinese state once more used brutal force to reassert its hegemony in the cultural and political domain. Neither Chinese medicine students nor their professors were known for their radical politics, however, and the events in Tiananmen Square did not cause visible ruptures within the field of Chinese medicine. Their after-effects, rippling across its apparently tranquil surface, continue to be felt today as the development of Chinese medicine mirrors that of the nation at large. The policy of paying equal attention to Chinese and Western medicine remained in place throughout the 1990s, as did the official rhetoric of "developing and carrying forward" the heritage of the Chinese medical tradition. From then on, however, that project was also joined to the establishment of a neoliberal economy, demanding that medical institutions become self-sustaining or even profitable, placing the onus to provide for health care needs to a significant extent back onto the individual, and seeking to insinuate Chinese medicine into the networks of the emergent global economy.

In terms of the politically orchestrated development of Chinese medicine, this meant that regularization and standardization—necessary for any practice seeking to escape the attachment to specific local contexts—acquired a new urgency. Beginning in the late 1980s, multiple directives were passed that sought to define standards for everything from diagnosis and treatment to technologies and management. As of January 2010, 305 standards have been issued and five professional technical national committees established. Increasingly, China is pushing to impose these standards internationally, culminating in 2009 in the submission of a proposal by the Standardization Administration of China (SAC) to the International Organization for Standardization (ISO) to establish a technical committee for the development of standards in Chinese medicine (Zaslawski and Lee 2010). Imposing its own standards globally is a tool not merely for globalizing Chinese medicine but also for maintaining control of that process, and for warding off the competing interests of other East Asian medical traditions.

Research and drug development constitute the second leg of the state-supported globalization of Chinese medicine. On June 4, 1997, the State Council decided to implement a national research program during the period from 1998 to 2010. Research into Chinese medicine formulas was listed as one of forty-two projects in the program and was allocated funding of approximately seven million dollars, the largest grant for Chinese medicine research ever awarded at the national level. This research program had, as its main objectives, enhancing the understanding of formula composition and efficacy, and advancing technologies of production for traditional pharmaceutical products in order to introduce them into the mainstream of international pharmaceutical markets ("Basic Research Program for Chinese Medicine Formulae" 2001). A decade later, this policy is beginning to reap its first rewards. Early in 2012 *Di'ao xin xue kang* (a patent remedy), produced by the Chengdu-based Di'ao Group, received marketing authorization from the Medicines Evaluation Board of the Netherlands, making it the first Chinese traditional drug to be identified as a therapeutic medicine in the European Union (Cheng 2012). Tasly Pharmaceutical Co., Ltd., based in Tianjin, is currently involved in Phase III trials to license a similar Chinese medical product with the FDA ("Tasly Pharmaceuticals" 2012).

More openly than ever before, standardization, pharmacological research, and efforts to define the effectiveness of Chinese medicine through randomized controlled trials and other techniques associated with evidence-based medicine define biomedicine as the gold standard to be emulated wherever possible. Not surprisingly, after half a century in which scientization was always the stated goal but Maoist dialectics and the importance of practice left sufficient room for self-cultivation and the development of personal styles of practice, younger physicians now openly suggest that the only logical conclusion of this development is for Chinese medicine to be gradually assimilated into a single and universal biomedicine.

At the same time, classical texts are more readily available than ever before, in bookshops as well as on CDs and the internet. In recent years, a movement has sprung up that vociferously criticizes the modernization of Chinese medicine over the past few decades, arguing for a return to more classical medicine or claiming that "true" Chinese medicine can no longer be found in the cities but remains intact only in the countryside. Local and regional medical currents are making a revival supported as in earlier eras by local money and local pride. Some of these local traditions have even become internationally recognized brands. One example is the "fire spirit current" (*huo shen pai*), a style of Chinese medicine that originated in Sichuan in the late nineteenth century and emphasizes the use of high dosages of warming medicinals such as aconite (*fuzi*), ginger (*ganjiang*), or evodia (*wuzhuyu*). It now has vociferous proponents throughout the world who hail it as one of the most effective forms of Chinese medicine (Lu 2008).

A third aspect of Chinese medicine's most recent history is its rediscovery by the state as a potential means of providing better access to health care in the countryside in an effort to remedy problems that ensued from the dismantling of the three-tier health care network in the 1980s. At the time, the existing comprehensive insurance scheme, based on a concept of shared social responsibility, was largely replaced by a cash-for-service system that pushed much of rural Chinese medicine into the private sector, with many previous barefoot doctors opening their own practices. Hospitals, meanwhile, forced to generate much of their own income, focused their development on biomedicine. Not only do biomedical interventions and drugs offer greater profit margins, but when given a choice, patients, too, consistently favor high-tech over traditional medicine, which they view as less effective (Köster 2009, 67). It is only quite recently that this trend has begun to change. In an effort to make health care available once more to a rural population that had simply been priced out of the market, the state is once more turning to Chinese medicine. In a movement harking back to Mao's creation of barefoot doctors, the recently passed Twelfth Five-Year Plan for Chinese medicine envisages the training of fifteen thousand Chinese medicine clinicians for hospitals at the county level by 2015, and thirty thousand Chinese medicine general practitioners for grassroots medical facilities. By the same year, every Chinese city at the prefecture level is planned to have a TCM hospital, while 95 percent of community health care centers and 90 percent of township health clinics will also provide Chinese medicine services ("China to Train 15,000" 2012).

In the cities, meanwhile, with an increasingly affluent middle class able to spend money on health care, famous Chinese medicine doctors are becoming, once again, sought-after providers of highly valued personal skills that can earn them fortunes. Riding on the back of the recent root-searching (*xungen*) movement, Chinese medicine professors like Qu Limei from Beijing or Liu Lihong from Guangxi have turned themselves into national media stars by writing best-selling books on how to employ ancient medical classics for the purpose of personal self-cultivation or acting as spokespersons for an authentic tradition beyond the urban state-controlled institutions. Buoyed by such indicators of enduring popularity at home and abroad, its most enthusiastic proponents thus boldly envision the twenty-first century as the century of Chinese medicine (Wang 1995a)—leaving us to wonder whether the laments of their elders regarding the loss of tradition from "traditional Chinese medicine" expresses instead a mourning for the loss of their own powers in a country that increasingly values youth over age.

We can certainly see them as such. More importantly, perhaps, they reveal enduring and ubiquitous tensions between contemporary Chinese medicine as a visible and highly valued embodiment of tradition (simultaneously national, regional, and local) and a product of the (post)modern that threatens to break into the open at any opportune moment. One such moment occurred in 2006, when Zhang Gongyao, director of the Technology and Social Development Research Institute at Southwest University in Hunan Province, openly attacked the Chinese medicine profession in an article entitled "Farewell to Chinese Medicine and Chinese Herbs" (*gaobie zhongyi zhongyao*), published in the reputable journal *Medicine and Philosophy* (*yixue yu zhexue*) (Zhang 2006b). The article criticized Chinese medicine for being unscientific and not worthy of being supported by a modern society. Encouraged by the widespread public support he received, Zhang created an online petition in October of the same year in which he demanded the removal of Chinese medicine from the national health care system. Only ten days later, the government felt forced to intervene, rejecting the proposal and declaring its unqualified support for Chinese medicine.

What this example demonstrates is the degree to which the survival of Chinese medicine throughout the Republican and contemporary periods has been intertwined with the state. At present, support for Chinese medicine by the state remains strong, though it is by no means unqualified. As throughout the Maoist and post-Maoist periods, it constitutes not a cultural essence but a resource to be utilized in the pursuit of wider economic and social policies. Adequately capturing the ongoing development of Chinese medicine in a context in which China is becoming enmeshed in global economics and politics will require of future historians that they move away from an emphasis on Western and Chinese medicine and their confrontation, interaction, and interpenetration, and turn instead toward a more fractured field of medical practice. This field is increasingly shaped by the global technocultural networks and markets to which it has sought access over recent decades, and by global disease vectors rapidly transmitting across borders. At the same time, by reconstituting itself as a market it is equally shaped by the needs, choices, and cultural histories of its local consumers.

Chinese Medicine in the Treatment of Menopausal Symptoms
Volker Scheid

Modern Chinese medicine textbooks claim that physicians in China have successfully treated symptoms associated with menopause for at least two thousand years. These claims are repeated by individual practitioners in their promotional materials as well as in the reasons clinical researchers give for seeking to evaluate the effectiveness of these treatments. The same textbooks provide model diagnoses and treatments that define menopausal symptoms as being caused by what Chinese medicine calls "kidney deficiency" (*shèn xū*). There is evidence that these textbook models consistently inform clinical practice and also clinical research.

There are several problems with these claims. There is no evidence that physicians in China or other East Asian countries considered the menopausal transition to be a medical problem much before the second half of the twentieth century. The kidney deficiency model of menopausal syndrome in Chinese medicine emerged in the early 1960s and is very likely a translation of the biomedical estrogen deficiency model into the idioms of Chinese medicine. This was then reconnected to older ideas about aging as well as to treatment strategies for kidney deficiency that had originally been used to treat disorders as varied as slow development in infants, tuberculosis, and infertility. However, this creative process of bricolage has been completely edited out of textbook discussions and it is simply accepted today that menopausal syndrome in biomedicine equals kidney deficiency in Chinese medicine.

Interestingly, during the same period in which Chinese physicians implementing a modernizing agenda directed by the Chinese state succeeded in globalizing a newly invented traditional understanding of menopause as a process that could be reduced to universal biological changes, Western anthropologists began to show that the experience of menopause significantly varies across cultures. They coined the term "local biologies" in order to draw our attention to the fact that the manifestations of a process like the menopausal transition are not determined by biology alone. Rather, they constitute the surface of a web of interactions among factors as varied as diet, individual constitutions, climates, life stresses, and beliefs. In other words, anthropologists critiquing disease arrived at an understanding of individualized patterns, while Chinese physicians were doing their best to make Chinese medicine match the biomedical understanding of disease.

Not surprisingly, perhaps, East Asian medical traditions less influenced by biomedical modernity, such as Japanese *Kampo* or Korean medicine but also Chinese medicine in Taiwan, do not generally equate menopausal symptoms with kidney deficiency. A survey of the mainland Chinese case record literature equally shows that how individual physicians, including physicians listed as authors of modern textbooks, treat menopausal symptoms in actual clinical practice is far more varied than textbook models and national standards.

Similar stories could be told about a whole range of conditions that Chinese medicine claims to have treated successfully for thousands of years: hypertension, for instance, which can only be detected by means of technologies not widely available in China prior to the twentieth century; depression, which only very recently has been accepted as an illness in China and whose clear and precise definition continues to elude the compilers of the International Classification of Diseases (ICD); or irritable bowel syndrome, another ill-defined disorder with roots in the nineteenth century, for which Chinese medicine textbooks, by and large, recommend a formula that treats painful diarrhea even though the syndrome is specifically defined as being characterized by alternating constipation and diarrhea.

This raises the question of what clinical researchers interested in the effectiveness of Chinese medicine should examine. Should they ignore the history of inventions as well as the diversity of medical practice on the ground and examine textbook treatments because there they can find clear diagnostic categories matched to model treatments? Should they consult experts in order to produce a consensus regarding best diagnosis and treatment, knowing that the experts will generally tend to reproduce textbook models? Should they simply select one of the many treatment models available on the ground? But if so, which one? These questions defy easy answers. They demand, above all, accepting and engaging with the issue of Chinese medicine's historical diversity rather than seeking to control it because it gets in the way of doing research.

One of the possibilities for doing this that we are currently exploring at the University of Westminster is action research. This allows a group of practitioners to treat menopausal women, to systematically pool their experiences and adjust treatment accordingly, and to seek to develop an understanding of how to best treat menopausal women in London with Chinese medicine. By seeking to facilitate the development of best practitioners, we simultaneously hope to generate the best practices that might then become the objects of more systematic clinical trials.

Note

This vignette draws on a long-term research project on Chinese medicine and menopause carried out at the EAST*medicine* Research Centre at the University of Westminster, funded by a Department of Health Research Capacity Development Grant to Volker Scheid. Initial findings have been published in a series of articles listed below.

Scheid, Volker. 2007a. "Acupuncture for Hypertension: A Tale of Two Trials; From the Perspective of the Anthropologist." *Forschende Komplementär Medizin* 14 (6): 371, 374–375.

———. 2007b. "Traditional Chinese Medicine—What Are We Investigating? The Case of Menopause." *Complementary Therapies in Medicine* 15 (1): 54–68.

———. 2009. "Globalising Chinese Medical Understandings of Menopause." *East Asia Science, Technology and Society: An International Journal* 2 (4): 485–496.

Scheid, Volker, Veronica Tuffrey, and Trina Ward. 2010. "Comparing TCM Textbook Descriptions of Menopausal Syndrome with the Lived Experience of London Women at Midlife and the Implications for Chinese Medicine Research." *Maturitas* 66: 408–416.

Scheid, Volker, Trina Ward, Wang-Seok Cha, Kenji Watanabe, and Xing Liao. 2010. "The Treatment of Menopausal Symptoms by Traditional East Asian Medicines: Review and Perspectives." *Maturitas* 66: 111–130.

Ward, Trina, Volker Scheid, and Veronica Tuffrey. 2010. "Women's Mid-Life Health Experiences in Urban UK: An International Comparison." *Climacteric* 13 (3): 278–288.

13 Barefoot Doctors and the Provision of Rural Health Care

Xiaoping Fang

Introduction

The year 1968 saw the publication of Ralph Croizier's *Traditional Medicine in Modern China: Science, Nationalism, and the Tensions of Cultural Change*, which would become one of the most cited books on twentieth-century Chinese medical history. It focused on one "central paradox and main theme": why twentieth-century intellectuals, committed in so many ways to science and modernity, insisted on upholding China's ancient "pre-scientific" medical tradition (Croizier 1968, 2). Through the perspective of cultural nationalism, Croizier argued that these intellectuals were influenced by "the interaction of two of the dominant themes in modern Chinese thinking—the drive for national strength through modern science, and the concern that modernization not imply betrayal of national identity" (Croizier 1968, 229). However, 1968 also marked the inauguration of a massive public health initiative in China, which would have far-reaching consequences for the medical development of the world's most populous country: a rural medical program that was inspired by the principles of revolutionary socialism and promoted nationwide. This new medical program pitted Chinese and Western medicine against one another and, more importantly, eventually determined the future of the two types of medicine in Chinese villages. This social transformation of medicine in Chinese villages has been largely overlooked by scholars of Chinese medical history. The centerpiece of the program was the introduction of "barefoot doctors" (*chijiao yisheng*) into Chinese villages at the height of the Cultural Revolution (1966–1976).

Barefoot doctors were health workers in Chinese villages under the people's commune system from 1968 to 1983. They were members of commune production brigades who were given brief, basic medical training so that they could provide treatment and perform public health work in their home villages. They formed the lowest level of a three-tier state medical system that comprised the county, commune, and brigade levels. The concept of barefoot doctors was first introduced to the public through newspaper pieces, particularly "Fostering a Revolution in Medical Education through the Growth of the Barefoot Doctors," an investigative report that was published on September 14, 1968, in the *People's Daily*, an organ of the Central Committee of the Chinese Communist Party. It described the work of barefoot doctors in Jiangzhen commune, Chuansha county, Shanghai municipality ("Cong 'chijiao yisheng' de chengzhang kan yixue jiaoyu" 1968). On December 5, 1968, the same newspaper carried a report with the headline "Cooperative Medical Service Warmly Welcomed by Poor and Lower-Middle Peasants." This article introduced the new cooperative medical service of Leyuan commune, Changyang county, Hubei Province ("Shenshou pinxia zhongnong huanying de hezuo yiliao" 1968). As one of the "newly emerged things" that reflected the political ideologies and rural development strategies of the Cultural Revolution, the barefoot doctors were rapidly popularized, and cooperative medical stations were set up in villages nationwide with revolutionary zeal. Villagers paid fees to form local "cooperative medical services" to cover the costs of establishing these medical service stations, which would be presided over by barefoot doctors. When villagers sought treatment at these stations, they were administered certain services and medicines free of charge. With the implementation of rural reform policies and the dismantling of the people's commune system after 1978, the barefoot doctor program began to gradually disintegrate. Barefoot doctors who passed medical examinations and continued practicing medicine in villages were renamed "village doctors." By 1983, cooperative medical services had basically ceased to function in most Chinese villages. Some medical stations were dismantled, while others were run by former barefoot doctors as private clinics.

From their first appearance, the barefoot doctors attracted the attention of scholars and social commentators. The barefoot doctor program has been regarded, both inside and outside of China, as "a low-cost solution built around easily available indigenous medicines" (World Bank 1992, 18; Sidel 1972, 1292–1300). Barefoot doctors presented a suitably revolutionary image: young people who waded undaunted through the mud of the rice paddies to provide medical services in answer to Mao's call to "stress rural areas in medical and health work." Their main equipment was popularly described as "one silver needle and a bunch of herbs," a reference to acupuncture and Chinese herbal medicine, but in practice they combined Chinese and Western medicine. Together with the three-tier rural medical system, barefoot doctors and cooperative medical services have been associated with improvements in basic health indicators under socialism after the founding of the People's Republic of China in 1949 (White 1998, 480–490). In the late 1970s, the World Health Organization promoted the Chinese system as a model of primary health care for developing countries (Worsley

1982, 340). It is widely argued that the rural medical system collapsed as a result of the reforms initiated in 1978, and that the commercialization and marketization of medical provision have reduced the accessibility, affordability, and equity of public health and medical care in rural China (Duckett 2010, 6–7). Meanwhile, in recent decades, both academic studies and public opinion have contrasted the current state of crisis in China's medical sector with the supposedly halcyon days of the barefoot doctor program (Klotzbucher et al. 2010).

This paper reaches beyond a nostalgic view of barefoot doctors and calls into question the orthodox interpretations that dominate present scholarship on public health and the provision of rural health in China. It retrieves Western medicine in rural China from potential historical oblivion through the perspective of the social history of medicine. It places barefoot doctors in the context of the history of debates concerning how the legitimacy of Chinese medicine has been challenged by Western medicine since the early twentieth century. Ultimately, it offers a carefully contextualized critique of conventional views on the role of barefoot doctors, their legacy, and their impact, both in rural areas and in China as a whole, while making theoretical contributions to the Chinese social historiography of medicine.

Village Healers, Medical Pluralism, and State Medicine

Paul Unschuld has argued that the "medical system" of a culture is made up of a spectrum of resources that meet the demand for health care services, and the distribution of possession and control over these resources (Unschuld 1979, 4). The government obviously plays an important role in resource distribution, and in Chinese medical history, the extent of this role has fluctuated over time (Scheid 2007, 37; Elman 2006, 209). Generally speaking, the imperial government did not show any real awareness of a modern state's medical responsibilities until the very end of the Qing dynasty (Croizier 1975, 25). However, since the turn of the twentieth century, the founding and development of a state medical system was clearly the main theme of medical modernization in twentieth-century China under both the Nationalist and Communist governments. As China had a largely rural population, the establishment of the state medical system in rural areas was highly significant. A rural medical system was proposed and implemented experimentally in the 1930s by the Nanjing-based Nationalist government and the Rural Construction Movement, which was represented by C. C. Chen in Ding county in northern China (Chen 1989, 423; Yip 1995, 76–77).

The development of the state medical system in rural China after 1949 was based on a constant reorganization of plural medical systems, including professional, folk, and popular medical systems. From the end of 1949, the Communist government began to investigate medical practitioners and register medical agencies in each county. Within this process, county hospitals were established by taking over existing county clinics, which had mainly been run by the Nationalist government, though their staff and facilities were quite poor. To form medical units below the county level, the various social medical and health workers, such as Chinese medicine doctors, Western medicine doctors, acupuncturists, and even itinerant healers, were "mobilized" and encouraged to "walk the collective road" and establish union clinics after 1952, following the principle of "one clinic per township." These clinics functioned as mini-hospitals beneath county hospitals—in other words, they formed the second tier of the three-tier medical system. As a socialist health and welfare entity under the ownership of a doctors' collective and established voluntarily by doctors under the leadership of the party and the government, union clinic personnel, finance, distribution, and management were all run by the medical collective, which established fees for services, undertook individual accounting, managed the facility democratically, and distributed salaries according to the contributions of each member (Yu 1998, 449–454). Thus, a two-tier state medical system was formed in the countryside, consisting of county hospitals and numerous township-level union clinics.

Union clinics established the basic form of the state medical system in China's villages from the early 1950s onward. Their creation also sparked a general differentiation and reorganization of the various healers in the villages. However, demand for independent professional medical practitioners' services began to decline as union clinics were further consolidated when the medical collectives owning the clinics signed health care contracts with agricultural cooperatives. The number of private medical practitioners therefore decreased, and more and more joined union clinics. In the meantime, with the beginning of agricultural collectivization, villagers were selected to become health workers within mutual aid teams and cooperatives as part of the program to enhance agricultural productivity. The selection criterion for these initiatives was the possession of both basic primary educational qualifications and the right political credentials. Selected candidates were required to follow an informal training program entailing the "Four Principles of Health Work," which pertained to basic first aid and preventive medical treatment (ZSDA 1954). Outside the state medical system, the lives and practices of other healers in the villages, such as bone-setters and acupuncturists, were largely unaffected. Even though healers from religious sects were affected to some degree by the social and political changes taking place, they continued to exist in Chinese rural society until the outbreak of the Cultural Revolution in 1966.

The emergence of the barefoot doctor program at the height of the Cultural Revolution in 1968 enhanced the establishment of the state medical system based on a constant reshuffling of the plural medical systems. Although there were no intrinsic changes to the role of health workers before the mid-1960s as they went from being "old things" to being "newly emerged things," the new contexts in which barefoot doctors worked within the cooperative medical service became institutionalized. Barefoot doctors and cooperative medical services addressed the needs for medical personnel and funding for health care in rural areas in a way that accorded with Mao's ideology and the strategy of the Cultural Revolution. In this way, the structure of the state medical system underwent a massive downward extension to the village level, as compared with the union clinic model. Meanwhile, through the changes to clinic names, the establishment of Communist Party organizations, financial investment, and the granting of "urban household" status to union clinic doctors, union clinics were comprehensively incorporated into the state medical system. As the second-tier medical units above the barefoot doctors in the villages, union clinics were strengthened, while barefoot doctors replaced the clinic model as the front line in medical and health work.

The Cultural Revolution had a tremendous impact on the plural medical systems of rural China. Private medical practitioners were criticized as being the "wind of individual work" and the "tails of capitalism." They were then either incorporated into the state medical system or forbidden from practicing medicine. For folk healers, it was pointed out that "in order to consolidate and develop the cooperative medical service and enlarge the medical group, the folk healers in the rural areas should be organized" ("Guangdongsheng Qujiangxian Qunxing dadui" 1969). The incorporation of folk healers into the barefoot doctor program consequently legitimized folk medicine. In theory, they became the barefoot doctors' instructors in folk (or indigenous) medical knowledge, while barefoot doctors became agents for continuing folk medicine in the villages. Meanwhile, local governments smashed temples and statues and denounced so-called "feudal" and superstitious behaviors. Healers from supernatural and religious sects were prohibited and their practices were eradicated for being "superstitious." Although "superstitious healers" and their practices did not disappear entirely from the villages upon the announcement of these policies, the villagers dared not seek treatment from these traditional sources openly. While religious and demonic ideas were being delegitimized, empirical folk healing, such as heatstroke acupuncture, was being endorsed by the government and was popular among villagers.

The barefoot doctor program and cooperative medical services fulfilled the design for "state medicine" that had been proposed by the Nationalist government and the Rural Construction Movement in the early 1930s. The difference between the policies of the Chinese Communist Party and the Nationalist government lay in their attitudes toward plural medical systems. For the Nationalists and the Rural Construction Movement, the goal had been to establish a new modern medical system in the villages without utilizing existing plural medical systems. This policy was based on Nationalist ideologies and strategies, as well as its capacity to impose reforms in the countryside. Likewise, followers of the Rural Construction Movement intentionally aimed to avoid conflicts with the existing system in order to sustain the operations of their social experiment. In contrast, the Chinese Communist Party constantly appropriated and reorganized the existing plural medical systems in order to build a new state medical system. The pace and nature of these changes depended on variations in coercive state forces and the impacts of various political campaigns.

Medical Knowledge, Pharmaceuticals, and Consumption

When the newly established state medical system reorganized existing plural medical systems, the state was seeking to replace the traditional family-based and apprenticeship-based ways of acquiring medical knowledge in order to meet the demands of a modern, integrated national health program with more numerous medical personnel (Leung 2003, 386). From the early 1950s the traditional family- and apprenticeship-based transmission modes, whose sources were mainly confined to the local community, started to change gradually. Meanwhile, Western medical knowledge had already entered Chinese villages and encountered Chinese medicine, mainly through vaccination. Chinese medicine doctors were agents of the dissemination of Western medical knowledge and techniques through Chinese villages in their daily epidemic prevention and treatment work, such as injections. A key impetus for change was the fact that the barefoot doctors drew a new type of person into positions of authority in villages. Those selected as barefoot doctors included the young, the moderately educated, and women—and as such, the program completely discarded the old knowledge transmission practices. Moreover, in contrast to the old-style village healers, the barefoot doctors absorbed both Chinese and Western medical knowledge, taking their information from both Western-style physicians and legitimate folk healers. The majority of the instructors were Western medicine–oriented doctors from outside the local community. The barefoot doctors' training was further facilitated by the appearance of unified medical textbooks. Nonetheless, the barefoot doctors' low literacy, limited training, and self-study made them more inclined to adopt the simple medical knowledge and practical skills of Western medicine, such as administering injections and preparing intravenous drips, and dispensing medicines according to the illustrated instruction labels on the medicine bottles. In contrast, as the reading of texts was the main method of traditional instruction in Chinese medicine, trainees needed high literacy and educational levels, especially as traditional medical books were written in classical Chinese. Learning Chinese medicine was therefore more complicated for the barefoot doctors, though it was acquired in both study and practice. The barefoot doctors who were introducing Western medicine quickly outnumbered the Chinese medicine doctors and folk healers in the local community, which exacerbated the decline of Chinese medicine that had commenced in the early 1950s. In each of these ways, the advent of barefoot doctors fundamentally transformed the village knowledge structures.

The dissemination of modern medical knowledge in rural China brought Western pharmaceuticals into the villages. Prior to the mid-twentieth century, although Chinese medicine shops had penetrated to the township level, villagers' access to medicine was still very limited. Villagers largely relied on self-medication. The gradual formation of the state pharmaceutical sales network, which depended on reforming the original network, facilitated the entry of Western medicine into villages by reducing the prices of Western medicine beginning in the mid-1950s. Then, in 1968 with the establishment of medical stations and the provision of medical kits through the barefoot doctors, the spread of a coherent pharmaceutical sales network into Chinese villages was consolidated. The price of medicine was another key factor. In the 1950s and 1960s, pharmaceutical prices were still high compared with villagers' incomes. For example, in 1957, bottles of tetracycline and terramycin (one hundred 2.5-gram tablets) cost 170.13 RMB and 177.88 RMB, respectively, yet the average annual income of villagers that year was less than 50 RMB (Zhongguo yiyao gongsi 1990, 274). As such, the reduction of prices was a crucial factor for villagers. On August 1, 1969, pharmaceutical prices were reduced nationwide "in obedience to the great leader Chairman Mao's glorious instructions to 'stress rural areas in medical and health work'" ("Weida lingxiu maozhuxi shenqie guanhuai guangda geming renmin" 1969). Prices for 1,230 kinds of antibiotics, sulphanilamides, fever-reducing medicines, pain-relieving medicines, vitamins, hormones, and other medicines were reduced by 37.2 percent. In this new system, Western medicine was not only available but also affordable to villagers for the first time because of the significant reductions in price.

Like Western pharmaceuticals for common diseases, vaccines (or biological products) were of great significance for combating acute epidemic diseases. From the early 1950s on, basic vaccines were applied to inoculation work, such as cholera and plague, while the range of available vaccines increased gradually thereafter. By the time the barefoot doctor program was initiated in 1970, fifteen vaccines had already been administered regularly. These vaccines covered all eighteen of the epidemic diseases that had occurred regularly in the rural Hangzhou area during the late 1960s (Yan 1985, 141–142; LWBW 1992, 257; Xu 1991, 15–16, 173–177). China had already invented vaccines for the most serious epidemic diseases—measles and epidemic cerebrospinal meningitis—and applied them between 1967 and 1970. As the mortality rates of measles and epidemic cerebrospinal meningitis were the highest of all the infectious diseases affecting rural China, the invention and application of vaccines for them were of great significance (Hangzhou shi weisheng fangyizhan 1982, 12). The mortality rates of infectious disease started declining after 1968 and dropped to their lowest-ever levels by 1970, where they have remained ever since because of the combination of new vaccines and the extended role of barefoot doctors.

Meanwhile, Chinese medicine received renewed official legitimacy and was promoted within a nationalist narrative, but it was also popularized because of its relative affordability compared to Western medicine. This formation of a nationwide pharmaceutical scheme, combined with the spread of barefoot doctors, meant that two kinds of pharmaceuticals appeared in village medical arenas on a large scale for the first time in the social history of China, which had great significance for the development of the pharmaceutical structure in the villages. This intermingling reveals that the intellectual and theoretical controversy over Chinese and Western medicines—in terms of the conferral of state legitimacy—started to appear in the Chinese countryside. During this process, Chinese herbal medicines, which had enjoyed popular acceptance and practical legitimacy before the arrival of the barefoot doctors in the villages, were seriously challenged by Western medicines, the spread of which was facilitated by their steadily increasing availability combined with their steadily decreasing prices. This situation also illustrates the dilemma inherent in the systematization of Chinese herbal medicine use when it was expanded from sporadic, small-scale use to regular, large-scale use within a national health program. In this sense, the barefoot doctor program provided the first real context in which Chinese and Western medicines would compete in the village medical arenas.

Together with medical knowledge and pharmaceuticals, the healing techniques of Western medicine gradually entered the village medical domain from the early 1950s onward. This accelerated after 1968 because the barefoot doctors had a preference for Western medicine in their daily practice. Although the barefoot doctors also employed Chinese medicine, they tended increasingly to apply modern medical instruments and prescribe Western medicine tablets. This trend resulted from a combination of their training and the greater availability and convenience of Western medicine as well as the revolutionary new knowledge structures that had emerged around health delivery since 1949. Meanwhile, the villager patients gained a greater degree of access to the new healing styles and techniques, and formed ideas about the comparative value of Chinese and Western medicine. For example, Chinese and Western medicine were considered to have different strengths and weaknesses in terms of treating "symptoms" and "roots," or being "quick" or "slow," or being better suited for some conditions rather than others. The interactions of healing styles and medical beliefs completely changed the structure of pharmaceutical consumption in Chinese villages. The result was that Chinese medicine was quickly marginalized, although it was still consumed and appreciated. According to the statistical data concerning thirty kinds of common Chinese *materia medica* in Jiande county, Zhejiang

Province, the average consumption rate per capita was under 0.06 *jin* (approximately thirty grams) before 1969. The consumption rate stayed the same in 1970 but suddenly increased to 0.08 *jin* (forty grams) in 1971, before settling at between 0.08 and 0.1 *jin* (forty to fifty grams) from 1971 to 1982 (Yan 1985, 110–111). This means that the average consumption rate of Chinese materia medica saw no significant change in conjunction with the Chinese herbal medicine campaign and the founding of the cooperative medical stations.

While the consumption of Chinese materia medica stagnated, that of Chinese patent medicines increased steadily. As prepared medicines, Chinese patent medicines solved the inconvenience of collecting and drying fresh herbal medicine and decocting materia medica. Meanwhile, increasing promotional activity by pharmaceutical companies, the state's efforts to standardize compound prescriptions, and patients' preference for easily consumable (and acceptable-tasting) medicine also contributed to there being more and more Chinese patent medicines on the market. These changes were reflected in the sales volumes of Chinese patent medicines. In Jiande county, Chinese patent medicines only accounted for 7.8 percent of the total sales income of various pharmaceuticals in the period 1961–1969, before rising to 8.7 percent in 1970, 12.7 percent in 1971, and 13.3 percent in 1971–1978 (Yan 1985, 116). The proportion of income from sales of patent medicines among total pharmaceutical sales exceeded that of Chinese materia medica for the first time in 1979, but this increase came mainly from sales of nutritional and tonic medicines rather than curative pharmaceuticals. According to statistical data for seventeen major Chinese patent medicines in the wholesale areas supplied by the Hangzhou Chinese and Western Pharmaceutical Station, Zhejiang Province, the sales incomes for nutritional and tonic medicines increased steeply, as did their percentage share of total Chinese patent medicines sales, growing from 33.3 percent in 1979 to 38.3 percent in 1980. Tonic sales eventually surpassed those of curative Chinese patent medicines, representing an average rate of 51.8 percent of total sales between 1981 and 1985 (HYSBW 1990, 88–89).

The increase in sales of Chinese patent medicine became the sole factor behind the increased percentage of Chinese medicine (including materia medica and patent medicines) in total pharmaceutical sales. In Jiande county, the average percentage of Chinese medicine of total pharmaceuticals increased from 24.2 percent in 1961–1969 to 31.6 percent in 1970–1978 before soaring to 40.8 percent in 1979–1983 (Yan 1985, 116). Though this increasing percentage of sales income represented by Chinese medicine indicates a decrease in the percentage represented by Western pharmaceuticals, the actual quantity of Western medicine consumed has been increasing steadily year by year. As discussed earlier, Western pharmaceutical prices were reduced by about 37 percent in 1969, with further reductions in 1974 and 1984. Therefore, increasing access and decreasing prices resulted in a significant increase in Western pharmaceutical consumption in villages throughout the 1970s (Zhongguo yiyao gongsi 1990, 273). Simultaneously, these changed practices also led to the abuse of Western medicine in rural China as a result of the unlimited prescription of medications and the widespread practice of self-medication.

The Formation and Evolution of a Rural Medical Community

After 1949, the world of village medicine was transformed through the gradual establishment of the three-tier medical system. This top-down process took over the Nationalist government's public county hospitals and renamed them county people's hospitals, formed union clinics in district and township seats after 1952, and established the medical stations presided over by barefoot doctors after 1968. Scholars have proposed a few interpretative concepts for this three-tier medical system. According to Ray Elling, the ideal structuring of any medical system includes the concepts of "medical regionalization" and "concertion." A regionalized system is a graded hierarchy of interdependent services with a two-way flow of patients and information between the periphery and the center of the system (Elling 1978, 107–115). These concepts have provided a macrostructural interpretation of the three-tier medical system, particularly in terms of public health campaigns. However, it is still worth exploring these new top-down institutions and the system itself from a bottom-up perspective.

In traditional Chinese village society, as in other premodern societies, medical encounters were usually based in the patients' homes. A medical community could not be said to exist in theory or practice because of the absence of hierarchical proficiency and cooperation. The lack of community was the feature that set Chinese medicine apart from Western medicine in terms of medical institutionalization. The establishment in the early 1950s of union clinics as mini-hospitals, which were renamed commune clinics in the late 1960s, indicated that a new medical community emerged in rural China based on the townships (or the communes, after 1962). This brought changes both for villagers, whose medical encounters started to move from their homes into clinics at a relatively slow pace, and for rural medical practitioners, who began to form part of a hierarchical system that stratified medical proficiency and coordinated the treatment.

However, the medical community was not mature and a coordinating scheme for medical practice inside and outside the local village community was basically absent. This situation would change in 1968 with the introduction of the barefoot doctor scheme. The establishment of medical stations presided over by barefoot doctors promoted the extension of the top-down medical system into a three-tier system. It not only strengthened the medical community based on each commune but also, for the first time in rural China, provided a coordinating mechanism for the new hierarchical medical system. Barefoot doctors played significant roles as participants, promoters, and guides during the process of institutionalizing villagers' medical encounters with doctors into the hierarchical medical system. As a result, villagers started to move beyond their home villages to access new medical services in modern medical settings, mainly county hospitals (Henderson and Cohen 1984, 95, 107).

More importantly, the fact that the barefoot doctors played dual roles was a key factor in the reshaping of the entire medical network. Some works of scholarship have argued that the barefoot doctors functioned in the same way as the health workers in C. C. Chen's experimental health program in Ding county in the 1930s (Yip 1995, 190–191; Yang 2006, 380–394). In fact, the barefoot doctors were quite different from Chen's health workers. Nor were they the same as the peasants who became "health workers" in the 1950s and 1960s under the union clinic model, even though this group formed a core recruitment base for the barefoot doctor program. In these two earlier programs, the health workers basically undertook auxiliary public heath work at the village level, such as administering inoculations and collecting stool samples (Chen 1989, 83; Li 1935, 108). In contrast, the barefoot doctors had their own medical stations and medical kits, and healing became an important part of their daily work, in addition to the epidemic prevention work associated with health workers. C. C. Chen also noticed a tendency among barefoot doctors in the 1970s and 1980s to overestimate their skills (Chen 1989, 161). In this sense, the barefoot doctors played a dual role throughout the 1970s, in that they were both health workers and physicians. However, the healing role of barefoot doctors was more significant than their public health duties because they started to take over medical practice in the local community, which had previously been provided by commune clinics. Their healing role therefore became a major influence on the structural evolution of the three-tier medical network.

In the meantime, the conditions of the commune clinics were embarrassing because they lacked the necessary equipment, supplies, and personnel to provide the medical services designated to them by the system. For example, there were a total of 309 commune clinics and forty-six district hospitals in the seven counties of Hangzhou prefecture, Zhejiang Province, in 1976, which was the peak year in terms of the implementation of the cooperative medical service. However, 23.6 percent of the commune clinics (73 clinics) had no clinic beds. As for medical instruments, only 8 percent (25 clinics) of the commune clinics had the five basic types of medical instruments. There were only sixty-nine X-ray machines and a total of 210 microscopes in the 309 commune clinics. As for surgical skills, only 5.5 percent of the commune clinics (17 clinics) could handle both acute abdominal disease and difficult labor operations (HPA 1976). The popularization of brigade medical stations, which had the authority to refer patients to the top of the medical hierarchy, resulted in villagers bypassing commune clinics altogether.

278 | Xiaoping Fang

Because of this situation, patients with relatively serious illnesses who could not be treated by the brigade medical stations could not be treated by the commune clinics, either. Instead, they had to be referred to higher-level hospitals, thus skipping the commune clinics. The decline of the commune clinics made the rural medical network take on a dumbbell shape: the middle part (the commune clinics) shrank, while the top and bottom (the county hospitals and the brigade medical stations) became increasingly important.

According to statistical data in Jiande county, Hangzhou Province, from 1973 to 1983, the number of patient visits to the county hospitals increased by 23.7 percent, from 321,786 visits to 398,117, while the number of patient visits to the commune and district clinics increased by only 0.22 percent, from 718,410 visits to 720,021. During the same period, the total population of Jiande county increased by 9.4 percent, from 404,800 to 442,700 (Yan 1985, 84). C. C. Chen, who strongly disapproved of the fact that barefoot doctors regarded themselves as physicians, also noticed the decline of the commune clinics in Shaifang county, Sichuan Province: "Some *xiang* (township) health centers received fewer patients than in the past" (Chen 1989, 169). By the early 1980s, the barefoot doctors and their village clinics (the former brigade medical stations) had replaced township clinics (the former commune and union clinics), thus achieving medical dominance in local communities. Meanwhile, the township clinics largely degenerated into administrative medical units. The dumbbell-shaped structure of the rural medical system therefore was further strengthened. This change in medical institutions occurred in tandem with an increasingly Westernized medical knowledge structure that resulted from the introduction of Western medicine into rural China (Leung 2007, 1). The fates of commune clinics were similar to those of Chinese medicine doctors. The clinics declined as traditional establishments evolved into modern medical institutions, while Chinese medicine doctors either gradually faded out of the village medical world or transformed themselves by adopting Western medical knowledge and techniques.

Legitimacy, Identity, and Profession

The emergence of barefoot doctors after 1968 occurred within the context of the concurrent penetration of state power and Western medicine into Chinese villages. As new kinds of village healers, barefoot doctors were inserted into the reshuffled and reorganized medical world of Chinese villages as one of the "newly emerged things" of the Cultural Revolution. They undertook medical and health work in the specific social environment of the people's commune system, which was an enclosed village society because of the implementation of the household registration system dividing urban and rural areas. The barefoot doctors' removal from agricultural labor meant that they gradually became a special category of commune member, distinguished by their professional knowledge and specialist work, which became the prime feature of their new group identity. Simultaneously, they demarcated themselves from "competitors" in the local community, including folk healers (legitimate ones like herbal medicine healers and illegitimate ones such as religious and supernatural healers) and other medical practitioners, and also forged links with medical station colleagues and their barefoot doctor peers. A steep career ladder and blocked social mobility facilitated their stability as a group and contributed to the formation of a sense of group identity. Meanwhile, the barefoot doctors' status and the respect they earned rose steadily in part as a result of their daily interactions with patients and because of the rapidity of the effects of Western medicine. The doctors' efficiency and availability contrasted with the shortage of medicine and medical knowledge among the villagers. When barefoot doctors made mistakes in their delivery of medical services, these were ignored by the state intentionally and neglected by the patients unconsciously. This further increased the barefoot doctors' power over the villagers. In this process, the state contributed to the formation of group identity among barefoot doctors and facilitated their ascendance in community power relationships.

The rural economic reform after 1978, in which medical proficiency was listed as a key requirement, redefined the medical legitimacy of barefoot doctors. In order to motivate barefoot doctors to improve their medical proficiency and thereby enhance the quality of the cooperative medical service, in October 1979 the State Council proposed holding examinations to certify barefoot doctors (LWBW 1992, 146). Concurrently, rural economic reforms began that would lead eventually to decollectivization and the fragmentation of the commune system. The barefoot doctor program disintegrated in the context of this dual process of new medical certification and the implementation of a new household responsibility system. The cooperative medical service, the core institutional context that had supported the barefoot doctors, also ceased to exist with the end of the people's communes (now known as townships). The barefoot doctors had to make a living from medicine on their own initiative rather than from work points allocated by the commune's production brigades (now known as administrative villages). On January 24, 1985, health minister Chen Minzhang announced during the concluding session of the National Health Bureau Directors' Meeting that the term "barefoot doctor" would no longer be used in China (Chen 1985b).

The reduction in barefoot doctor numbers that resulted from the inability of individual doctors to meet new medical proficiency standards during the 1980s was highly significant for both the state and the barefoot doctors themselves. This process raised the barefoot doctors' expertise as a group, because those remaining had necessarily attained these qualifications. This increase in expertise simultaneously contributed to the consolidation of their authority among their fellow villagers. As a result of this process, the barefoot doctors increased their legitimacy in the eyes of both the government and their fellow villagers. The rise in their social and economic status further separated the barefoot doctors from their fellow villagers and positioned them as a professional group in possession of specialist knowledge to which they had privileged access. In this sense, the medical examination and group differentiation had a positive impact on rural health because of the increasing professionalization of the field. The development of barefoot doctors presented a special path toward the formation of a medical profession. It was initiated by a political campaign, developed in an enclosed village society, and strengthened through the doctors' having survived profound social changes.

Rural Medical Reform in the New Millennium

The basic structure of the rural health care delivery system did not undergo much change from the early 1980s until the implementation of medical reforms called the "integrated management of rural health" (*nongcun weisheng yitihua guanli*) in 2008–2010. These regulations required each former township clinic or hospital to be converted into a community health service center. Extant village clinics were abolished, while county governments established new health service stations or converted extant village clinics into health service stations. Each station was to have an outpatient room, treatment room, pharmacy, and transfusion room (for intravenous drips). The locations of health service stations were set according to the "twenty-minute service circle," a distribution principle that ensured that nobody should be more than twenty minutes away from a health service station by foot. Village doctors were incorporated into these health service stations, but the majority of them had to leave the home-based clinics from which they had been operating since the early 1980s because they were assigned to neighboring villages or even other townships. Instead of the twenty-four-hour service that village doctors previously provided, they were to work according to a strict timetable at the new community health service centers and stations. The regulations specify that these centers and stations must provide "six-in-one" services to villagers (now called rural residents), which encompass prevention, treatment, promotion of health and well-being, rehabilitation, health education, and family planning advice.

At the same time as this major restructuring of the rural medical system, the National Basic Pharmaceutical Catalog (*guojia jiben yaowu mulu*) was put into effect. It regulated that doctors at rural health centers could prescribe 307 pharmaceuticals (205 types of Western medicines and 102 types of Chinese patent medicines). As economic conditions vary nationwide, local governments are authorized to complement the national catalog with extra pharmaceuticals. For example, Zhejiang Province added 150 types, while Hangzhou prefecture added 50, bringing the total types of basic pharmaceuticals for some counties within Hangzhou prefecture up to 507. These pharmaceuticals are supplied to health service centers through a collective bidding system. The centers implement ze-ro-profit sales in which there is no difference between the wholesale and retail prices.

Meanwhile, since the majority of current village doctors (*nongcun shequ yisheng*) will be retiring soon, in 2009 each county government started train-ing rural community doctors to fill these forthcoming vacancies. Senior middle school students who sit for the national college entrance examination were se-lected and sent to study clinical medicine for three years at medical colleges, and will be assigned to health service stations after graduation. Without any doubt, the barefoot doctors of the Cultural Revolution era will completely disappear from the medical world of China's villages in the near future.

Conclusion

The barefoot doctor program, which lasted from 1968 to 1983, represented a piv-otal stage in the displacement of Chinese medicine by Western medicine in rural China. Actually, the program was one of a series of landmark events that occurred in the long-term historical development of rural health and medicine in China since the early twentieth century, including the initiation of the experimental ru-ral health programs in the 1930s, the founding of the Communist regime in 1949, the popularization of the barefoot doctor program in 1968, the disintegration of the barefoot doctor group around 1983, and the recent rural medical reform. The essence of this developmental trend has remained constant: the introduction of Western medicine (i.e., modern medicine) profoundly influenced the scientiza-tion, institutionalization, and professionalization of medical practice.

The introduction of Western medicine into the villages was not only a top-down process dependent on the power of the state, but also a bottom-up process of acceptance and adaptation. As Volker Scheid has argued, while political pro-cesses have been an important factor in these changes, they are by no means the only factor that has shaped contemporary Chinese medicine. He contends that "grassroots pressure for a more modern Chinese medicine expressed locally by patients through such mechanisms as practitioner selection, demand for cer-tain kinds of diagnosis or treatment, or simply through bringing to the clinical encounter certain kinds of problems cannot be ignored" (Scheid 2002, 128). As the villagers experienced their health care providers' transformation from "old things" to "newly emerged things," they necessarily experienced a dramatic shift in their health worlds and underwent significant changes as citizens and patients. Their participation in public health campaigns fully reflected the features of body politics in socialist contexts, such as submitting stool samples in the morning and allowing doctors to take blood samples from their ears in the evening. The villagers quickly formed their own comparative medical beliefs about Chinese and Western medicines, as a result of which Chinese medicine was soon relegated to a secondary position. Thanks to medical institutionalization, the scope of the villagers' medical encounters was greatly expanded and extended beyond their home village boundaries. The establishment of the state medical system and the formation of a socialist medical profession also diversified their relationship with doctors. With the advent of barefoot doctors, villagers enjoyed a relatively equal relationship with their medical service providers in the enclosed societies of their home villages. But the advent of medical commercialization under the market economy not only brought more plentiful medical resources, but also worsened the doctor-patient relationship, leading to both holding negative images of each other.

Undoubtedly, as the performers of state policies and providers of medical service to villagers, the barefoot doctors played the most important role in this transformation. The foundations laid by the barefoot doctors in rural medical health—scientization, medical institutionalization, and professionalization—are still the key themes of rural medicine in present-day China. Meanwhile, the recent radical medical reform has intended to tackle a few thorny challenges, including ending the abuse of pharmaceuticals, demolishing the dumbbell-shaped structure of the medical system, and improving the proficiency of rural medical personnel. These main challenges are similar to those faced by modern medicine today throughout the world. Therefore, even the challenges that now face medicine in rural China—and will continue to confront it for the foreseeable future—are further evidence of the great transformation in rural health that was brought about in large part by the barefoot doctor program.

Part IV
Professional Transitions

14 A Case Study of Transnational Flows of Chinese Medical Professionals

China Medical Board and Rockefeller Foundation Fellows

Mary Brown Bullock

COMPELLING QUESTIONS ABOUT human health have motivated the transnational flow of physicians for millennia. Egypt was seen as the font of medical knowledge by the Greeks, Persians, and Turkic kingdoms from the thirteenth century BCE to the Roman era. Egyptian physicians were dispatched to the ancient courts of Europe and the Middle East while medical writers plumbed ancient Egyptian texts for knowledge of ancient Egyptian pharmaceutical formulas. In the first millennium AD, Arabic physicians first retrieved and then reinterpreted the classical Greek medical traditions of Hippocrates and Galen. In Asia, trade routes between the Middle East, the Indian subcontinent, and China facilitated the flows of medical practitioners and ideas from west to east and east to west. In her book *Needles, Herbs, Gods, and Ghosts: China, Healing, and the West to 1848*, Linda Barnes (2000) details the multiple Chinese influences on European medicine in the early modern era. During the sixteenth and seventeenth centuries the Jesuits included medicine in the intellectual repertoire they brought to the late Ming and early Qing courts.

It was not until the nineteenth century, however, that medicine emerged as one of the most important avenues of cultural encounter between China and the West. Earlier chapters in this volume describe the multiple international influences on medicine in China. With regard to education, during most of the nineteenth century medical missionaries trained Chinese assistants as apprentices in missionary hospitals. Statistics indicate that 268 students had been trained up until 1898, with 194 still in training at thirty-six missionary hospitals. The first medical schools were constituted in the 1890s in Hong Kong, Tianjin, and Beijing. By 1930 there were twenty-four medical schools, eight of which were missionary-sponsored (Choa 1990, 80–94).

Relatively few Chinese students studied abroad during the nineteenth century, but among the few were medical students. The first Chinese to study medicine in the West appears to have been Huang Kuan, who obtained his medical degree from the University of Edinburgh in 1853. Four notable Chinese women graduated from American medical schools in the last quarter of the century: Jin Yunmei (Women's Medical College, New York Infirmary), Hu Kim-eng (Philadelphia College for Women), and Shi Meiyu and Gan Jiehou (University of Michigan). All returned to China for active medical careers. But by the end of the century Chinese students were traveling to Japan, Europe, and the United States for foreign study; engineering was the most prevalent field but medicine was also important (Choa 1990, 80–94).

These individuals were the vanguard of China's Western-educated medical profession. During the first two decades of the twentieth century most medical students studied abroad for their primary medical degrees. Early key destinations were Japan and Germany, followed by the United States, the United Kingdom, and France. When they returned to China these physicians constituted subgroups by virtue of their international training, and they often affiliated with institutions sponsored by their host country. The Japanese-returned group, for example, was largely based in northeast China while the German-educated group concentrated in Shandong and Shanghai. Subsequent study-abroad cohorts, especially after the early 1920s, were usually graduates of Chinese or missionary medical colleges who sought advanced training abroad. They returned to China, bringing updated knowledge of Western medicine, especially the specialized professions which were becoming part of the landscape of American and European medicine.

Chinese studying medicine abroad joined a much larger cohort of individuals who sought scientific and medical expertise in Europe and the United States during the twentieth century. There is a considerable body of literature which explores this transnational flow of people, including analysis of specific disciplines, countries, or time periods. Other studies explore the challenge of "brain drain" or cultural and social adaptation. Still others assess the intellectual, professional, or technological impact of returned scholars in their home country. Since Asia has been the source of some of the largest flows of students to study in Europe and the United States there have been numerous case studies and books that explore different facets of these intellectual migrations. A particular focus has been on Taiwan, South Korea, and India. There have also been many studies of Chinese students and scholars studying abroad, both prior to 1949 and since 1980 (Ye 2001; Bieler 2004; Levine n.d.; Li 2008a). There does not, however, appear to have been any study of Chinese medical personnel who studied in the United States and returned to China.

As their numbers grew, foreign-trained returning Chinese physicians began to replace their missionary forebears on the faculties of medical colleges, as leaders of hospitals, and in new public health institutions. Their international training positioned them well for higher-level positions. While there has been some interest in the growing professionalization of practitioners of traditional Chinese medicine, there has been less focus on these Western-educated Chinese who began to shape the directions of modern medicine in China, assuming responsibility for China's medical and public health institutions (Xu 2001). Sonya Grypma and Cheng Zhen's chapter in this volume contributes to this vacuum in its review of the history of nursing. This chapter focuses on the medical fellowship program sponsored by the Rockefeller Foundation and the China Medical Board as a case study of Chinese medical personnel who studied abroad, primarily in the United States, during the Republican period. From this admittedly selective cohort we gain some insight into the transnational influence of secular American medicine in Republican China and its longer-term influence in China.

Between 1905 and 1954 approximately 35,931 Chinese students trained in the United States, of whom 2,455, or 7.8 percent trained in medical fields (Wang 1966, 510–511). Of these, approximately 350 were sponsored by the China Medical Board and the Rockefeller Foundation. One distinguishing feature of the CMB/ RF fellows was that they were graduate students, not undergraduates. Nearly all of the CMB/RF fellows had already completed their medical study in China before studying abroad: they were older than many of their Chinese colleagues and were seeking advanced degrees or specialized medical or public health education. If Y. C. Wang was correct in his 1969 study, *Chinese Intellectuals and the West, 1982–1949*, this means that the medical fellows were likely to have a successful career experience upon their return to China. For Wang writes, "Foreign study has a maximum chance of success only if the students are mature in age, have definite objectives in mind and limit their sojourn to fairly short periods" (Wang 1966, xiii).

A second distinction was that individuals were selected with the specific goal of building institutional capacity in their home institution. This differed from the better-known Boxer Indemnity Program or the Chinese government–sponsored scholarship program, which relied on examinations for the selection of promising individuals, not their future institutional roles. Peter Buck's *American Science and Modern China, 1876–1936*, which is otherwise very critical of the Rockefeller project, made this comparative observation:

> The proponents of the Boxer scholarships presumed that individual Chinese could be outfitted with a science so powerful that they could revivify their government and then reorder their society without additional assistance. By

Table 14.1. Source institutions for Chinese medical grants awarded
Rockefeller Foundation Fellowships to the United States

Institution	Number of Fellows 1917–1950
Peking Union Medical College	35
Changsha: Yale-China	14
Shantung Christian College (Qilu)	8
Shanghai National Medical College	8

Note: This is an incomplete records of PUMC medical fellows. My earlier records indicate that sixty-four PUMC graduates studied abroad before 1937 (Bullock 1980, 127).

contrast, the China Medical Board found in a similarly potent body of knowledge evidence that the prerequisites for effective social, scientific, and medical practice were irreducibly organizational and institutional rather than personal. (Buck 1980, 48)

For the CMB/RF, strengthening medical institutions in China meant a commitment to advanced training in the United States *and* successful reintegration into scores of home institutions in China. Nominees were carefully selected with a view to both what training was needed and what position each individual would assume upon return to China. Staff in Beijing and New York kept meticulous records of each individual's course of study, with particular focus on their preparation for return to China.[1] The records also note what institution (or institutions) and what position the individual returned to in China. For in fact almost all returned. Immigration laws were highly restrictive throughout this era and very few Chinese scholars found placement in American universities or other institutions (*A Survey of Chinese Students* 1954; Wang 1966).[2]

Medical Fellows

An analysis of the CMB/RF medical fellows reveals a network that linked an extensive number of Chinese institutions with a targeted group of medical educational institutions in the United States. More than fifty home institutions are identified for the CMB/RF Chinese fellows in public health, medicine, and nursing. Adding the Chinese home institutions of CMB/RF missionary fellows would bring the number to well over one hundred.[3] In the United States the Rockefeller Foundation relied on about twenty institutions to provide advanced medical training for Chinese fellows. As we shall see, however, more than 56 percent of all medical and public health fellows went to three institutions: Harvard, Johns Hopkins, and the University of Chicago.

Looking first at the home institutions of medical fellows, a predictable pattern of home institutions is observed: from a total of eighty-three fellows for

Table 14.2. Destination institutions for Chinese medical grants awarded Rockefeller Foundation Fellowships to the United States

Institution	Number of CMB/RF Medical Fellows 1917–1950
Harvard	21
Johns Hopkins	16
University of Chicago	10

whom we have records, the Peking Union Medical College (PUMC) garnered the lion's share of fellowships, followed by three prominent medical colleges.

The remainder were scattered across eleven additional medical colleges or hospitals, including the Japanese-sponsored Mukden Medical College, West China Medical College, and the Shanghai Red Cross Hospital. This group includes prominent Chinese medical leaders of the Republican era, including Zhang Xiaoqian, Liu Juiheng, Marion Yang, Shi Meiyu, Yan Fuqing, Lin Kesheng, and Wu Xian. Their careers are discussed elsewhere in this volume.

The American host institutions were somewhat predictable as well—they were dominated by Harvard, Johns Hopkins, and the University of Chicago.[4] Each had established distinct medical relations with China during the early years of the Republic: Harvard had started a medical school in Shanghai, Johns Hopkins was the model for PUMC, and the first director of PUMC (Franklin McLean) returned to be the first head of the University of Chicago Medical School.

The Chinese CMB/RF fellows usually had an MD degree, either from abroad in the early years or from PUMC or another Chinese institution in later years. They stayed for one or two years, strengthening their specialization or conducting research. All had senior American faculty mentors. Nine received doctorates in medicine (this was during an age when PhDs in medicine were not common). It was this in-depth advanced training abroad that set the CMB/RF fellows apart from their domestically trained colleagues, enabling them to become leaders in their medical fields in China.

Public Health Fellows

Public health was not a formal institutional focus of the Rockefeller Foundation in China but China was the origin of the largest group of Rockefeller public health fellowships from Asia: a total of ninety-eight, primarily sponsored by the International Health Board, a division of the Rockefeller Foundation. These public health fellows appear to have constituted almost all of the Chinese students who studied public health in the United States during the Republican period. The China Institute in America's *Survey of Chinese Students in American Universities and Colleges in the Past One Hundred Years,* a comprehensive questionnaire sent to all American colleges and universities and published in 1954, only lists a total of sixty Chinese public health students overall. This obviously low number may be because Johns Hopkins did not participate in the survey; also it is highly likely that some public health specialists are subsumed under the medical category. It should be noted that missionary medicine gave little attention to public health (Andrews 2013), and PUMC was the only medical school that included a department of preventive medicine. This was a relatively new field and domestic training institutions were just beginning to emerge, primarily under government auspices and at a technical level.

A review of seventy-two of the CMB/RF fellowship files reveals that about one-third came from various units of the Guomindang's National Health Administration in Nanjing, while others came primarily from provincial health administrations in other cities and provinces. The years covered (1917–1950) included the transition from the Beiyang to the Nanjing government and then to the great dislocation during the Sino-Japanese War, discussed elsewhere in this volume by Nicole Barnes and John Watt. An analysis of the Chinese sending institutions illustrates the dominant role played by the Nanjing government in supporting national and provincial institutions which required public health specialists. While significant concentrations were in Nanjing, Shanghai, and Peking, the home institutions also included China's far-flung emergent public health programs during the Republican period—from Inner Mongolia and Gansu to Guizhou and Yunnan, and, in the late 1940s, Taiwan. Attention to Gansu and Inner Mongolia was directly linked to the Guomindang military efforts. Rockefeller fellowship funding certainly stimulated these government nation-building efforts. As in most countries there were relatively few, if any, nongovernment public health institutions.

Twenty-five specific institutions were included in the home institutions, and the majority were national or provincial institutions such as the National Epidemic Prevention Bureau (which changed location several times), Shanghai's Department of Health, the Guiyang Provincial Health Administration, or the several different (and changing) institutions which comprised Nanjing's National Health Administration itself—the National Institute of Health, the Central Field Health Station, and so on. Indeed, of eighty-seven individuals, twenty-seven, or 30 percent, came directly from some Nanjing-based institutional component of the National Health Administration. (Most of these moved to the southwest after 1937.) The individuals who received fellowship grants reads like a who's who of public health during the Republican period, and include Wu Lien-teh, Jin Baoshan, Hu Houki, and Chen Zhiqian.

What at first seems most surprising is where these individuals studied in the United States: 85 percent studied at either Johns Hopkins (forty-three fellows) or Harvard (thirty-one fellows). The remainder were scattered among six other American institutions, including the University of North Carolina, Columbia University, and the University of Michigan. The overall predominance of Harvard and Johns Hopkins for CMB/RF fellows reflects the elite educational orientation of Chinese students in many fields of study in the United States. We do not have the comprehensive figures for Johns Hopkins because of its nonparticipation in the *Survey of Chinese Students,* but Harvard ranked fourth (behind Columbia University, the University of Michigan, and MIT) in the numbers of Chinese students in all fields between 1854 and 1954 (*A Survey of Chinese Students* 1954). Since the largest group of Chinese students were in engineering and Harvard did not have an engineering program, the significance of this concentration is more notable.

Nature of the Sino-American Medical Connections: Johns Hopkins, a Case Study

In the early decades of the twentieth century Harvard and Johns Hopkins both reflected the revolution in American medical education promulgated by the Flexner Report of 1910, which emphasized the premedical natural sciences, research laboratories, clinical research, and full-time teaching in a university setting. Both universities also created new schools of public health that epitomized a new American, as opposed to European, approach: the European curricula tended toward laboratory-based science and sanitary engineering, with a focus on disease control. The Flexnerian reforms reinforced a hospital-based curative medicine and a science-based, instead of sanitary engineering–based, approach to public health. This emergent American medical style differed very significantly from the missionary internships of the late nineteenth century, the basic medical education of the early Chinese and missionary medical colleges, and European sanitary engineering programs. Given its prominence in educating Chinese students in medicine, public health, and nursing, and its serving as the model for PUMC, a brief analysis of the Hopkins model and its China connections suggests the nature of this secular, scientific American influence on medicine in Republican China.

In the late nineteenth century the creation of Johns Hopkins University, hospital, and medical school coalesced into one institution the varying European influences on American medical education. The integration of the basic sciences and clinical medicine into an educational model which emphasized both laboratory research and hospital clinical care transformed American medicine, and ultimately global medicine as well. A School of Nursing, essential for a hospital-centered medical system, was included as part of the Johns Hopkins biomedical complex. Enshrined by the 1910 Flexner Report and funded by the Rockefellers as *the* reform model for medical education, Johns Hopkins set the standards for American medicine.

The creation of the Johns Hopkins School of Hygiene and Public Health in 1916 added the "Hopkins model" of public health as well. This was the first professional school of public health that integrated scientific investigation into disease causation, with such fields as epidemiology and sanitary engineering. It sought to create a new multidisciplinary medical profession that would no longer be dominated by either sanitary engineers or physicians. William Henry Welch, trained in laboratory science as a pathologist in Germany, became both the first dean of the Johns Hopkins Medical School and the first dean of the Johns Hopkins School of Public Health and Hygiene. Welch traveled to China twice, in 1915 and 1921, and was the key advisor in structuring PUMC's curriculum along the lines of Johns Hopkins'. He also retained a strong interest in China, serving as a mentor for Chinese students who studied at Hopkins and American faculty who taught in China. Welch personally selected Hopkins faculty or recent graduates to teach and do research in China, monitored their progress, and assured their professional return, if not to Hopkins then to other elite institutions such as Harvard or the University of Chicago. An intellectual map of American medical professionals with experience in China, primarily at PUMC, who also had Hopkins, Harvard, or Chicago connections would be very revealing.

As early as the 1910s and 1920s, Johns Hopkins played an active role in educating Chinese students. By 1925, sixty of them had matriculated in various fields, including thirty who had received an MD degree. This early China interest was reinforced by Rockefeller funding which supported the Johns Hopkins Medical School, and it was also Rockefeller funding, after a national competition, that created the Johns Hopkins School of Public Health and Hygiene. It was thus quite natural for both the Rockefeller Foundation and its China Medical Board to use Hopkins as an American institutional base for their international fellowship programs. The connections between the Johns Hopkins School of Public Health and Hygiene and Rockefeller personnel were especially close: except for Victor Heiser, all of the senior International Health Board's public health personnel in Asia, including John Grant, had been trained at Hopkins (Bullock 2011). It is likely that a review of Rockefeller Foundation fellowship recipients from other Asian countries would also reveal that a disproportionate number trained at Hopkins. An institutional history describes the small classes and international character of the Johns Hopkins School of Public Health during the 1920s and 1930s. In the 1920s one-third of the students were international—long before the late twentieth-century "globalization" of higher education (Fee 1987).

It should also be emphasized that the flow of ideas across the Pacific was not one-way. John Grant's Peking urban health station—a community-based concept of preventive medicine which integrated curative and preventive medicine in a single model—was emulated for a time in an experimental program at Hopkins. Also, a recent Hopkins undergraduate honors thesis by Alexandra Zenoff describes the similar institutional structures and the many collaborative research projects between Johns Hopkins faculty and PUMC, sometimes in Beijing, sometimes in Baltimore. Key Hopkins faculty who played a critical role in China included Adrian Taylor (surgery), Francis Dieuaide (medicine), and William Cort (parasitology) (Zenoff 2010).

Significance of CMB/RF Fellowship Program

As noted earlier, Chinese medical students went to the United States under many auspices; this analysis includes only the small cohort under the Rockefeller Foundation and the China Medical Board. Most of the others who went to the United States would have experienced some variant of the Hopkins model outlined above: after 1911 American medical education across the country began to adopt the Flexnerian reforms. The growing range of medical professional opportunities in China would have been open to them—ranging from hospitals to private practice to research and professorships. One difference between the CMB/RF fellows and other Chinese medical professionals was that CMB/RF fellows overwhelmingly spent their careers in institutions rather than in private practice.

Compared with other medical professionals, the participants in the CMB/RF medical fellowship program were further along in their careers and were located at the more privileged institutions with which Rockefeller personnel worked. Their American research experience deepened the biomedical background of an elite group who returned to positions of some influence. For example, we know that seven of the ten presidents of the National Medical Association from 1915 to 1937 had received a China Medical Board or Rockefeller fellowship to study abroad (Wong and Wu 1936, 612, plate 43).[5]

We do have some data on the careers of the CMB/RF contingent after they returned to China, at least until 1949. The majority of the medical fellows returned to their former institutional base—medical colleges—and often to higher positions. Absent case-by-case detailed analysis, there are several ways to project their subsequent roles. Given the reward structure in higher education in Republican China, specialized study abroad undoubtedly enhanced their individual professional careers. Their return also reinforced the American medical influence—with its emphasis on biomedicine—on these already elite medical colleges. We know that many of these individuals became prominent in the Western medical associations of the era, whether the Chinese Medical Association or the growing number of specialized societies. We can surmise that these individuals were influenced by the research and institutional norms they experienced, which included an emphasis on full-time institutional roles (not private practice) and clinical research.

While detailed information on the role of this entire cohort after 1949 is not available, data on the medical careers of PUMC alumni (many of whom were represented in this group) suggests that the majority would probably have remained at their original institutions and in positions of increasing leadership even after the establishment of the People's Republic of China. Many suffered severely during the anti-American campaigns of the 1950s and the Cultural Revolution. The imported Soviet model of medicine, which also drew from continental influences in the Republican period, rejected the Flexnerian model with its eight-year curriculum that included a liberal arts premedical program. During the Maoist period, medical training varied from three to five years. But the primarily Flexnerian model of medical education which had prevailed in most Chinese medical colleges by the 1940s was not forgotten. The Peking Union Medical College repeatedly tried to resurrect it. After Deng Xiaoping's "reform and opening" the longer eight-year curriculum, with its emphasis on premedical education in the natural sciences and clinical research, became the aspirant model for China's top medical colleges.

One component of the Flexner and Johns Hopkins model which many Chinese medical institutions (including PUMC) lacked in both the Republican and the PRC periods was integration with comprehensive universities. They were primarily stand-alone medical institutions, and this did not change in Maoist China. This has isolated medical schools in China from their sister disciplines in the humanities and the natural, social, and engineering sciences. During the last ten years the Chinese government has attempted to merge medical schools into comprehensive universities. These mergers, however, were not intellectually driven but were rather "forced" mergers: a comprehensive research university with an integrated medical school has yet to evolve. Intellectually this means that medical education in China throughout these past hundred years has been intellectually separate from the natural and social sciences and the humanities.

If medical education was significantly altered, the curative hospital-based system of medical care delivery in urban areas was not dismantled. This emphasis on institutions of curative rather than preventive medicine is a lasting Flexnerian influence. Michelle Renshaw's chapter in this volume reveals the persistence of the hospital model in China to this day. The urban hospitals of the late Republican period, many of which were started as missionary hospitals, are often the key urban hospitals in China today. Some institutions have museums which reach back to the early Republican period, often highlighting the careers and institutional influences of those who studied medicine abroad.

The influence of the CMB/RF public health specialists is quite different. There is no question that this cohort, who also primarily returned to China, were among the only public health specialists trained in the United States. (China also trained public health specialists in Europe, especially the United Kingdom and in some eastern European countries, but detailed data is not available.) Their ongoing influence is directly tied to the fate of China's National Health Administration and its provincial outposts. Here there are also direct linkages between the Guomindang's public health institutions and those of the People's Republic of China. The National Health Administration's Central Field Health Station merged with the National Personnel Training Institute in 1941 to create China's National Institute of Health (*Zhongyang weisheng shiyanyuan*). After 1950, most of the functions of that institute and its personnel were moved to Beijing. By 1958 the government had consolidated them into the Chinese Academy of Medical Sciences, co-housed with the Peking Union Medical College. The institute of public health went through several iterations but eventually became China's Center for Disease Control in the 1990s.

Although many of the American-trained public health specialists continued in research and administrative positions, the most prominent (with the exception of Chen Zhiqian) were too closely tied to Chiang Kai-shek's government to remain in the People's Republic of China. While a few went to Taiwan, a significant number found positions in the newly created World Health Organization. One of the most prominent, Jin Baoshan, did return to China in the 1950s and led Peking Medical University's Department of Preventive Medicine.

Unlike the Flexnerian model of medical education, the American public health education model, well represented by the Johns Hopkins College of Public Health and Hygiene, did not have an institutional impact in China. China did not develop a university-based model of public health education during the Republican era. The governmental National Health Administration, including its training institutions, assumed responsibility for training in many public health disciplines. After 1950 the Soviet model of public health education, a second-tier system of primarily vocational and engineering training, prevailed. These public health institutions continue today, augmented by newer schools of public health within medical colleges which generally lack the prestige of other medical disciplines.

This analysis of the CMB/RF medical fellowship program augments previous studies of the Rockefeller Foundation and the China Medical Board. It reveals that the Rockefeller patronage network in China was far broader and deeper than hitherto realized. While PUMC received the lion's share of funding, Rockefeller medical fellowships contributed to scores of other Chinese institutions. Many of these individuals came to know each other as Hopkins or Harvard alumni, reinforcing existing professional relationships. It is also clear that the elite American medical institutions gained experience and became vested in the training of Chinese physicians and public health specialists, creating additional networks across the Pacific. One additional thing is quite clear as well: the patterns of transnational medical education during the Republican period were quickly renewed after President Richard Nixon's trip to China. Indeed, medical diplomacy led the way in the rapid normalization of scientific relations between the two countries.

The first Chinese delegation from the People's Republic of China to visit the United States was a medical delegation in 1972. Within a few years the transnational flow of medical specialists (primarily visiting scholars, not matriculating medical students) from China to the United States resumed.

Notes

Michella Choa reviewed the CMB/RF fellowship records at the Rockefeller Archive Center and prepared summary sheets of the individual records. Pan Jiening prepared a summary database of the medical and public health fellows.

1. In her review of the CMB/RF fellows' grant records, Michella Choa indicated that most note cards kept track of the course of study of each fellow.

2. Very few Chinese were in teaching positions in the United States prior to 1945. It is unlikely that many were in hospitals either.

3. Many of the CMB/RF medical missionary fellows were based at hospitals in China's hinterland, greatly expanding the geographical reach of the program. They are not included in this study.

4. Most of the primary host institutions were in the United States, although a few students studied in Europe. Fairly typical was a pattern of study abroad that included travel to European medical institutions at the end of a stay in the United States as well as multiple American institutional hosts. For convenience the first host institution has been chosen for this analysis.

5. These individuals were F. C. Yen, Wu Lien-teh, W. L. New, Liu Ruiheng, Lin Kesheng, W. S. New, C. E. Lim, and H. P. Chu.

15 The Development of Modern Nursing in China

Sonya Grypma and Cheng Zhen

The need for Chinese nursing leaders is great and can be met only through upholding high standards in nursing education.

—Lin (1938, 8)

In the introduction to her thesis submitted to the Department of Public Health at the Massachusetts Institute of Technology in February 1944, Chinese nurse Zhou Meiyu lamented that the China Ministry of War had not yet agreed to her proposal that army nurses be granted regular ranks (MCANYP 1944).[1] The following year, in a booklet geared toward garnering Western support to "help China train enough nurses to safeguard the health of her people," Zhou observed with satisfaction that "the people in military hospitals no longer consider nurses merely as privates or civilian guests. Nurses have won respectable positions among them" (Chow 1945, 16). Tacitly appealing to supporters of the American Bureau for Medical Aid to China for financial aid to develop the Army Nursing School to include postgraduate training of nursing teachers, Zhou noted that although the war was over, of the 6,400 nurses in China, scarcely 300 were qualified for teaching. "Since the army alone has asked for 2300 additional nurses," she wrote, "the preparation of sufficient teaching staff to handle the job [is] a serious problem" (Chow 1945, 15).

This snapshot of army nursing hints at three enduring themes in the early development of modern nursing in twentieth-century China: adaptation (adapting Western missionary and philanthropic nursing models to Chinese aims), status (seeking social acceptance and professional recognition), and crisis (responding to war and humanitarian disaster). We use the career of Zhou Meiyu as a springboard to discuss how these themes were expressed during three periods of nursing before 1949: nursing as Christian service (1873–1914), nursing as a profession (1914–1937), and nursing as patriotic service (1937–1949). We then examine how China developed new iterations of nursing after 1949 as seen through the (re)development of the Chinese Nursing Association, nursing higher education, nursing publications, nursing theory, and professional standards. Recognizing that nineteenth-century China had well-established traditional systems for healing and caring for the sick that were not well understood by the Western missionaries who introduced professional nursing (Liu 1991), we identify early modern (hospital-based) nursing in China as a transnational phenomenon involving the flow of nursing knowledge between nations.

Early Development of Nursing, 1873–1949

Zhou Meiyu was among the most influential Chinese nurses of the early twentieth century. A brilliant woman deeply committed to addressing the enormous health needs of wartime China, she embodied the complexities of a transnational profession. By leveraging her considerable social capital with both Western and Chinese decision-makers, Zhou advanced a vision of nursing as a highly organized, essential service comprised of well-educated men and women recognized for their expertise. The granddaughter of a Yale graduate and fully bilingual, Zhou attended Christian missionary schools in Beijing. She graduated at the top of her nursing class at the Peking Union Medical College (1930) and was awarded two Rockefeller fellowships to the United States (to study at MIT in 1933 and at Columbia in 1948), where she earned master's degrees in public health and nursing education, respectively (Chang 1993).[2] She served as chief nurse with the Mass Education Movement (1931–1938) and as director of the Army Nursing School (1938–1948) before moving to Taiwan in 1949, where she led nursing education reforms well into the 1980s. In 1958, Zhou became the first Chinese woman to achieve the rank of major general (*shaojing*) (Lo 2003). Today she is regarded in Taiwan as the mother of modern military nursing (*minguo junhu zhi mu*) and the "Chinese Florence Nightingale" (Zhang 2009a; "Tenth Medical Care Dedication Prize" 2000). Her personal links with some of the key players in nursing in both China and the West before 1949 expose the interrelatedness of those who were most influential in the development of modern nursing in China—the earliest of whom were Christian missionaries.

Nursing as Christian Service: Establishing Missionary Ideals (1873–1914)

When American missionary nurse Elizabeth McKechnie arrived in China as the first "trained" nurse in 1884 there was no equivalent in Chinese culture to the conceptualization of nursing popularized by Florence Nightingale—that is, a noble profession suitable for unmarried, God-fearing ladies (Grypma 2011). In the traditional healing system in China, "caring" (always undifferentiated from "serving") was a family responsibility with well-established gender norms and a status hierarchy in which care (particularly care of the body) could only be performed by a family/household member of the same gender and lower status than the patient (Liu 1991). In late nineteenth-century China it was inconceivable that Chinese ladies "of good family" would care for the sick, or that Chinese men would be cared for by women (Liu 1991). The earliest medical missionaries provided rudimentary training for young men from lower classes to assist them as attendants. While it is not clear whether male assistants worked with female patients, it is unlikely; a significant impetus for the recruitment of female medical missionaries was gender segregation in China. Although the goal of missionaries before the twentieth century was less to develop a profession than to find expedient ways to assist medical missionaries in their dual pursuit of healing bodies and souls, the outcome was the same: a cadre of nurses was necessary to support the increasingly hospital-based missionary work.

Female medical missionaries from American medical schools were the first to introduce modern nursing to China. China was a place where female American physicians could find career opportunities and status that eluded them at home. Dr. Lucinda Coombs (1873) and Dr. Elizabeth Reifsynder (1881), both American graduates from the Philadelphia Woman's Medical College, started the earliest nursing schools at women's hospitals they founded in Beijing (1881) and Shanghai (1886) (DCM 1881; Warrick 2005–2012 [1998]). Reifsnyder's decision to support missionary nurse Elizabeth McKechnie was closely related to the practicalities of establishing a hospital: nurses were needed to staff hospitals and to teach the next generation of nurses. Following the Western model of hospitals as the site of both training and service—where students provided much of the day-to-day care of patients—female physicians were the first to create a space for Western-style nurses. Gender played a significant role in this regard: in China, female doctors could carve out a professional niche for themselves that was socially acceptable in both China and the United States—that of women caring for women. Because nursing in the West was almost exclusively a female domain, it is not surprising that the earliest site of modern nursing in China was the "woman's hospital"—a place focused primarily on obstetrics and gynecology.

Like gender, religion also played a significant role in the early development of nursing. An understanding of nursing as Christian service extended into China where, for example, nursing textbooks translated into Chinese were imbued with Christian ideals—such textbooks included the seminal *Nursing Ethics* (1901), by Isabel Hampton Robb of the Johns Hopkins School of Nursing, which describes nursing as a "ministry [that] should represent a consecrated service, performed in the spirit of Christ" (Robb 1901).

Following on the gendered and religious model of sick care exemplified by the first female missionary physicians, American-educated Chinese physicians Jin Yumei (May King), Shi Meiyu (Mary Stone), and Kang Cheng (Ida Kahn) also started training schools for nurses. Associated since childhood with missionaries (Kang and Jin had been adopted by American missionaries as young girls), these women studied medicine at women's medical colleges in the United States before returning to China under the auspices of American missionary boards

(Chow 1998). They viewed their work as an expression of their Christian faith and piety (Ye 1994). By extension, the nursing schools they established—Jin Yumei in Tianjin (1907), Shi Meiyu and Kang Cheng in Jiujiang (1896)—were also imbued with Christian values. The congruence between early nursing and Christian ideals cannot be overstated: it was a belief in nursing as God's work that shaped the way it was introduced and adapted in China. Indeed, Western religious ideals proved more enduring than gendered ones: while most nursing programs in the West did not admit men until the 1970s, hospital-based training schools in China began admitting men in the early 1900s.

The development of modern nursing in turn-of-the-century China was largely dependent on the support of physicians, foreign missionary boards, the geographic location of the mission, and the local Christian community from which prospective nursing students were drawn. This is perhaps best illustrated by the comparatively slow development of nursing at Canada's first mission, in Henan Province (Grypma 2008). Although Canada's first missionary nurse, Harriet Sutherland, arrived only four years after Elizabeth McKechnie, the first nursing school in Henan was not established until thirty-five years later, in 1923. Unlike the American nurses recruited to work alongside female physicians, the earliest Canadian nurses were recruited to assist a male physician, James Frazer Smith. When Smith was invalided home in 1894, the remaining physicians displayed no interest in nursing assistance. Margaret McIntosh, the sole nurse in Henan between 1894 and 1914, turned her attention to evangelistic work. When subsequent missionary nurses later criticized McIntosh for her inattention to the development of nursing (Grypma 2008, 33), they overlooked a critical point: without evangelistic efforts, there could be no pool of Christian converts from which to draw student nurses. For example, Zhou Meiyu attended Peiyuan Primary School and Bridgeman Girls High School in Beijing and retained a lifetime reputation as a devout Christian (Lo 2003).

The theme of nursing as Christian service would underpin nursing development in China well into the 1920s. By the time, as Feng Qiuji notes, "we struck out their religious shadow," Christian missionaries had developed a scaffold of standards and values upon which subsequent nursing leaders built (Feng 2010). The earliest (American-sponsored) nursing schools were established in treaty ports like Beijing, Shanghai, Nanjing, and Fuzhou, where prospective students had more exposure to Western ideals. Still, while missionaries developed nursing schools across China between 1886 and 1914 (Chen 1996a), the actual number of schools remained small until the post-1911 Republican period when, as we shall see, Chinese nurses came into their own (Liu 1991, 320).

Nursing as a Profession: Developing a Chinese Nursing Elite (1914–1937)

Two organizations played a key role in the transition of nursing in China from a predominantly missionary enterprise to a fully nationalized one: the Nurses Association of China (established in 1909) and the Rockefeller Foundation's China Medical Board (established in 1914). Although both had missionary roots (Ferguson 1970, 20), their role in the Nanjing Decade (1927–1937) was characterized by a secular aim: the pursuit of an academically rigorous educational system for Chinese nurses in line with the highest international standards. The Rockefeller Foundation supported nursing through the creation of a first-rate nursing school at the Peking Union Medical College ("Johns Hopkins in the Orient") while simultaneously providing nursing fellowships for highly qualified Chinese nurses to study at prestigious universities in the West (Chen 1996b, 78). The NAC, in turn, sought to establish the status of nurses in China by enrolling all in a full course of training, and to protect standards by regulating the curriculum and minimum requirements for a diploma (Simpson 1922).

The NAC and PUMC were related in other ways: leaders in the former were frequently graduates of the other and both used English as their primary language of business. PUMC students were criticized, however, for their condescending attitudes toward graduates from various local hospitals of the country—something that was particularly evident during the PUMC evacuation to the "backwoods" of Chengdu during wartime (Watt 2004, 72). Yet PUMC graduates, who accounted for less than 2 percent of all nursing graduates in 1936, were sought out for their advanced knowledge of teaching and administration (Chen 1996b, 88).

In 1923 all nursing schools in China, "whether under missionary, government or private control," were invited to join the NAC ("Registration of Schools of Nursing" 1923). To be registered, hospitals housing the schools had to have at least twenty-five beds, and be able to provide obstetrical experience for female students. In 1926 the NAC reported 112 registered nursing schools across China (Simpson 1922, 7–10). Most prominent were Hunan-Yale in Changsha, Margaret Williamson in Shanghai, and Sleeper Davis and PUMC in Beijing (Lin 1938, 5–6).

In the absence of governmental oversight of nursing education in China before 1927, the NAC took responsibility for setting the criteria for all nursing schools in the country, formulating a model curriculum based on American standards, and holding certification examinations (Chen 1996a, 134). Initiated during an auspicious period of social change during which it became increasingly acceptable for female nurses to care for male patients (Stanley 2010, 282), the cumulative effect of NAC and Rockefeller Foundation initiatives was the development of a Chinese nursing elite, poised to take up leadership roles that emerged during the Nanjing Decade.

According to the NAC, the Chinese nurse was named into being at the 1914 national NAC conference in Shanghai, when Elsie Mawfung Chung (later the wife of Bayard Lyon), a graduate of Guys Hospital in London and the first Chinese nurse to be trained abroad, proposed the Chinese term *hushi* (caring scholar) to represent the emerging role for Chinese women (Simpson 1922, 15; Breay 1937). In 1915 the first NAC diplomas were granted to three students—two men and one woman who had passed the NAC examinations (Breay 1937, 137). Between 1909 and 1928 the number of registered nursing schools in China grew from 4 to 126 (Liu 2009). The appointment in 1928 of Wu Zheying (Lillian Wu), the first Chinese NAC president, marked nursing's potential as and transition to a thoroughly Chinese profession (Liu 2009, 34–35). Not incidentally, this shift to Chinese leadership occurred at the threshold of a new political era in China—the establishment of a new central government in Nanjing. The relative peace of the Nanjing Decade paved the way for the development of organizational structures to support a national program for nursing education and registration.

China's admittance into the International Council of Nurses in 1922 was a milestone for nursing in China. To be accepted into the ICN, member countries were required to have a national nursing association (with paying members) and a national program for nursing education. They also had to have a nursing journal. Beginning in 1920 the NAC published its own quarterly journal, the *Nursing Journal of China,* which carried each article in both English and Chinese (Chen 1996a, 138). Missionary nurse Nina Gage, who served as NAC president from 1912 to 1914 and as chair of the NAC Committee on Nursing Education in 1922, was elected as ICN's president in 1925. Notably the ICN quadrennial conference was set to be held in Beijing in 1929 (this plan was, however, later aborted).

In 1930 the Nationalist government invited the Nurses Association of China to move its headquarters from Beijing to Nanjing. The proximity of the NAC to the central government reflected the significance being placed on nursing education in China (Watt 2004, 72). In 1933 the minister of education established a subcommittee to register and supervise nursing education. In 1934 the Ministry of Health required nursing schools to have Chinese principals as a condition of registration (Lin 1938). This regulated preference for Chinese leaders sent an important message to the nursing community, still largely comprised of foreign nurse educators and administrators: Chinese nursing would no longer be dependent on foreign missionaries for its future direction (Watt 2004, 76). PUMC became an important source of well-educated nursing leaders; by 1937 it had graduated ninety-nine nurses who were specialists in teaching or administration.

The appointments of Nie Yuchan (Vera Nieh) and Zhou Meiyu to leadership positions during the Nanjing Decade illustrate the interrelatedness and relative influence of the China Medical Board, PUMC, and the NAC on nursing innovations encouraged by the new Nationalist government. Nie Yuchan was appointed by the Ministry of Health as the first secretary of the Central Board of Nursing Education in Nanjing (part of the NAC) ("News about Nursing" 1940). She was a PUMC graduate (1927) who received Rockefeller fellowships to study public health nursing at the University of Toronto (1929) and Columbia Teachers College (1929–1933) and then supported herself during her graduate studies at the University of Michigan (1937–1938) (Davis 1983a; CMB 1938). After war broke out

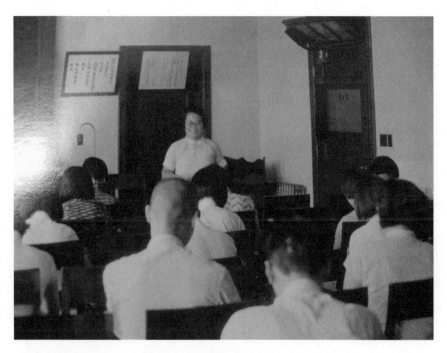

Figure 15.1. Public health classroom, Ting Hsien (Dingxian), 1935.
Source: Courtesy of Rockefeller Archive Center.

in 1937, both Nie and Zhou Meiyu were identified by the Nationalist government and the Rockefeller Foundation as among the best qualified to lead and address new nursing challenges that emerged during the war. Their responses to wartime trials would lay the groundwork for new forms of nursing that were more directly linked to the on-the-ground health care needs in China. Just as the Crimean War, the American Civil War, and World War I are considered catalysts for the development of nursing leadership in England, the United States, and Canada, respectively, the Second Sino-Japanese War (1937–1945) and Chinese Civil War (1945–1949) shaped the nature of nursing leadership in China. It was during this period that Chinese nurses would, for the first time, play a primary role in determining the most urgent nursing needs and creating new programs and structures to support them.

Nursing as Patriotic Service: Developing Wartime and Emergency Nursing (1937–1949)

Both Nie Yuchan and Zhou Meiyu played prominent roles in China nursing during wartime. Each was invited in 1938 to become the first Chinese dean of the

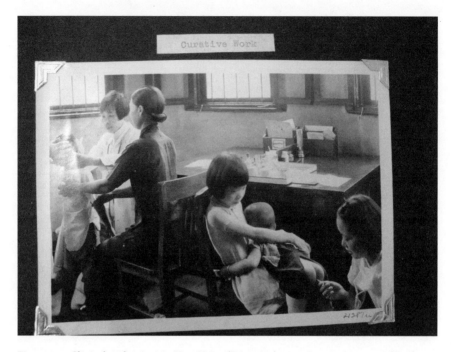

Figure 15.2. Clinical evaluations in Ting Hsien (Dingxian), 1935. *Source:* Courtesy of Rockefeller Archive Center.

PUMC School of Nursing when Gertrude Hodgman went on furlough in 1940; Nie was approached after Zhou declined the position. Both desired to work in the interior as part of the direct effort against the war; Zhou refused the PUMC deanship in order to do this.

At the outbreak of war in 1937, Nie Yuchan was in Michigan studying for a master of science degree in public health nursing (Davis 1983a; CMB 1938). In 1938 she decided to return to China rather than continue studies at Michigan, where she had intended to pursue a PhD. "Of course I am rather patriotic," reflected Nie in a 1983 interview. "I couldn't study anymore and I thought it was my duty to come back as a nurse and come back to join the war and do something" (Davis 1983a). Her hope was to work with the Red Cross in China's interior. But when she returned to Beijing to visit her mother, she was asked by Dr. Henry Houghton, director of PUMC, to take the position of dean of the PUMC School of Nursing. Although her first reaction was to decline since "I'm patriotic [so] I liked to join the war and not work in this invaded area [Beijing]," Nie agreed to take over the deanship when Hodgman went on furlough, in November 1940 (Davis 1983a).

When Nanjing fell into Japanese hands, the Nurses Association of China in Nanjing was reconstituted as the Chinese Nursing Association in Chongqing

(*Zhonghua hushi xuehui*), with new statutes that aimed to avoid political dilemmas associated with the Japanese occupation (80 percent of the nursing schools in occupied areas were closed or under puppet governments) (Watt 2004, 77). The trajectory of PUMC was suddenly altered after the December 7, 1941, attack on Pearl Harbor brought the United States into the Pacific war. Japanese soldiers entered PUMC in February 1942, and ordered the closure of the PUMC hospital and school. Nie made arrangements for the nursing students to be transferred to other nursing schools around China. Not willing to work under the Japanese—and believing that the best war efforts were to be found in Sichuan—Nie made the decision to go with her younger brother to Chongqing, site of the provisional wartime government capital. Ten of her colleagues—almost the entire PUMC nursing faculty—accompanied her (CMB 1946). A mass emigration of Chinese institutions to free China had already taken place, involving thousands of students and hundreds of professors traveling by boat, bus, or foot over hundreds of miles of dangerous territory—something C. H. Corbett called "one of the most astonishing phenomena in the struggle against Japan" (UCC n.d.). Partway through the two-month journey from Beijing to Chongqing, Nie's brother was killed by Guomindang soldiers (Davis 1983a). In Chongqing Nie became involved with plans to reopen PUMC under the aegis of the West China Union University nursing program in Chengdu (Davis 1983a). Although Nie took in three classes of PUMC students who had been studying in other universities in 1943 (Davis 1983a), Dr. Y. T. Tsur, chairman of the PUMC Board of Trustees, was clear that the nursing program at Chengdu was not to be considered a continuation of PUMC, but rather "a contribution of the College towards the war effort" (CMB 1945). After the victory against Japan in 1945, sixty PUMC students and staff returned to Beijing (CMB 1946); the hospital and nursing program officially reopened in 1948. By most accounts the level of nursing education achieved in Chengdu was extraordinary. As Dr. I. C. Yuan wrote in 1946, "What Miss Nie and her faculty have achieved during the war has shown the finest quality of Chinese professional women. We all are very proud of them! It may be of interest to you to know that the authorities of the West China Union University have decided to establish a school of nursing having the same standard as that of ours" (CMB 1946). That same year Nie Yuchang was elected president of the Nurses Association of China.

Wartime also tested and opened up new opportunities for Zhou Meiyu. She left PUMC in 1931 to work with the Mass Education Movement in Dingxian. As a result of the outbreak of the war in July 1937 and the rapid Japanese conquest of regions in northern and eastern China, nurses fled occupied regions and hospitals and nursing schools were closed, while the demand for emergency care of wartime wounded increased. The first wartime priority was to assist refugee nurses by arranging for their employment in existing hospitals or encouraging them to join military units. In September 1937 Zhou and her nurses fled Dingxian as Japanese soldiers advanced. She relocated to Changsha with the rest of the

Mass Education Movement (MEM) group, where Yan Yangchu worked to convert the MEM to national defense work for the central government (RAC 1937). This meant the conversion of nursing, too. When Zhou declined the deanship at the PUMC School of Nursing in 1938 (RAC n.d.b), it was to join Dr. Lim Khosheng (Robert Lim) at the newly formed Emergency Medical Service Training School at Guiyang (CMB 1939).

Concerned mostly with the dire need for emergency care, Zhou Meiyu trained all levels of health students, from ambulance workers to hospital orderlies to nurses. Her goal was for each of these individuals to be responsible for spreading health principles to the Chinese soldiers and others whom they came in contact with.

As large cities like Shanghai, Nanjing, Beijing, and Tianjin fell to the Japanese, well-equipped hospitals and nursing schools (including PUMC) were closed. During the war the number of nursing schools fell 80 percent, from 183 in 1937 to 35 in 1945. By 1946 the number had recovered to 150 (Watt 2004). Although 784 nurses graduated between 1940 and mid-1943, this had a negligible impact on the total number of nurses, which hovered at around 6,000 from 1936 until the end of the Republican period.

Only a comparatively small number of nurses were successful in evacuating to free China to carry on nursing work there. In 1942 the lack of facilities, books, supervisory personnel, and funds contributed to a growing shortage of prepared nurses. As a result, the government launched a large-scale educational program for the training of medical and nursing personnel. A committee comprising Rockefeller fellows Zhou Meiyu, Xu Aizhu, and Zhu Bihui (Bernice Chen-Chu), together with missionary nurse Cora Simpson, was struck to administer an NAC program subsidized by the American Bureau for Medical Aid to China to establish three new schools in three state hospitals—at Guiyang, Lanzhou, and Chongqing—and to offer graduate studies to make the profession more attractive (Watt 2004, 78). On July 1, 1943, Zhou Meiyu helped to establish the first National Army Nursing School in Guiyang, under the auspices of the Emergency Medical Service Training School. Fifty students were admitted.

While little has been written on the Japanese influence on Chinese nursing, it is worth noting that Chinese women drew from Japanese sources to help shape nursing as patriotic service. For example, female democratic revolutionist Qiu Jin translated and published a Japanese nursing textbook, *Kanhu jiaocheng*, in 1907 (Andrews 2001). The Red Cross Society of Japan (founded in 1886) had established nursing as a highly respectable profession there (Checkland 1994). While the extent to which the Chinese Red Cross Society (founded in 1905) modeled its nursing after Japan's is unknown, it seems likely that Zhou Meiyu's experience with the Red Cross Medical Relief Corps, and her subsequent development of military nursing, was informed by both Japanese and Western ideals.

In 1944, and with the encouragement of Yan Yangchu, Zhou completed a thesis on the development of an army nursing school in China (MCANYP 1944). She sent the thesis to MIT to fulfill the requirements of a master's degree in public health. When the war against Japan ended in 1945, Zhou argued that the army school was still necessary as a way to provide regular training for the thousands of young men and women who had served the army as nurses' aides. Given the necessary training, Zhou insisted, many of them would gladly embrace nursing as their life's profession (Chow 1945). In 1945 Zhou estimated that there were 6,400 nurses in China, including those in occupied regions. In a pamphlet published by the American Bureau for Medical Aid to China, she appealed to readers to support the education of nurses. Indeed, the American Bureau and the British United Aid to China Fund sponsored Zhou to travel to England and the United States to promote the Red Cross's work in China (CMB n.d.). It was successful. In addition to collecting cash and material donations from England, New York, Boston, Chicago, and Los Angeles, Zhou also managed to secure the donation of twenty trucks to be used for the transportation of the wounded in the ongoing civil war (Chang 1993, 65). Zhou was studying at Columbia Teachers College in New York under her second Rockefeller fellowship when the Nationalist government (and army) relocated to Taiwan in the wake of the Communist victory in 1949. Rather than returning to Shanghai, Zhou moved to Taiwan, where she was eventually promoted to the rank of general, and continued as director of the Army Nursing School for the rest of her career.

The intersecting careers of Nie Yuchan and Zhou Meiyu illustrate the interrelatedness of key people and organizations in the first half of the twentieth century. As students at PUMC and Rockefeller fellows, Nie and Zhou developed reputations as bright and capable nurses in China and abroad. Both perceived nursing as a way to provide patriotic service to China, were offered leadership roles in PUMC and the NAC, and made career decisions in response to wartime needs. Yet they had differing ideas about the best form of education for nurses. Whereas Nie followed the American model of (baccalaureate) nursing education established at PUMC and recreated at the West China Union University, Zhou responded to urgent army needs by creating a modified version of the Ministry of Education nursing curriculum, along with a series of shorter courses for emergency technical personnel (X-ray technician, sanitary engineering, laboratory technician) (MCANYP 1944, 24). While PUMC, Rockefeller fellowships, and the NAC provided the educational and other preparation and advancement opportunities for a small number of highly capable nurses—a Chinese nursing elite—it was wartime that helped transform Chinese nursing from a form of Christian and professional service administered by foreigners into a patriotic, nationalized service administered by highly qualified Chinese nurses. Although it would not be until after the Republican era that nursing would move beyond its scope as a small "modern urban outpost in a patriarchal rural culture" (MCANYP 1944, 87), the progress since 1911 was nonetheless remarkable.

Development of Nursing as a Profession in New China, 1949–2010

Changing Nursing Education

In the early years of the People's Republic of China (PRC), nursing education followed national foreign policy by copying the Soviet model. The Ministry of Health proposed that nursing would no longer require a college-level education. Instead, a secondary school–level education would be available from three sources: professional nursing in secondary health schools, hospital nursing schools, and independent nursing schools.

In 1950, the First National Health Conference proposed that medical education should contain three levels: primary, secondary, and higher medical education. The emphasis was to be on training medical workers at the secondary-school level; nursing education was to be one aspect of this, in which nurses would receive two years of training. In 1952, all nursing schools associated with medical schools were closed and were replaced with technical training programs. In 1954 the Ministry of Health issued trial teaching plans for all health professionals, including doctors, nurses, and midwives. The technical school system of nursing and child care nursing was extended to three years. In 1958, the Great Leap Forward had a great effect on nursing education. The number of national secondary health schools jumped from 182 in 1957 to 1,333 in 1960, and the number of students increased from 19,737 to 120,878 (Wang 1999, 339). Accelerated secondary nursing education deemphasized research and academic training, reducing education to concrete skills such as providing injections and medications. Nurses were to refer questions to doctors, which made patients lose confidence in the knowledge and capability of nurses, whose status fell accordingly. Nurses lacked the chance to continue their education—for example, through graduate training—and with the uncertain development of the nursing profession could only be doctors' assistants. Because nursing emphasized "giving injections and holding bedpans, cleaning beds and carrying things," the slogan "doctors' mouths, nurses' legs" reflected the most vivid portrayal of the Chinese nurse. In the late 1950s, China canceled hospital-based nursing schools, allowing health schools to offer a nursing major. The hospitals undertook the later clinical teaching of nursing students, which led to a separation of theory and practice. The result was that after graduation, nurses could not work independently. Because the government-determined quotas of places at hospital-based nursing schools was not stable or predictable, there was wide variation in the age structure and level of education of students. Most students were graduates of junior middle schools, coming from rural areas, whose main purpose in applying to nursing school was to qualify for urban residency and acquire urban household status (*hukou*). These changes had a negative effect on nursing as a profession.

During the Cultural Revolution (1966–1976), the development of all careers was thwarted in China, and nursing education came to a standstill. After the reform and opening up of China in the late 1970s, initiatives were taken to improve secondary nursing education.

Because higher nursing education had been canceled in 1952, China lost a generation of highly trained nurses and nursing leaders. After the 1970s, as the Chinese economy began to recover from the chaos and international isolation of the Cultural Revolution period, nursing education and practice were reestablished. In 1971, the PRC government took the Chinese seat at the United Nations (it had been held by Chiang Kai-Shek's Republican government-in-exile since World War II). As a result, China became a member of the World Health Organization, which in 1978 proposed the global strategy of "Health for All by the Year 2000." The development of primary care nursing was an important component of this strategy. The object of nursing was to be extended from patients to healthy people and the range of nursing services was broadened from hospitals to families and communities. As in other parts of the world, nursing in China expanded from a focus on disease and hospital-based acute care to a focus on primary health and community-based health promotion and illness prevention.

Nursing had two big breakthroughs: the range of nursing was enlarged from within the hospitals (acute care nursing) to outside the hospitals (primary and community nursing), and from physiology to psychology. In 1984, the Ministries of Education and Health held a nursing professional education symposium in Tianjin. Following this, some higher education medical schools established nursing majors and formally recruited students. These included Peking Medical University, Peking Union Medical College, Shanghai Medical School, China Medical University, Shandong University School of Medicine, Faculty of Medical Sciences of Sun Yat-sen University in Guangzhou, Tianjin Medical University, and Nanjing Medical University (Yan 1986). In 1984 the Beijing Institute of Traditional Chinese Medicine (Beijing University of Chinese Medicine) first established a department of traditional Chinese nursing, thereby establishing advanced education in traditional Chinese nursing. Since then, ten traditional Chinese medical schools have opened junior college classes of traditional Chinese nursing. In 1997, the Ministry of Health established independent four-year schools of secondary nursing education. The guiding ideology was to "emphasize nursing, stress unity, strengthen humanity, and reflect community" (Chen 1999). Humanities courses concerned with the needs of the society and medical service were added to the curriculum. In addition to teaching these courses in the humanities, this new secondary nursing education taught nursing specialties such as geriatric nursing, community nursing, and spiritual nursing, to reflect the health needs of the community (Ma et al. 2001). This form of education began to narrow the gap between Chinese and international advanced nursing educational models.

Graduate nursing education gradually developed. Beijing Medical University got the first warrant from the Ministry of Education to offer a master's degree in nursing in China in 1990, and began to recruit students in 1992. By the year 2000, according to incomplete statistics of the Ministry of Education, there were 67 undergraduate schools, 50 junior colleges, and 19 graduate schools of nursing in China. By May 2004, the number of schools with advanced nursing education programs had increased to at least 110 (Yu 2001). In 2003, the Second Military Medical University in Shanghai was credentialed to award a PhD in nursing. Presently, the level of Chinese nursing education is consistent with that offered abroad (Jiang 2004). With the rapid development of Chinese higher nursing education, graduate education has gradually become the main channel for cultivating teaching, research, and clinical talent.

In response to these international movements and to changes in the Chinese health care delivery system, Chinese nursing education has changed from secondary nursing education to junior college, college-level undergraduate, graduate, and postgraduate multilevel education. Nursing education is provided in specialist schools and as continuing education and adult education. In 2010, 0.1 percent of registered nurses in China held a graduate degree, 8.7 percent held a bachelor's degree, 42.5 percent had an associate's degree, and the remaining 48.7 percent held secondary education qualifications in nursing (Ministry of Health 2011b, 32).

Spreading Nursing Knowledge

Most nursing books published before 1949 were translations of English works. Few Chinese nurses wrote scholarly nursing books; what books they did write were brief, popular texts for the education of the general public. In 1953, the Textbook Compiling Committee of the Ministry of Health published the first Chinese nursing textbook, *General Nursing,* which was used until the Cultural Revolution. From 1950 to 1960, nursing books took the form of rules and manuals, such as *Basic Nursing Practice Rules, Nurse Manual for Emergency Rooms, Prevention Manual of Tuberculosis, Clinical Experience and Common Sense,* and so on, which played an active role in popularizing nursing and medical common sense. Since 1970, nursing books have gradually increased in number, and now include works on nursing theory, nursing education, comparisons between Chinese and Western nursing, the progress of foreign nursing, and so on, which reflect the continuous development of Chinese nursing as a career.

After the founding of the PRC, the first task of the Chinese Nursing Association was to facilitate academic communication. In 1953, after its move to Beijing, the CNA printed the first two issues of *Nursing Communication* for internal circulation only. *Nursing Journal,* first published on May 1, 1954, was the first academic nursing journal of the PRC. In the early issues, this journal included articles on disease management, clinical nursing techniques, and health policies, as well as the opinions of nurses. From its founding in 1954 until its first suspension in 1960 (due to the crisis in government funding as a result of the famine caused by the policies of the Great Leap Forward), its focus was on developing hospital-based clinical nursing and head nurse management skills. In 1963, the journal resumed publication, but in 1966 publication was suspended again because of the Cultural Revolution. It has been in continuous publication since resuming in 1977. In 1981, its name was changed to the *Chinese Journal of Nursing,* reflecting its status as the state-approved journal of the nursing profession. In order to adapt to the rapid development of nursing education and the management of clinical nursing, the journal set up more than twenty additional columns, covering both Chinese medical nursing and integrated Chinese-style and Western-style nursing care. As Lin Juying has noted, articles before 1980 were mainly retrospectives and summaries, but after 1990, articles have emphasized forward-looking research, which reflects the overall improvement of nursing and the establishment of advanced and continuing nursing education (Lin 2004).

The number of journals has also increased since the 1980s. The *Nursing Journal of the Chinese People's Liberation Army* was founded in 1984 with the main aim of serving the troops and introducing new theories and technologies. The *Journal of Practical Nursing,* founded in 1985, places special stress on clinical and basic nursing research ("Ganwu lishi" 2005). Since the journal's academic level and its circulation met state-level requirements, it was awarded a name change to the *Chinese Journal of Practical Nursing* in 2003. The *Journal of Nurse Training* was founded with the support of the Guizhou provincial government in 1986. At that time, Chinese nursing quality could not meet the nursing need because the majority of nurses had only received a secondary education. Wang Xiuying, nursing scientist, wrote that the "*Journal of Nurse Training* proposes a timely education program to improve the level of nursing with characteristics of multi-channel, multi-level and multi-form" (Wang 1986). This rather cryptic formulation meant that nurses should learn from journals as well as from formal training programs; that nursing education should continue to be provided at several levels, from secondary school to graduate school and beyond; and that nurse training should occur in several forms, including self-study, continuing education classes, and mentoring in addition to nursing school education. At present, there are dozens of national and local journals of nursing. These journals provide a platform for communication and nursing trends, indirectly promoting professional development.

Infectious diseases threaten human health, and one of the important measures to prevent infectious disease is to publicize health knowledge. The First Health Office of Peiping, founded in 1925 by John B. Grant of PUMC, was a model for the development of Chinese public health professionals and also an important base for public health nurses to play a role in community health. Ruth Ingram and Gertrude E. Hodgman, the second and third deans of the nursing school of PUMC, began the work of public health nursing education and practice in the 1920s. Wang Xiuying graduated in 1931, and was awarded the twenty-ninth Florence Nightingale Medal by the International Red Cross in 1982 for her contribution to public health nursing. Public health nurses took charge of home care, maternal and child health, infectious disease care, school health, factory health, and the treatment of common diseases. After the founding of the PRC, the First Health Office of Peiping was enlarged and changed its name to the Beijing Dongcheng District Health Bureau, and further municipal and district Health Prevention Stations were set up in Beijing. In 1957, the Beijing Municipal Health Bureau held a public health nursing continuing education course. At around the same time, the PUMC nursing school added preventive medicine courses. China thus experienced the stages of visiting nurse, public health nurse, and community nurse. The community nurse replaced the public health nurse beginning in the 1970s.

Most Western developed countries had been exploring new nursing models since 1950. By the 1960s, the nursing professions of the developed world were proposing functional nursing in which patients were the core. By the 1970s, this had developed into holistic nursing (that is, concerning body and mind), which aimed to go beyond treating only disease to also considering the psychological, social, and cultural factors that might influence a patient's ability to recover (Zhen 2008, 122–126). After the reform and opening up of China in the late 1970s and '80s, and especially the adaptation of collegiate education for nursing, the Chinese nursing establishment became increasingly interested in American nursing theories that had become hugely popular in English-speaking educational programs. With the shift of nursing education from hospital to university settings and a concurrent increase in PhD-prepared nursing educators, American nursing had become focused on developing a body of nursing knowledge that was distinct from medical knowledge. The resultant "nursing theories" became the cornerstone of nursing philosophy, education, and research, and made household names of nursing theorists like Sister Callistra Roy (Roy's Adaptation Model of Nursing), Dorthea Orem (Orem's Self-Care Deficit Theory), and Betty Neuman (Neuman's Systems Model of Nursing). Indeed, in the 1960s and '70s it was a common expectation that nursing programs in the United States and Canada would adopt a particular "theory" or "model" upon which to base the entire nursing curriculum. China was among those nations that also took up nursing theory as a foundation for nursing education.

In 1994, with the assistance of the United Nations Development Program, Wu Jianyun of George Mason University in Virginia set up study classes in systematized holistic nursing and pattern ward construction in Beijing and some other cities, including Shanghai, Jinan, Binzhou, and Hangzhou. In this model of holistic nursing, people were to be the focus of service, nursing processes were the framework, and modern service views were the guide. The task of modern nursing is now to research the relationship among society, psychology, behavior, and many other factors in the appearance and development of diseases. During medical work, the task of nursing staff is mainly to understand the influences of these factors, to regulate people's psychological responses to help them be optimistic and stable and cooperate with treatment, and to carry out holistic nursing as well as cooperate with doctors (Yan 1986). In the late 1990s, with the new developments in community nursing, geriatric nursing, family nursing, and palliative nursing, nursing theory research and practice entered a new phase of development. In recent years, the government and international foundations such as the China Medical Board have provided funds and support for the development of modern nursing in China.

After the founding of the PRC, China issued some regulations concerning nurses, but specific nursing rules did not appear until 1993. A Code of Ethics for Nursing was proclaimed in 2000. In order to strengthen the basic quality of nurses, to ensure the quality of nursing and the safety of patients, and to prevent people without professional nursing training from practicing, the Ministry of Health also issued a new law, the Nurse Management Method of the PRC. In 2008, the Central People's Government issued the Nurse Management Regulations of the PRC. This legislation protected the right of nurses to get equal pay for equal work, increased the ratio of nurses to patient beds, promoted registration for nurses, and modified the criteria for admission to the profession, enabling nurses to take the licensing examinations separately from their college educations. This change effectively regulated the nursing profession by means of law, which was beneficial to protect nurses' legal rights, and clarified the responsibility of health care institutions to maintain high standards of nursing (Li 2008b).

Current Nursing Issues

In China, the ratio of nurses to doctors has risen from 0.61:1 in 2000, to 0.97:1 in 2005, to 1.16:1 in 2010 ("Yihu bili" 2011). In 2001, the ratio of the national average number of nurses to hospital beds was 0.4:1, while many other countries' ratio was above 1:1 (Zhang 2004). In China, there were 2.048 million registered nurses in 2010 (Ministry of Health 2011b, 30). However, according to international standards, this indicates a shortage of about 1 million nurses.

In the 1990s there were 530 secondary nursing schools in China. Thirty-three higher academic schools had established junior college nursing education, nineteen colleges set up undergraduate nursing education, and four college nursing schools provided graduate nursing education. By contrast, the United States had more than nine hundred associate degree nursing schools, more than five hundred bachelor's degree nursing schools, more than three hundred master's degree nursing schools, and more than thirty doctoral degree nursing schools (Zhang 1997). From this comparison it is evident that the higher levels of nursing education in China still need to be strengthened.

In recent years, although Chinese advanced nursing education has developed rapidly, economic efficiency has been paid so much attention that the comprehensive cultivation and capacity training for nursing staff has been ignored. In concrete terms, what this means is that too many students have been admitted in order to meet targets at the expense of student quality and access to teaching resources. In addition, because providing employment was the short-term goal of nursing education, the cultivation of social consciousness in nursing staff has generally been overlooked. This situation has emerged because even though nursing education is a public function, students pay tuition. This commercialized undergraduate nursing education has paid the price by sacrificing educational quality, which needs to improve (Xu 2005).

The notion of holistic nursing has become a presumed norm in international nursing standards. Holistic nursing refers to an interest in caring for biological, psychological, social, and spiritual dimensions of a patient's health. Originating in American nursing, holistic nursing developed as a way to differentiate nursing from medical approaches to care. Whereas a "biomedical approach" focuses on treatment of disease (the domain of physicians), a holistic approach takes into account the whole person, their family relationships, and other social influences on their health (the domain of nurses). Holistic nursing presumes a level of independent decision-making on the part of the nurse, apart from physician's orders. This notion of holistic nursing has been introduced but not fully realized in China. Rather than nurse-directed patient care, clinical nursing in China is still largely physician-directed, with nurses playing a functional role in the division of labor.

For nursing in China to progress further toward implementing holistic nursing as the norm, the government and nursing leaders will need to accept that every country's health care system has its own particular characteristics. Holistic nursing can only be implemented as part of a broader array of health care reforms that take the features of nation and location into consideration (Yin 2006). One of the development goals for the future is to explore Chinese characteristic nursing, especially the application of traditional Chinese medicine and acupuncture in nursing work and the application of nursing in health care.

Conclusion

Nursing in twentieth-century China has experienced a number of transitions. Prior to the establishment of New China in 1949, nursing was characterized by its ties with the West. Established by missionaries, modern nursing was introduced to China as a form of Christian service. Following World War I, nursing became increasingly professionalized and nationalized through the establishment of the Nurses Association of China, the nation's acceptance into the International Council of Nurses, the Rockefeller Foundation's support for undergraduate education and its provision of fellowships for graduate nursing education, and government support for national standards and networks for nursing education and registration. Wartime stimulated new forms of nursing, including army nursing under the leadership of Chinese nurses. Following the establishment of the PRC, nursing education and progress stalled for three decades. Since the (re)opening of China in the late 1970s, nursing has resumed a trajectory of development that has included graduate education, the publication of nursing journals, the advancement of nursing specialties, and the establishment of nursing-related research.

In 1949, the ICN recognized the Republic of China on Taiwan as China's only legitimate government, with the result that the PRC was removed from ICN membership (Chan and Wong 1999). Although the Chinese Nursing Association was reorganized in the early 1980s, by 2012 it had still not been readmitted into the International Council of Nurses ("International Council" 2012). According to Splane and Splane (1994), readmission might be possible "were it not for the membership in ICN of Taiwan." The complex "Taiwan issue," a continuing legacy of the Cold War, involves China's claim that Taiwan is part of China, and the counterclaim of the government in Taiwan that it is the legitimate government of all China. In 1983 CNA president Lin Juying noted that she hoped the CNA would have more international ties (Davis 1983b). In 2001 China began working to rejoin the ICN in order to be part of the world nursing community (Davis 2001). The persistence paid off. On May 19, 2013, the ICN announced the inclusion of the Chinese Nursing Association. They were admitted by a unanimous vote of the assembled delegates at the meeting of the ICN's Council of National Representatives (International Council of Nurses 2013).

It is noteworthy to see the connection between the evolution of nursing in China after the 1980s and nursing before 1949. Among the earliest nursing leaders of the 1980s and 1990s were PUMC graduates and others who had been educated in the old system. For example Lin Juying, who was president of the Chinese Nursing Association from 1983 to 1991 and director of Nursing and dean of the School of Nursing at Beijing Hospital for many years, was also a PUMC graduate. Lin also received honorary doctorates from the University of Missouri and the University of Michigan (Davis 2001, 485). After the civil war that brought Mao Zedong to power, China was isolated from the rest of the world for about thirty years; nurses could not participate in professional activities. During the Cultural Revolution, when the worker was considered the model citizen, the government sent professional people to the countryside. According to Lin, the usual norms and standards were not maintained and "we experienced much confusion" (Davis 2001, 485). Those like Lin who had become nurses before all these social changes had a vision of professional nursing. "When the moment came," Lin noted, "we began to influence nursing education and practice according to that vision" (Davis 2001, 485). In 1981 China's first bachelor of science in nursing (BSN) degree was awarded at Tianjin Medical College. Twenty years later, in 2001, there were sixty-two BSN programs and over ten master of science in nursing programs (Davis 2001, 485). According to Lin, in the 1980s nursing returned to a prewar emphasis on virtues and behaviors such as being kind, compassionate, and truthful. Over time this evolved into a more complex model of ethics that went beyond virtue ethics to a more comprehensive understanding of economic, political, and transcultural influences on nursing practice. Lin Juying's 1983 assertion that China should double the number of nurses from 60,000 to 124,000 echoed Zhou Meiyu's assertion forty years earlier (Davis 1983b).

Today, nursing education remains a hallmark of the development and progress of nursing in China. With the advent of nursing specialities, master's and doctoral programs, and exchange and cooperation agreements with nursing programs globally (e.g., the Johns Hopkins nursing doctoral program partnership with PUMC) ("Nursing Doctoral Program Partnership" 2012), China is poised for another transition—this time toward a vision of nursing that is at once Chinese and global.

Notes

Sonya Grypma wrote the section titled "Early Development of Nursing, 1873–1949," and Cheng Zhen wrote the section titled "Development of Nursing as a Profession in New China, 1949–2010."

1. Zhou Meiyu is also known as Chow Mei-yu or Chou Mei-yu.

2. In 1933 Zhou Meiyu was awarded a certificate in public health (CPH) from MIT. In 1944 she sent her master's thesis to her supervisor, C. E. Turner. In 1948 MIT voted to replace the CPH with a master of public health (MPH) degree, awarding the latter to all its graduates, including Zhou Meiyu. She earned a master of arts degree in nursing education from Columbia University (RAC 1948; RAC 1948–1949).

16 The Evolution of the Hospital in Twentieth-Century China

Michelle Renshaw

In 2010 CHINESE hospitals consumed 76 percent of national health spending, whereas in the United States 31 percent was spent on hospitals and in Australia, 33 percent. The first port of call for most Chinese patients is a hospital outpatient department staffed by specialists, while for 80 percent of Americans and Australians it is a general practice physician. The hospital is so dominant an institution in the Chinese health care system that 90 percent of all in- and outpatient services in the country occur in one—a remarkable feat for an introduced institution with no indigenous counterpart.

Like a successfully introduced plant species, the hospital found its niche in nineteenth-century China and was well-established by the turn of the century. As dramatic changes in the political, economic, medical, and social environment have played out over the past hundred years, the institution has proved remarkably adaptable. It has both outperformed and crowded out potential competitors.

But the "hospital" in China should not be confused with the "hospital" in the United States or Australia or Britain. In China, "hospital," or *yiyuan*, is an imprecise term used to encompass everything from a medical missionary's clinic with a few beds, to a military facility set up on the battlefield, to a commune or town hospital with twenty to forty beds, to a vast complex organization with specialists employing expensive technology serving millions of outpatients per year and hundreds of thousands of inpatients. This ambiguity makes using statistics to describe the pattern of hospital provision or utilization over time and space problematic. Official Chinese health data since the early 1980s has used two terms, "hospital" and "health center" (*weisheng yuan*), for facilities where the main focus is on curative medicine (as opposed to "preventive" health), which can accommodate patients overnight, and which are manned by professionally qualified staff. This definition would serve equally well in the United States or Australia, but it misses an essential feature of the institution: the way in which a patient relates to it via outpatient clinics. American outpatient departments might look the same as they do in China (i.e., staffed by specialists using high-technology apparatuses), but in the United States patients are referred there by another physician. In contrast, Chinese patients interact with hospital outpatient departments in a manner more akin to how the urban poor used nineteenth-century stand-alone American dispensaries (Rosenberg 1974) or today's uninsured Americans use the emergency room. Not only do Chinese patients visit the hospital outpatient department for all manner of ills, but it is the patient, not a primary care physician, who decides which specialty unit to register with.

This difference in the scope of the hospital's role goes some way toward explaining the disparity in the share of each country's health budget spent on hospitals. But why is the hospital so prominent in China, or, to frame it another way, why did China not inherit a complementary general-practice, primary-care system? In this chapter I will tell the story of the Chinese hospital's evolution, hypothesize on why it has been so successful, and, using past and present-day examples from Suzhou (Jiangsu Province), briefly speculate on its future.

Protestant Missionary Hospitals

We start at the beginning, with the hospitals that Protestant medical missionaries brought to China in the nineteenth century. Before coming to China the early missionary doctors would have treated the vast majority of their patients at home, not in a hospital. They would not have worked as permanent staff in a hospital, let alone run one, but (if they were lucky) they might have had visiting or operating rights in one. Even their medical training did not necessarily include clinical experience in a hospital. Nevertheless, medical missionaries chose a novel approach by combining two institutions which at home operated separately: the stand-alone dispensary and the (relatively unfamiliar) hospital. Necessity was one reason for the choice. Before the treaties which afforded them access to all of China, missionaries' movements and activities were severely circumscribed by Chinese law: they had neither access to people's homes to treat them nor the right to evangelize. Secondly, Western medicine was hardly more efficacious than Chinese medicine at the time, but missionaries could exploit the one advantage they had in the marketplace: they performed surgery while Chinese practitioners did not. Surgery necessitated a place to prepare patients, operate, and provide postoperative care, i.e., a hospital. Missionaries believed that the longer patients stayed in the hospital the more likely they were to embrace Christianity, which, after all, was the missionaries' main purpose for being in China (Renshaw 2005, 167–171). And lastly, the evangelizing preachers of the United States' Second Great Awakening who went to China needed an audience. Attaching a dispensary to the hospital meant not only that large numbers of Chinese could be treated but also that the waiting patients would provide that audience. A missionary preaching to several hundred outpatients and their families assembled in the hospital courtyard evokes the image of a snake-oil salesman of the American West as well as the itinerant Chinese healer in the market square.

While missionary physicians might have been competing with Chinese practitioners for patients, there was no competition for their hospitals. Charitable institutions which took in old folks, foundlings, orphans, and the afflicted such as the deaf and the blind existed in China, but the institution known as the hospital—a place where sick people are gathered together under one roof for a period of time to be ministered to by medical staff—did not. By the turn of the twentieth century Western-style medicine and hospitals had been conflated in people's minds for more than sixty years. They would have seemed to be one and the same thing. Western medicine in China was hospital-based medicine, and a hospital had two sets of clients: relatively few inpatients and lots of outpatients.

By 1905 there were, by one count, 164 missionary-run hospitals in the country. By 1919 this number had almost doubled to over 310 (Fowler 1923), which was still woefully inadequate to the health needs of the estimated four hundred million Chinese if China was to adopt Western medicine as a norm. China's modernizing reformers, who would take over from the imperial government of the Qing dynasty, favored such a move. So, while missionary-run hospitals remained dominant throughout the first half of the century, Chinese players now entered the field of hospital-based medicine.

The First Employment-Based Hospitals—Railways and Mines

One of the problems the new nineteenth-century mining and railway companies faced both in China and in the United States was how to care for workers in dangerous occupations in remote areas. Hospitals fit the bill. Like those which had been set up along the transcontinental railroad in the United States, they were intended to care for both passengers and wounded or sick railway employees and their families (Gillespie 2006). China's railway system expanded once the First Sino-Japanese War ended in 1895; as rails were laid, hospitals followed. The Chinese Government Railways established hospitals at either end and along the line completed in 1908 from Tianjin to Pukou near Nanjing. And, according to one source, in 1927 fourteen medical districts, each with a "fully staffed and equipped hospital," sat along the 1,821 kilometers of the Chinese Eastern Railway (Wong and Wu 1936, 569–570). University of Chicago graduate and sanitation expert Huang Tse-fang painted a not-so-rosy picture in 1935. He described the situation faced by the newly appointed managing director of the "Two Railways" Medical Service (Nanjing-Shanghai and Shanghai-Hangzhou-Ningbo) in 1931. The service was in bad shape: the sole hospital, at Chinkiang (Zhenjiang) was inadequately equipped, poorly administered, and staffed with unqualified doctors and nurses. The railway doctors' role had been reduced to providing minimal first aid to "lowly labourers, minor clerks and 3rd and 4th class passengers." Employees with more resources used the doctors to get a mandatory sick-leave certificate before seeking treatment from a local practitioner or a more distant hospital. But by 1935 the Chinkiang hospital had been remodeled and equipped, a seventy-five-bed hospital had been established at Hangzhou, and a new thirty-five-bed hospital at Shanghai provided service-wide coordination, specialist services, and training facilities for doctors and nurses. Arrangements had also been made with hospitals in towns along the line to admit emergency cases.

The service's budget increased by 27 percent between 1932 and 1936, reflecting a broadened role that, in addition to the free curative services for railway employees and their dependents, included preventive services, educational activities, sanitary supervision, factory hygiene, and school health. As a result, family members' use of the service almost doubled, from 11.7 percent of all clinic visits in 1932 to 22.5 percent in 1934, and it was planned to make services available to "communities along the line." As Huang pointed out, the effect of improved sanitary and health services extended to the "hundreds of thousands" of inhabitants of these communities as well as "some 15 million passengers [who] travel on the Two Railways" every year (Huang 1935). In addition, exposure to hospitals would have reinforced the link between hospitals and "modern medicine" in people's minds.

Central Government Hospitals (Ministry of Civil Affairs)

In the dying days of the Qing, the so-called "New Policies" era (1900–1911), the Chinese government had become involved in health care provision and, with it, hospitals. In 1912 a medical missionary, John Mullowney, described one of three government hospitals he had visited in Peking. They had been established six years earlier by the Ministry of Civil Affairs, and Mullowney understood that other hospitals that were similar in plan and operation had been set up in a number of large cities. Patients in these government hospitals could choose between doctors who practiced Western or Chinese medicine (Mullowney 1912). Chinese medicine for the first time since the Song was being provided in an institutional setting (Renshaw 2005, 22–23, 33).

Isolation—Plague Hospitals

The 1910–1911 Manchurian plague epidemic further stimulated government involvement in hospital-based care, and the already established railway hospitals played a role. At the beginning of 1911, railway and provincial authorities set up "hospitals and segregation camps, each capable of holding from 400 to 2000 persons" at the principal railway stations of North China and Manchuria (Wu 1913,

238). By late 1912, the Chinese government had taken charge and established the North Manchurian Plague Prevention Service under the direction of Cambridge University–trained, Malayan-born Chinese physician Wu Lien-teh (1879–1960). In addition to undertaking research, public education, and sanitary measures, the service established permanent plague hospitals at Harbin (哈尔滨), Tsitsihar (Qiqihar 齐齐哈尔), Sansing (Yilan 依兰县), Taheiho (Hehei 大黑河), Newchwang (Yingkou 营口), Manchouli (Manzhouli 满洲里), and Lahasusu (Tongjiang 通江) (Wu 1920, 1203). The hospitals were intended not so much to treat the afflicted (in fact none were cured) as to hinder the spread of disease and protect the well. They were, however, intended to be dual-purpose in that suspected and confirmed cases of plague could be isolated when necessary and the general population treated in the absence of an epidemic. It is hard to imagine that the Harbin Hospital, with its individual cells designed to allow a patient to be observed without contact and a compound with two crematoria and burial pits, was the most inviting health facility (Chun 1923, 11).

Teaching Hospitals

By the beginning of the Republican period, hospitals internationally were occupying an increasingly central role in society. Major European and American city hospitals with large contingents of patients suffering a wide range of ills were indispensable for the new scientific medical training and research. Chinese hospitals followed this trend. In 1900, Jiangsu Province had been ranked a close second to Fujian in the number of (missionary) hospital beds per thousand people (Witte et al. 1900). In 1911 the Qing government established a city hospital, medical school, and outpatient clinic in the Jiangsu city of Suzhou, a city with a proud and long history of producing famous physicians and medical texts and which had experienced hospital-based Western medicine: the Methodist Episcopal Mission (MEM) had opened a hospital there in 1883. By the end of the century, at least another three missionary hospitals, including the Mary Black Hospital for Women headed by Shi Fumei, a graduate of the Suzhou Medical School, were operating in the city (Wong and Wu 1936, 522). This familiarity would have smoothed the government's entry into the field. In 1914, the Jiangsu Medical School started taking in new students whose clinical experience was gained in the "first government-run large-scale Western hospital," the Jiangsu Provincial Hospital (SLRO 2009d).

Private Hospitals—Western and Chinese

By the 1930s Jiangsu matched top-ranking Fujian's availability of hospital beds (Lennox 1932, 487), and Suzhou was particularly well-served with both public and private hospitals. When the MEM hospital celebrated its fiftieth anniversary in 1933 it reported having treated over one million patients in fifty years while graduating twenty-six doctors and thirty-seven nurses. It had forty-three medical staff (twelve doctors, eighteen nurses, and twenty-three "pupil nurses") and had become Suzhou University's teaching hospital. The hospital's nursing school had started in 1913, originally training only men; after closing in 1920, it was reopened in 1922 for women only (Snell 1924, 11). The hospital was the first "general hospital to advocate and use only female nurses" and, in the words of the superintendent of nursing, Marian Babb, "We can truthfully say that never at any time have we regretted it" (Li 1928, 12).

After relocating to a new purpose-built, architect-designed building partly funded by the China Medical Board in 1922, the hospital had, in line with international trends, increasingly departmentalized into specialties (Renshaw 2005, 36–39, 78–81). By 1924 there were four medical departments: medicine, surgery, gynecology and obstetrics, and EENT (Snell 1924). The makeup of the management and staff was also changing. Since at least 1919 the board of management had included Chinese members, two of whom were elected by the Suzhou Chamber of Commerce. Chinese board membership was formalized in 1930: three members were to be elected by the mission, three by the annual meeting of the MEM South China Conference, and three by the Suzhou gentry. In 1931 Pai Tsai An replaced Bishop W. N. Ainsworth to become the first Chinese president of the board. Six of the nine members of that board were Chinese, and the hospital staff was predominately Chinese. Dr. Li Guangxun had become the first Chinese superintendent in 1927 and all but two staff members—the head of the surgical department, John Abner Snell, a Minnesotan who had arrived in 1909, and Marian Babb—were Chinese. Snell's Chinese colleagues had been trained variously at the University of Pennsylvania, Yale, the North China Union Medical College for Women, Yale-in-China (Hsiangya) in Hunan Province, and the Peking Union Medical College (PUMC) (Thoroughman 1938).

While they dominated the market, missionary hospitals did not have the private field to themselves. A number of Western-trained Chinese doctors who had furthered their studies in Germany, Japan, or the United States returned to set up shop. The earliest among these was Yu Shengjia, a graduate of Beijing National Medical School, who had qualified in Germany. An appreciative financier brought Yu to Suzhou to treat his wife and children and subsequently subsidized the establishment of Yu's Wufeng Garden, a fifty-bed hospital, in 1917. This hospital boasted an operating room, laboratory, electrotherapy room, and X-ray machine, and survived (with a short break due to war) until 1952. Zhang Boxiong, a Harvard graduate, started out at Suzhou in 1925 offering only surgical outpatient services but soon expanded into new premises with forty-five beds and a full range of specialist services, including the one for which he became most famous: obstetrics (SLRO 2009a). In all, forty private Western medicine establishments began operation in Suzhou between 1920 and 1949. Most were short-lived—victims of war or occupation—and not all were "hospitals." However, seven of the eight that opened during the 1940s had inpatient accommodations of between five and forty-two beds (SLRO 2009d).

Doctors trained in Western medicine were not the only ones to found hospitals. While the majority of doctors of Chinese medicine in Suzhou in the Republican era offered no inpatient accommodations, many used the term *yiyuan*. The first in Suzhou to "emulate a Western hospital" was Zhu Yaoqing, who opened the Suzhou Chinese Medicine Hospital (*Suzhou Zhongyi yiyuan*), in 1928. While the number of beds is unknown, there were wards (*bingfang*) and a range of specialty clinics, as well as rudimentary nursing and someone to prepare medicines. The following year Zhu expanded his operation by opening an associated outpatient department to treat women and children, those with venereal and skin diseases, and those addicted to opium (SLRO 2009c). The fifty-bed Suzhou Hospital of National Medicine (*Guoyi yiyuan*), founded in 1939, employed eleven physicians and could call on ten "special physicians" for consultation; it listed its medical departments as "internal medicine" (*neike*), "external medicine/surgery" (*waike*), women and children, acupuncture, and traumatology (SLRO 2009c). Whatever the reasoning behind adopting both the form and the name, it is clear that the concept of the "hospital" had expanded beyond Western notions.

Public Hospitals

Once the Nationalists were established in government in 1927, conditions should have improved for contemplating a more comprehensive health system to cater to those outside the metropolitan areas. In late 1929, the Ministry of Health sought the League of Nations Health Organization's guidance on how to proceed. It recommended a hierarchical three-tier network of health services, with a provincial hospital at the apex, able to "extend health activities to the *xian* [county] level," a structure based on those being adopted for "rural reconstruction and state medicine" after World War I in war-ravaged European countries (Lucas 1980; Borowy 2009). But the new government's focus was military, not social change, and progress was slow. Nevertheless, the numbers of *xian* centers, essentially small thirty-bed hospitals, rose from 17 in 1934 to 181 in twelve provinces in 1936 and, dramatically, to 751 in thirteen provinces in 1942 (Ministry of Information 1943, 674).

Wartime Hospitals

As Nicole Barnes and John Watt demonstrate so well elsewhere in this volume, the legacy of the war years was a body of trained health care leaders and workers, a network of highway health stations with thirty-bed hospitals, and a county health care system with hospitals at its core. The role of missionary hospitals during this time depended on whether they were located in so-called "Free China" or in cities under Japanese occupation. The Chinese government subsidized the former to treat wounded or sick soldiers—two dollars per day per inpatient and forty cents per outpatient visit for soldiers (Ministry of Information 1943, 669).

The Suzhou MEM Hospital was one of the latter, so, before the city fell to the Japanese in November 1937, the hospital staff were evacuated and handed over to the National Health Administration to work further inland. By the time John Snell's successor as head of the surgical department, J. C. Thoroughman, could return to the city in January 1938, the hospital had been "well looted" and a few days later the Japanese authorities took it over and ran it as "a hospital for civilians in spite of our expressed desire to reopen it ourselves." In late June the occupying Japanese military allowed two foreign members of staff to reside again in Suzhou, and they regained control of the hospital in October 1938. They had lost all their instruments; their diagnostic, treatment, and laboratory equipment; books, linen, drugs, and many of the beds, but they felt the loss of all patient records most keenly. Within two months some of the old staff had returned and, joined by new recruits, were looking after eighty inpatients. The conditions in wartime Suzhou meant that "clean" surgical cases had given way to gunshot and burn victims, and the number of wounded inpatients rose from 35 in mid-August 1938 to 172 a month later, and to 183 by the beginning of November (Thoroughman 1938). The Japanese again seized the hospital after the attack on Pearl Harbor in 1941 and operated it for their own nationals stationed in the city, though some local residents were also treated. The hospital was finally returned to church management after the Japanese surrendered in 1945 (SLRO 2009b).

Several missionary hospitals that had been abandoned when war broke out were brought back into operation by the joint British-American Friends Ambulance Unit (FAU). The unit had originally planned to transport medical supplies into Free China from a base in Burma and to set up a medical team to work alongside the Chinese Red Cross in military hospitals. But when Burma fell, they entered China and set to rehabilitating mission hospitals that had been devastated by "flood, famine and war," including three one-hundred-bed hospitals in Henan Province (AFSCA 1950). A member based in Yunnan described one of their "biggest sources of patients" in the bombed city of Tengcheng (Tengchong, Yunnan) to be the many dangerous undischarged missiles "which only need a slight tap to set them off. . . . [C]hildren, in the usual way of Chinese children are full of curiosity, and have a way of banging things on stones to see what they contain. In the case of mortar shells, the revelation is usually the last of its kind. We have one or two emergency cases nearly every day here." The FAU member had tried prevention by "blowing some of the duds up" but he had "run out of TNT!" (McBain 1945).

Once the Japanese had been defeated and World War II ended, the Guomindang (GMD) and the Communists (CCP) resumed hostilities. Both armies had established mobile medical teams to carry out emergency treatment near the front and send the wounded back to more permanent base hospitals. Some of these were custom built but more often old temples or other communal buildings such as local guild quarters were adapted to suit (McBain 1945). Reports by the

American Communist sympathizer Agnes Smedley claimed that, other than in a few in big cities, a tiny fraction of the doctors attached to the (GMD) Chinese Army Medical Service had "any semblance of modern medical training" and the "nurses" were "soldier-coolies trained to change dressings" (Smedley 1939).

Six years later, FAU member Alan McBain suggested that Nationalist Army hospitals had improved since Smedley's visit. He describes one, operating as "the first Casualty Evacuation Hospital for the whole area," as having "been made as a Hospital and not extemporised out of old houses or temples." There were two dispensaries (one Chinese, from which "come weird mixtures at times for other patients than ours") an operating theater where chief surgeon Bob McClure "carried out his usual rapid-fire surgery," a sterilizer room, and a surgical ward which held "17 men in traction apparatus" (McBain 1945).

The first Communist hospital, *Xiao jing yiyuan* (Little Well Hospital), set up in the Jiangxi Soviet in late 1927, was described as having almost no resources. But in 1931 Dr. Ho Ch'eng (He Cheng) established the General Medical Department of the Worker-Peasant Red Army. Within three years the department was running "ten rear-area hospitals" (*houfang yiyuan*) (Lampton 1977, 11–12).

Smedley contrasted a Communist base hospital with the Nationalist's military facilities: it was orderly and clean, with all four doctors trained in modern medicine in China or abroad and "twenty modern-trained women nurses." She saw her "first scientific laboratory," an "excellent operating room," and, for the first time, records of patients, operations, and examinations being kept in a Chinese hospital. The hospital also had a supply section which packed and distributed "sanitary dressings and medicines" to all units in the field (Smedley 1939). Associated Press reporter Gunther Stein described a hospital he visited in Yan'an in 1944: "rows of caves in a steep, yellow hillside are its wards, with over 200 beds" (Stein 1945). As pacifists, members of the FAU worked on both sides of the conflict. They had first visited the political and military capital of the Chinese Communists, Yan'an, in early 1946, carrying a load of medical supplies aboard the first "outside trucks" to enter the area since 1940. Later that year they established a medical and surgical team to work in the First International Peace Hospital (AFSCA 1950).

When they came to power in 1949 the Communists, like the Nationalists, had considerable experience with Western medicine and hospitals. While their main emphasis was on mobilizing the people for vaccination campaigns, sanitation, and general public health activities, a hospital was always at the apex, providing coordination, administration, training, and support, as well as treatment, recuperation, and, when necessary, isolation. The majority of doctors working in these army hospitals had been trained in Western medicine. They used modern drugs.

War not only kills and wounds the warriors and civilians; the chaos of war encourages the spread of disease. Surgeons in the field, supported by base and mobile hospitals, were able to save many lives because of their skill, but also because they had access, for the first time in the history of medicine, to antimicrobial drugs which could treat infections inside the body. Sulfonamides, the so-called "sulfa" drugs, patented in the early 1930s, were being mass-produced by the end of the decade. John E. Lesch's definitive book on the subject describes their discovery as "a pivotal moment in the history of twentieth-century medicine" (Lesch 2007). Not only did sulphonamides prevent postoperative infections, such as erysipelas, but they were also rapidly deployed to treat pneumonia, gonorrhea, meningitis, bacillary dysentery, hemolytic streptococcal infections, wounds, and burns. The antimalarial drug quinine and its equivalent, atabrine (synthesized in the 1930s), were also shipped to wartime China in large quantities. Literally tons of drugs were sent to China. Alan McBain describes driving a charcoal-fueled truck along the Burma Road from Kunming to Tengcheng carrying "over three tons of drugs, apparatus, and electrical equipment." Another shipment contained twelve tons of quinine bound for Kunming (Davies 1947). According to the FAU, at one time they "were responsible for transporting 90% of the medical supplies into China for civilian use" (AFSCA 1950).

Missionary and publicly run hospitals were all using these new drugs; a hospital drugstore inventory from 1949 includes many different sulfa drugs as well as quinine, atabrine, and penicillin (AFSCA 1949). If the failure of traditional physicians to control the Manchurian pneumonic plague had "changed the attitude of some Chinese towards Western medicine" (Yip 1992, 397), there can be little doubt that the reputation of modern medicine, practiced in hospitals, was enhanced during the war. Nevertheless, the wholesale embrace of Western pharmaceuticals has not been an unalloyed boon, as we shall see.

Communist-Era Government Hospitals

The basic three-tier structure which the Nationalists had developed in the 1920s and '30s provided the scaffolding for the health system established by the Communists when they prevailed in 1949. As Xi Gao has discussed elsewhere in this volume, the CCP had been working with the Soviet Union since before Liberation and much of its thinking on health services had been reinforced by the Soviet model of hospital-based medicine. It is worth noting that hospital-trained Western-style doctors filled the upper and middle echelons of the various manifestations of China's health bureaucracy from 1949. It is not surprising that they retained the hospital as the foundation of the urban health care system.

The Communist government's first move was to take over and expand existing missionary hospitals and, where possible, keep the staff. In Suzhou, for example, the MEM Hospital continued operating as usual until November 1951 when all missionaries were ordered to leave China. It was handed over to the government and became known as the First People's Hospital of Suzhou City in

1954 (SLRO 2009b). New hospitals were also built, such as the Suzhou Municipal Hospital in 1952. The notion of the "iron rice bowl" meant that as well as being housed, employees of state-owned and collective enterprises, universities, and the military would be treated on-site in clinics or hospitals just as their counterparts on the railways had been.

Official data shows that by 1960 some 3,580 hospitals (at the county level and above) had been added to the 2,600 reportedly in existence throughout the country in 1949—a rise of close to 140 percent in that decade. Despite political upheavals and policy changes, the number of hospitals continued to increase steadily and numbered 9,478 by 1980. However, not all practiced Western medicine. Responding to Mao Zedong's 1950s call to integrate Western and Chinese medicine, *zhongxi yi jiehe* (so-called "integrated Chinese-Western medicine" hospitals) and TCM (Traditional Chinese Medicine) hospitals joined the system. Specialist hospitals more than quadrupled between 1949 and 1960 and have proliferated at an accelerating pace ever since. The range of specialties also rose, from a handful before the economic reforms of the 1980s to more than twenty in 3,716 facilities in 2009 (Ministry of Health 2010).

A Catastrophe in the Making—Economic Reform

Xiaoping Fang's chapter on barefoot doctors details the rise and fall of the cooperative medical service and its impact on rural health care provision. I will limit myself to the effect of the post-1978 economic reforms on urban hospitals.

Rural folk who could afford to pay for health care, who were now free to choose, eschewed the private clinics established by former barefoot doctors in favor of the higher-level urban hospitals they considered to be superior. So by 1991 the occupancy rate of urban hospitals averaged 85 percent while in rural hospitals it had fallen to less than 50 percent (Liu and Wang 1991, 109). Greater demand was not the only effect on urban hospitals; the new requirement that enterprises become financially self-sufficient, the "household responsibility" system—a euphemism for "you're on your own"—also applied to them. Their hands were tied, however. The government not only reduced funds for salaries; they also continued to regulate the prices (at below cost) for certain services and introduced a bonus system for doctors depending on the hospital's profits. To cover costs, hospitals came to rely on profits made through drug sales and new diagnostic technologies. This was not a new phenomenon: as early as 1919 the MEM Hospital in Suzhou had increased the range of services attracting a fee. By 1940, anesthetics, X-rays, diagnostic tests, and tissue examinations, which were all charged separately at different rates depending on the patient's class, contributed 45 percent of total revenue and drug sales a further 25 percent (Snell 1919; Thoroughman 1940). The bonus system worked as a bonus system is designed to: it influenced behavior. If doctors were to be paid according to the profitability of the hospi-

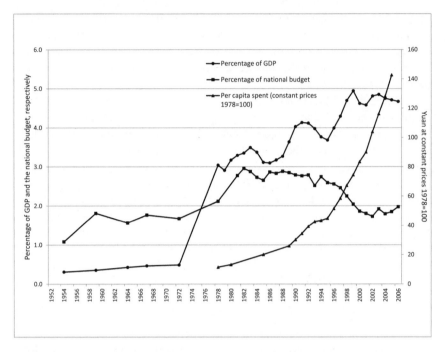

Figure 16.1. Percent of GDP and of national budget and per capita spending on health in China. *Sources:* Post-1978 data constructed using tables in Ministry of Health (2010). Pre-1978 data is less reliable and is compiled from a number of sources, principally Lampton (1972).

tal, they worked to increase profits. The easiest way to do this was to prescribe more Western than Chinese drugs—which had a greater allowed markup—and to order more diagnostic tests and treatments than might have been called for. Today, China's per capita consumption of antibiotics is more than ten times that of the United States, according to China's Ministry of Health. Antibiotics, the majority being expensive "second-line" drugs, are prescribed for 70 percent of Chinese inpatients—more than twice the WHO recommended rate—and 50 percent of outpatients. The dangers posed by overprescribing—increased prevalence of drug-resistant disease forms and, because the most common mode of delivery is intravenous infusion, infection—has led to government action. New regulations placing "unprecedented restrictions" on antibiotic prescription by hospital doctors came into force as recently as August 1, 2012 (Zhou 2012). Overprescribing contributed to the escalation of total health care and per capita costs (see figure 16.1), while structural reform—the dismantling of state-owned enterprises and the migration of workers to cities—resulted in an increase in the number of urban residents with no health insurance (Liu 2002, 135). As direct government

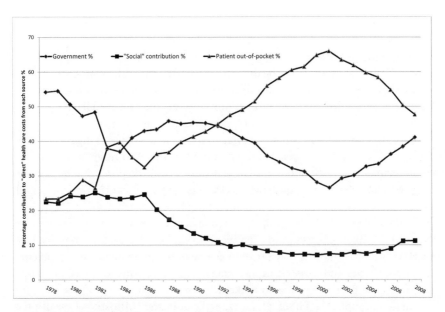

Figure 16.2. Direct government, insurance, and individual patient out-of-pocket shares of health care costs. *Source:* Ministry of Health (2010). I have used "Price Indices" from National Bureau of Statistics of China (2011) to convert published current prices to constant prices.

support also declined, the burden increasingly fell on the patient, whose out-of pocket costs rose dramatically (see figure 16.2).

Politically the situation was fraught. People's frustration with high prices, growing inequity of access to affordable care, and the belief that doctors were corruptly influenced by greed and pharmaceutical companies were all starting to seriously threaten political stability. Between 1998 and 2001, the Chinese Medical Association reported over 1,500 cases of serious conflict between patients and medical staff in Beijing hospitals alone; patients or their families used weapons or corrosive liquids in one-third of the cases (Hui 2007). In response, the government has undertaken a series of reforms since the late 1990s to redress some of the harm done by economic reform. Initially they focused on health insurance policies, and the reversal (in 2002) of earlier trends can be clearly seen in figure 16.2; the patients' out-of-pocket contribution declined and the health insurance component increased.

By 2009, medical insurance coverage was again almost universal in China, and most of the population had access to health care facilities. However, coverage was generally shallow, costs continued to rise and there were wide disparities in resources. So, in April 2009, the government announced a three-year concerted effort to tackle the twin problems of cost and access—regionally and between urban and rural areas. They planned to double government spending on health care (an extra 850 billion RMB) over three years in a multipronged approach to achieve "affordable, equitable health care for all by 2020." The plan concentrates on five key areas: lowering health insurance premiums; redistributing resources to poorer areas; directly financing community health centers (CHCs) in cities and township centers in the countryside to deliver basic primary and public health care; controlling the price of pharmaceuticals; and improving the efficiency of public hospitals by streamlining governance. The most recent assessment of the reform is that "China has made great strides towards providing its population with affordable and equitable access to basic health care" (Yip et al. 2012, 840). The targets for primary care infrastructure are being met, and a "no-profit" policy on drug sales has been implemented in health centers and will be extended to hospitals. Pilot schemes have been set up to explore strategies to improve hospital governance, but this may prove to be one of the more intractable problems. Seven ministries and three insurance plans, with competing agendas, priorities, and interests, have the power to make decisions directly affecting the running of public hospitals. As Yip et. al. (2012, 835) put it, the "Ministry of Health has the responsibility for health care but no means to control the provision of health services."

Hospitals Today

In 2010 Jiangsu had 1,157 hospitals: 65 percent general hospitals, 9 percent either TCM or integrated Western/Chinese, and 25 percent specialist, along with 3,500 CHCs or township centers (Jiangsu sheng tongji ju 2011, 504). In Suzhou there were fifty-three hospitals, thirty-six neighborhood medical service stations, seventeen township hospitals, and fifty clinics (Suzhou tongji ju 2010, 527). During a 2012 visit, I found, tucked away in a corner of fifty-four acres of what is now the First Affiliated Hospital of Suzhou University, the building the MEM Hospital had opened in 1922. The old dispensary/outpatients building is long gone, as is the Chinese tile–covered gallery that used to connect it to the hospital proper. In accord with Chinese traditional practice, the northernmost building of the campus is symmetrical, faces south, and is reserved for the "senior, expert doctors" and VIPs. And here I found the missing gallery—not the same one but a facsimile—leading to the building with the highest status. The multistory outpatient building, located at the southern end of the campus nearest the main road, houses dozens of specialty clinics and treatment rooms. There are no long queues to register—each of the six floors has its own registration office and cashier. People appear confident that they know where they are going, but a nurse stationed at the "One-Stop Service" in the main foyer is there to advise them if necessary. In addition to a full range of specialist clinics, there are departments of integrated medicine and TCM surgery; incongruously, the small room for decocting herbs (*jianyao shi*) sits alongside the building housing PET/CT equipment; a father leads his adolescent son by a simple infusion pole from the "shopfront," standing-room-only, twenty-four-hour infusion room to a waiting car; a couple of young men squat down near the pharmacy checking two dozen boxes of medicines against a prescription list.

The new Eastern Branch of the Suzhou Municipal Hospital, a beautiful two-story building in the "modern Suzhou" style exemplified in the city's I. M. Pei–designed museum a ten-minute walk away, caught my attention. The emergency department was strangely quiet on a Sunday morning, and I discovered that "emergency" in China means what it says, unlike in the United States where the ER is often the refuge of the uninsured. The triage nurse even had time to leave her desk to find someone to direct me to the old Suzhou Hospital. Next door in the Outpatients Department it was a different story. Evocative of a modern hotel or airport, the large atrium foyer with its highly polished marble flooring, three-story-high decorative screen, and full-size trees was busy but not crowded. Signage ranged from the huge banner exhorting people to "save energy, treasure resources, protect the environment" to electronic message and direction signs in English as well as Chinese. Staff photographs and qualifications, arranged by department on three double-sided screens near the entrance, helped would-be patients select a doctor. Suzhou Municipal Hospital patients do not have to queue for hours to register; they can make an appointment by phone or the internet and, when they arrive, register using their hospital identity card (linked to their medical record) in the ATM-like machines that line one wall.

Later, I turned a corner into a street filled with young women, accompanied by girlfriends, mothers, or husbands, walking proudly belly-first past the maternity and baby-wear shops toward the Maternal and Child Health Care Institute. The "Children's Center" invites children in with large-scale McDonald's-like play equipment, and new mothers can join the "Mommy and Baby Club." The family planning clinic, housed in a domestic-scale traditional Suzhou-style building accessed through a small gate in a wall, is suggestive of the gardens for which Suzhou is famous. To my Australian eye, while all these establishments were unmistakably hospitals, like an exotic introduced plant species they had successfully "naturalized" and thrived in the Chinese environment. Perhaps too successfully?

Beijing's Dongcheng Community Health Care Station appeared to be comprehensive and accessible. It offered a general practice clinic, community and preventative health, education, rehabilitation, and family planning services. It was open from eight o'clock in the morning to six o'clock in the evening on weekdays and eight o'clock to noon on weekends, and it had a twenty-four-hour hotline telephone service. When I was there in 2012, I watched from my hotel window, but saw no patients between ten o'clock and noon. The outpatient department of the nearby PUMC Hospital, however, was swarming with patients. A constant stream of them studied the modern-day *dazibao* posted at the entrance listing times and names for dozens of specialist clinics. Despite potentially long waits, it seemed that most patients were choosing the hospital over the health station. What I was observing in Suzhou and Beijing was the "disequilibrium" which characterizes China's current health care system (see chapter 1).

Increasing medical insurance coverage—held by over 90 percent of rural residents, up from the 10 percent who had it between 1980 and 1986—was easy compared to the challenge involved in reallocating capital and manpower resources in order to right the top-heavy inverted pyramid that is China's health care system. To this end, in 2011 the government directed approximately one-third of the health budget to rural institutions and primary health care facilities. According to government reports the targets set for infrastructure and training were "close to completion" by mid-2011. However, as my observations confirmed, "no shift in the flow of patients from high-level institutions to primary health-care facilities has been recorded" (Yip et al. 2012, 836).

I cannot pretend to be able to identify all the factors operating in China's political and economic environment which account for the failure to affect people's health care–seeking behavior, but it seems there are two important ones which, together, militate against change: an elevated trust in high-level hospitals (with corresponding low trust in clinics and their staff) and the Chinese patient's high degree of autonomy. China still lacks appropriately trained and respected primary health care practitioners to fulfill the intended dual role of health centers: service provider and "gatekeeper." While hospital-based medicine thrived in China, the complementary Western tradition of general practice never developed. As we have seen, a limited number of missionary-run medical school graduates established private general practices in the first half of the twentieth century, but any chance that a general practice system would evolve was foiled when private practice was effectively outlawed by the 1951 State Council Decision directing doctors to "take the road of collective organized medicine." In 1952, Chinese surgeon Chen Mingshan (陈明山), with a member of a family of famous acupuncturists, You Haomin (尤嗥民, 1896–1959), heeded the call and opened the first "joint clinic" in urban Suzhou. With a staff of thirty-six and six specialty divisions it was essentially a small hospital. By 1963, seventeen such TCM clinics operated in Suzhou (SLRO 2009c). Furthermore, elite medical schools led by PUMC, and encouraged by the China Medical Board, had trained specialists suited to hospitals, not to generalist primary care. The legacy of this practice is evident today in the design of most medical schools' curricula, which is premised on and encourages early adoption of specialist training.

China's health system was not unique. The Soviet health systems of countries of Central and Eastern Europe were similarly segmented into narrow medical specialties. Just as Russia had initiated a plan to develop an "integrated primary care system centred on general practitioners" in 1992 (Rese et al. 2005), the Chinese government announced a plan to develop a similar system serving the whole country by 2020 ("General Practitioner System to Take Shape" 2011). The scheme is facing many challenges, not the least being recruiting and training candidates who perceive the lowly paid job as lacking the opportunities for promotion enjoyed by hospital-based doctors. And once they are trained, these general practitioners (GPs) face the hurdle of winning the patients' trust, for in China it is the patient who decides which medical service to access. Xiaoping Fang has shown elsewhere in this volume how the Chinese authorities' best-laid plans of the 1960s were thwarted by people bypassing the (middle-tier) commune clinic in favor of village health stations run by barefoot doctors and the county hospitals. Thus the rural health system came to more closely resemble a dumbbell rather than the intended three-tier pyramid.

Chinese patients have demonstrated time and again that they are not passive consumers of health services; they have been choosing among increasingly specialized medical practitioners for generations. One example of the remarkable autonomy of Chinese patients is their use and management of medical records. Unlike in the United States, Australia, or the United Kingdom, where the health provider owns a patient's medical record, Chinese patients not only own their medical records, but are responsible for their maintenance and safekeeping. The *bing li,* or "record of illnesses," contains all professionally generated clinical information such as diagnoses, prescriptions, treatments, and tests (including printouts, if a hospital stores information electronically). Between hospital visits, patients also record information such as blood-sugar levels, blood pressure, diet, and emotional states, and they bring these records to the consultation. The record is the starting point for the discussion between patient and doctor, and vicariously between the doctor and other practitioners who have treated that patient. The long tradition of patients' maintaining their own medical records provides University of California medical records software developer Yunan Chen with the perfect laboratory in which to study their value. In a large Beijing hospital she has observed that the records "allowed patients to integrate their health information in a patient-centric way [and afford] a strong sense of ownership and control over their own health information" (Chen 2011a; Chen 2011b).

Exercising agency as a patient is not always so straightforward. Chen watched a man wanting a second opinion "hide previous records so that the doctor could provide him with fresh insight." The wealthy female patients in Stefani Pfeiffer's study of the PUMC Social Work Department during the Republican era did not accept the doctors' advice uncritically. But rather than initiate direct confrontation they used the strategy of bargaining over the price of specific treatments to select between hospital therapies (Pfeiffer 2005). Choosing a physician, though, has always been the Chinese patient's most important decision.

In the absence of practitioner registration before the 1920s, Chinese patients became expert at judging a Chinese doctor's competence. They learned as much as they could about medicine to effectively "test" the doctor, or they might hide their symptoms and judge him by his diagnosis; often they relied on recommendations from friends and family (Chang 1998, 55–83). All doctors in China are registered today, but the length and quality of tertiary medical education is highly variable. Anecdotal evidence suggests that today's patients feel as confident in differentiating between a good and a bad doctor as their predecessors did; for instance, a good doctor is likely to recommend a "modern" caesarean section, an MRI, or antibiotics by infusion. The status of the hospital is also a guide: Chinese hospitals are graded into three classes and further into three levels. Patients believe, with some justification, that doctors in Class III hospitals are "better" than those in lower-class units, and so they choose them (Dyckerhoff and Wang 2010). Their choice is reflected in the statistics: in greater Suzhou, for example, the rate of utilization of available beds in general hospitals was 83 percent in 2009, whereas in township hospitals it was almost twenty points lower, at 64 percent, and at community medical service stations was still lower, at 53 percent (Suzhou tongji ju 2010, 528).

In line with global trends, the Chinese patient has added the internet to his arsenal. According to a recent survey (admittedly among more highly educated, middle- and upper-income patients) more than 80 percent of the sample group conduct research on the internet "every time or most of the time before they consult a doctor" (Huang and Li 2011). The Suzhou Municipal Hospital hosts a "Specialist Online" service where patients can ask questions ranging from the practical ("When is Dr. Hu on duty?" "Thursday morning.") to the reassurance-seeking ("I have been breastfeeding for eight months but menstruation has not returned. Is this normal?" "Yes, it is normal."). Many describe symptoms to ask whether they need to visit a clinic and, if so, which clinic. Others provide detailed medical information, such as the patient with hyperthyroidism concerned that his hormone levels have changed and his heart is racing; he is given the phone number to make an appointment with the endocrinology department. These knowledgeable patients are actively engaged in their own health care and, for the past hundred years, they have preferred to seek medical care in a hospital.

The Future for Hospitals—Speculation

The main building of the Suzhou Municipal Hospital was being completely rebuilt during my visit there, and major construction work was underway at each of the hospitals I visited. Hospitals are clearly here to stay. But, as noted earlier, the flow of outpatients has not yet diminished significantly. Even if they are adequately staffed it is hardly surprising that health centers are not fulfilling the gatekeeper role expected of them; as the citizens of walled cities know, a gatekeeper is only useful if there is only one way in. Taiwan, for instance, has a GP system but also allows direct patient access to specialists (Wu, Majeed, and Kuo 2010). Like their Taiwanese counterparts, without a strong referral system Chinese patients will continue to choose hospitals—the bigger the better. If the burden on outpatient department specialists is to be shifted, then a different strategy is called for, one that works with (as opposed to against) the characteristics of today's Chinese health care consumers: trusting in and preferring hospitals and having the confidence to exercise their autonomy. Patients in China are not accustomed to having an ongoing relationship with a generalist physician who takes responsibility for all their health care needs, including coordinating their use of other elements of the system. Furthermore, they view the clinic and the generalist based there as inferior. Trust is built on experience, so any policy designed to build it needs to first introduce the participants in a setting which can engender trust. A gatekeeper does not fit the bill. Rather than providing primary care in the first instance, health centers today would seem to be better suited to relieving the burden on hospitals caused by affluence-linked chronic diseases which increasingly plague China: a "refer down" as opposed to "refer up" strategy.

This approach would see patients suffering from chronic diseases—cardiovascular conditions, stroke, cancer, and diabetes—being diagnosed and treated in hospitals but referred to local health centers for ongoing management by GPs and nurse practitioners. What's more, comorbidity—the existence of more than one disease—is common in patients with chronic diseases, and GPs and nurses are ideally suited to treat and monitor the "whole" patient. As with the relationship that evolved between villagers and barefoot doctors, it is reasonable to expect that mutual respect would develop between patient and GP, leading in time to a bolstering of the status of GPs as their all-important "reputation" spread throughout the community by word of mouth. The words of one medical missionary are as true today of hospitals as they were in 1915 of physicians: "The particular branch of medicine in which the . . . physician individually excels becomes speedily known among the Chinese. Probably there is no country where a man's reputation spreads faster than in China" (Barton 1915). It seems to me that, while Chen and Chen's "revamping of the health professional education system" is essential (see chapter 1 of this volume), the shape of China's health care system will not change until the Chinese family discovers by experience that their local GP is their best and, thus, first port of call.

Conclusions

The History of Medicine in Twentieth-Century China

Bridie Andrews

At the start of this project, we knew we were attempting something unusual in scholarly terms, for at least three reasons. Firstly, we asked historians who were specialized in one half of the twentieth century—either before or after the foundation of the Peoples' Republic of China in 1949—to consider their topics across the "long" twentieth century. We were interested to see the contours of continuity and change over the longer time frame in order to avoid the teleologies of any one political regime. Secondly, we asked scholars from different scholarly communities to collaborate, so that our synthetic project would make visible the importance of different national and cultural perspectives on the interpretation of medical history. Fortunately, the last few decades of relative open exchange between China and the West means that we were able to call on experts based in China, Hong Kong SAR, Singapore, Taiwan/Republic of China, Britain, Canada, Australia, and the United States. Lastly, we decided not to limit ourselves to the development of "modern" medicine in China, even though that was the original remit of the China Medical Board. The engagement of the state with Chinese medicine was most pronounced during the Maoist era (1949–1976), but the whole history of modern medicine in China has been framed by the contrast and competition with indigenous medicine. We felt that any survey of medicine in twentieth-century China needed to take this encounter into account.

All three of these initiatives have yielded interesting new results, and the juxtaposition of topics and approaches has also brought several themes into newly sharpened focus. Additionally, our contributors have reminded us that culture and location are important variables in the writing of history. Those of us based in the United States would probably never have wondered why the North American–style hospital continues to be the dominant site of biomedical care delivery in China. Michelle Renshaw, coming from an Australian tradition in which most doctors operate in private practices, and with her own rich knowledge of the history of hospitals in China, was able to explain why this particular institution has proved so enduringly well adapted to the vicissitudes of political and medical changes in China. For the authors of our chapter on nursing, it was self-evident that the development of nursing as a respected and independent career path, mainly for women, was an objective desideratum. For Sonya Grypma, a nurse, scholar of nursing history, and dean of a major nursing school, and Cheng Zhen, a historian who has been writing the biographies of nursing pioneers in China, it is natural to measure the development of nursing in China against international norms set by the International Council of Nurses (ICN). Other scholars might have asked why the presence of unmarried women as medical workers came to be seen as a good thing when it ran so counter to societal norms, and might have written a chapter that focused more on exploring changing domestic and workplace gender roles.

The importance of the *lieu de savoir* is also evident in Daqing Zhang's study of the changing health of Beijing. As the director of the Institute of Medical Humanities at Beijing University, Zhang finds it natural to focus on the health gains reflected in official statistics, where scholars working outside the PRC might have wanted to spend more time understanding how such statistics were compiled. It is nonetheless clear that enormous health gains have been achieved in the decades since 1950, and Zhang does not hesitate to indicate that much remains to be done. For example, he notes that the disproportionate consumption of public health resources by political elites has been eroding public confidence, and the 2003 outbreak of SARS showed that the old way of relying on political and social motivational campaigns to ensure compliance with public health initiatives is inadequate. He also engages directly with the Thomas McKeown thesis and argues—in accordance with McKeown's many recent critics—that declines in mortality cannot be cleanly adjudicated between rising living standards and public health interventions. For the successful control of tuberculosis in Beijing, both these factors were in play (and, one might add, both were supported by direct government action).

The view from Beijing in Zhang's chapter is offset in Miriam Gross and Kawai Fan's chapter on schistosomiasis. Their view from Hong Kong and the United States combines investigative rigor with a desire to understand how policies affected ordinary people's lives. By collecting and comparing reports from many different sources, Gross and Fan have concluded that even though the mass public campaigns to eradicate the snail vectors of schistosomiasis did reduce infection rates in the short term, they were massively expensive in terms of human labor and thus reduced agricultural productivity and rural livelihoods, and that farmers soon lost enthusiasm for tackling recurrent snail populations. Chairman Mao's close interest in this particular disease meant that public support for snail eradication closely mirrored the chairman's own popularity. Lasting gains from the anti-schistosomiasis movements were not achieved before the anti-helminthic drug Praziquantel became available in the mid-1970s.

In the control of both schistosomiasis and tuberculosis (described for Shanghai in detail by Rachel Core as well as by Daqing Zhang in his description of Beijing public health activities), developing the political and social infrastructure of socialist work units and production brigades during the 1950s turns out to have been key to the success of public health efforts. While the socialist infrastructure was a necessary precondition, the Communist government was also fortunate to be able to capitalize on the arrival of new and effective therapies, such as the BCG vaccine and new antibiotic treatments for tuberculosis and sexually transmitted diseases, all widely available only after World War II, and Praziquantel against the nematodes of schistosomiasis. This reminder that collectivization was essential to the health gains of the PRC is also borne out by Xiaoping Fang's work on the history of the barefoot doctors. Collectivization made it possible for the cooperative medical system to provide the new vaccines and antibiotics to rural populations for the first time, and the nationwide implementation of the barefoot doctor system extended the health care delivery system to the village/production-brigade level.

Thus we see that even though some of the Communist public health campaigns—against schistosomiasis in particular—may have been primarily effective at extending party control further than ever before, the success of the party in penetrating to all levels of society was also a prerequisite for the distribution of the new and effective drug treatments. The fact that these findings are robust enough to emerge from different ends of our contributors' political and historiographic spectrum is a reassuring testament to the rigor of the scholarship presented here.

Back to the Future?

One observation that emerges clearly from our collective studies is that many of the issues first debated in the 1930s have started to recur as unintended consequences of the decollectivization and market opening of China's economy, a process that began under Deng Xiaoping's leadership in the 1980s and has been accelerating ever since. Then, as now, there were large income disparities, leading to great inequity in access to health care; new initiatives were and are being developed to try to bring affordable health care to rural populations in the face of physician preference for lucrative urban clinics (Yip 2010); and the issue of whether the state should support Chinese medicine was and remains hotly debated (see Scheid and Lei in this volume). China today is open to foreign exchange with scientific and technical personnel, and has been consulting widely with foreign health economists, just as occurred in the 1930s. There is an obvious difference in emphasis, though: as Liping Bu and others note, in the 1920s and 1930s, John B. Grant was working to persuade the Nationalist government that health care delivery was an essential duty of the state and that social medicine was the most efficient way to provide it; now, although the state is in charge of much of the health care delivery system and is currently directing a huge overhaul of the entire sector, there is a new emphasis on ways of returning control of health care to the individual. For, as several of our authors acknowledge, the state is now widely held to have overreached in its use of mass health movements for political ends, and to have abrogated individual rights in the process. Still, the model of primary health care remains similar to that developed for Dingxian and Gaoqiao townships in the 1930s, and to the barefoot doctors program of the Cultural Revolution. As Yip et al. (2012) write, "China's long-term strategy to improve efficiency of resource allocation involves building a strong delivery system based on primary health care, anchored in community health centres in cities and township health centres in rural areas." It will be interesting to see, going forward, whether the limitations of the barefoot doctor movement described so vividly here by Xiaoping Fang will be corrected in the new primary care reform as it is extended into rural China.

There are other continuities, too. For example, nurses within China are still struggling to establish themselves as legitimate health care providers rather than hospital housekeepers, and it is remarkable that it has taken until 2013 for the China Nursing Association to be admitted to the International Council of Nurses (ICN) (see Grypma and Zhen in this volume). Mental and emotional disease statistics remain hard to come by, and even though the most reliable recent survey suggests that up to 17.5 percent of Chinese may have mental disorders at any one time, the stigma of working with this group of patients remains so high that it is still extremely difficult to train or employ sufficient numbers of mental health professionals (see Pearson in this volume).

The second standout theme is clearly the enormous symbolic importance of health and scientific medicine. Several of the chapters here have emphasized how keenly sensitive Chinese elites were to the perception of China as "the sick man of Asia" in the early twentieth century. This was interpreted both as a political metaphor in the context of what Ruth Rogaski has termed the "hypercolonialism" of the treaty port system (Rogaski 2004, 11), and also as a literal description of the majority of Chinese people. With sick bodies, how could China have a strong army, and without a strong army, how could China defend itself? Many Chinese (including Mao Zedong) felt that their nation, their race, and their own bodies were all under threat from invasion by foreign forces, both microscopic and macroscopic. Returning individuals to health and establishing a healthy environment thus became patriotic imperatives early in the century.

Women continue to bear the extra burden of responsibility for the health of the next generation, even though much has changed in the fields of maternal and child welfare. In the late nineteenth century, calls for women's education and the abolition of the practice of footbinding were made primarily by men and not for the purpose of liberating women but to promote better-educated, healthier mothers of future generations of Chinese men. As education rates for young women (and men) increased in the early twentieth century, the Chinese version of the 1920s "modern girl" appeared, with a bobbed or curled haircut, high heels, and a high-necked *qipao* dress. Unmarried women were the preferred factory workers in the burgeoning textile industry, but their freedoms as workers in the new capitalist industries were constrained by the expectation that they would remain chaste until marriage, at which point their work lives would be controlled by their in-laws in the service of continuing the family patriline (Judge 2011). Similarly, much of the impetus for the establishment of modern midwifery as a profession came from a rhetoric of the need to strengthen the nation and the race: "The so-called 'sick man of Asia' (*dongya bingfu*) could become healthy again with good prenatal care and aseptic childbirth" (Johnson and Wu, this volume). The eradication of venereal diseases was high on the list of priorities for both the Nationalist and the Communist governments in Beijing, but where the Nationalist government quickly ran out of funds with which to run penitentiary sanatoria for STD-infected prostitutes, and resorted to fining them instead, the Communist government closed down brothels with revolutionary zeal in the final months of 1949, almost immediately after taking office (see Zhang in this volume). The existence of a market for sexual services is an embarrassment to the Communist government, and was also one of the reasons it took China so long to admit to having an HIV/AIDS problem in the late 1980s (Liu 2011).

The international context also colored debates about the value of Chinese medicine for a modernizing China. Nicole Barnes and John Watt note that wartime exigencies led the Nationalist government in Chongqing to issue state licenses to many traditional physicians, something the state had previously been reluctant to do. The same is true of the Communist leadership in its wartime base in Yan'an, where severe manpower shortages led to the inclusion of acupuncturists and herbalists on the mobile medical teams sent into the countryside as part of the party's commitment to rural welfare. Xi Gao notes that after the war, during the 1950s period of Soviet tutelage, the CCP advocated Pavlovian neurophysiology, which operated on the body as an integrated system. This allowed supporters of Chinese medicine to assert its scientific nature on account of its own systemic approach to physiology. In the highly charged ideological environment of the 1950s and 1960s, it even became possible to reinterpret the Chinese-medical theory of yin-yang duality as an indigenous anticipation of dialectical materialism.

Chinese medicine's popular appeal among less educated Chinese, combined with its value to Mao as a tool with which to discipline the bourgeois intellectualism of Western-style physicians, meant that by the late 1950s, it was accorded status as an essential part of the new "world medicine" that China set out to create. The period of Soviet tutelage also saw the Chinese government commit itself to creating a single, unified health administration with a national education network in medicine. Chinese medicine was therefore incorporated into the new collective insurance systems, and a network of state-run colleges of Chinese medicine was also operating by the end of the 1950s.

After the Sino-Soviet split in the early 1960s, Chinese medicine continued its institutionalization, while at the same time still being subject to strong pressures to assimilate modern medical ideas and practices. This is seen most clearly in Xiaoping Fang's study of the barefoot doctor movement, which was one of the "newly emerged things" of the Cultural Revolution period. Although much of the rhetoric around the barefoot doctors stressed the unification of "old" and "new" in medicine, Fang is able to show decisively that the movement borrowed ideas and technologies from Chinese medicine mainly in order to smooth the acceptance of Western medicine. A great example of this was the giving of vaccinations at specific acupuncture points that would supposedly exert a helpful synergistic effect. When James "Scottie" Reston visited China in connection with Richard Nixon's 1971 visit and was given acupuncture for his postsurgical pain after an appendectomy, his *New York Times* account of the procedure launched a new phase of international enthusiasm for Chinese medicine, with multiple study tours of Western physicians coming to observe major surgery carried out using acupuncture analgesia alone. In the increasing openness to the West that has characterized the period since Mao's death in 1976, Chinese medicine has become a major source of foreign revenue to China in terms of exports of drugs, fees from foreigners wishing to study Chinese medicine, and World Health Organization funding to support research into Chinese medicine. Even though some sectors of Chinese society are once again embarrassed by Chinese medicine and are agitating to have its state support reduced or even cut off, Chinese medicine is now a globalized cultural export commanding an enormous and profitable market. The state is unlikely to withdraw its support anytime soon.

There are, of course, many great changes that are thrown into stark relief by observing the whole arc of twentieth-century medical history. At the beginning of the century, only a few people visited the mainly missionary-run hospitals and clinics to receive medical care. By 2000, as Michelle Renshaw observes, such institutions had a virtual monopoly on professional medical practice. This evolution, born from a need to create recognizable spaces for modern medicine that would allow both teaching and research and would also be transparent to suspicious patients, was expanded at different periods by both Nationalist and Communist governments. The governmental motivations included showing that China had a medical infrastructure that met international standards, achieving economies of scale in patient care, and creating spaces where medical professionals could be trained, controlled, and disciplined. At the same time, neither patients nor caregivers were passive in the face of governmental actions. The shrinking of the rural township clinics in favor of either local care by village doctors or expert care at county hospitals is another strong piece of evidence that patients did not simply follow directions. More evidence is provided by Tina Phillips Johnson and Yi-Li Wu, who describe both the resistance of women to the state's various attempts to control reproduction, and also the insistence of Communist Party women cadres in 1953 that they had a right to contraception if they were to be expected to participate in socialist reconstruction work.

Of all the changes, the most striking is the enormous increase in life expectancy achieved in the second half of the twentieth century. China's average life expectancy is now on par with many developed nations, at seventy-one years in 2000, having been only forty-six years in 1900. It is hard to know how much of this improvement can be attributed to relative political stability and how much to the development of effective medicines, particularly antibiotics for use against communicable diseases. Nonetheless, the Chinese government's effective management of environmental sanitation and the development of a local pharmaceutical industry capable of supplying the population with essential drugs were clearly key transitions. Whether or not the great mass health campaigns such as those waged against schistosomiasis were significant depends on what one considers the desired outcome to be. Clearly they demonstrated the power of the Chinese Communist Party to mobilize the massive Chinese population in the service of nationalism, as evidenced by the Patriotic Health Campaign of the Korean War era. They also used mutual surveillance in communities to identify cases of disease and bring them to the attention of the medical authorities. Because these health campaigns provided greater state penetration into the private lives of citizens and also improved health outcomes, medical work has had a uniquely important role in perceptions of party effectiveness.

Rachel Core's study of the history of tuberculosis in Shanghai reminds us that not all health initiatives came from the state—the Chinese and Shanghai Anti-Tuberculosis Associations began as voluntary groups. With the backing of the Communist Party, by the mid-1950s they were using X-rays to screen over a million residents a year, and conducting widespread BCG vaccination drives. Even though treatment initially offered only uncertain outcomes, there seems to have been little opposition to it. When DOTS treatment ("Directly Observed Therapy, Short-Course," using a cocktail of different antibiotic drugs) was developed by WHO in 1989, China became one of the earliest recipients in a control project that rapidly produced a doubling of cure rates. Here again, we see that drug availability played a key role, even though improved living conditions were doubtless also key to the ongoing epidemiological transition discussed in our first chapter by Lincoln Chen and Ling Chen.

It is fitting to end this survey of medical transitions in twentieth-century China by paying tribute to the enormous resourcefulness of the Chinese people in finding solutions to their health care challenges. Nicole Barnes and John Watt describe how "the war years marked the apogee of the process, begun in the late nineteenth century, of imprinting individual bodies with national concerns." The widespread belief that the fate of the nation was closely bound up with the health and survival of each individual Chinese led to heroic efforts in medicine and public health work unparalleled anywhere in the world. Marion Yang's modern midwifery schools and training courses for teaching old-style birth attendants how to avoid tetanus neonatorum and childbed fever, John B. Grant and C. C. Chen's efforts at creating affordable rural health centers, and the efforts of several generations of Chinese-style physicians to incorporate hygienic principles into their practice illustrate just some of the efforts made during the Republican era. Add to this the convergence of government propaganda efforts and marketing literature in favor of hygiene (which even extended to the "hygienic cigarettes" described by Carol Benedict), and it can truly be concluded that many Chinese grew up believing that personal hygiene and contributions to the cleanliness of their environments were expressions of patriotism and good citizenship. Mao's use of mass campaigns such as the Patriotic Health Campaign of the Korean War era and the anti-schistosomiasis movement may have abused the goodwill of the citizenry in their excesses, but it is beyond doubt that these campaigns achieved remarkable results in short order. During the second half of the twentieth century, the scourges of tuberculosis, syphilis, smallpox, polio, and cholera were all brought under control as a result of vast extensions in the state's ability to access and monitor its population and deliver treatment. The one-child policy, put into effect in 1979, has been mainly understood as a measure to control China's population, but it was preceded by the highly effective and much less coercive campaign of "later, longer, fewer" in the early 1970s, which encouraged young people to marry later, space their children at longer intervals, and have smaller families. The propaganda for this campaign as well as its predecessor in the 1950s, which advocated "one pregnancy, one live birth; one live birth, one healthy child," was couched much more in terms of the health and well-being of mother and child as essential aspects of a future healthy nation. And indeed, infant and maternal mortality rates dropped precipitously.

During the war, with little support from the state and with no guarantee of a future, many physicians trained paramedics to extend their own reach and cut medical expenses. Such work built on blueprints developed in the Republican era with collaboration from League of Nations Health Organization experts, and in turn provided the inspiration for the primary health care structures of Communist China, which retained these wartime command-and-control structures. Since decollectivization began in the 1970s, collective health insurance schemes have shrunk or disappeared, leading to a large disparity in access to health care between the wealthy and the working poor. Once again, towns and villages are experimenting with collective insurance schemes, and the state is also in the process of reinventing state medical insurance in ways that will give individual citizens more control.

Now, in the early twenty-first century, China is faced with a new set of health challenges, and new medical transitions will be required to deal with them. Environmental pollution has created a frightening disease load in terms of cancers and lung conditions such as asthma; the rapid economic development of China's maritime provinces has led to an unprecedented increase in chronic conditions such as diabetes, heart disease, and high blood pressure; and the incidence of mental health disorders is not only very high, at nearly one-fifth of the population at any given time, but also remains stigmatized, poorly treated, and widely misunderstood (see Pearson in this volume). While the Chinese government and the Chinese Medical Association are consulting widely, just as they did at the start of the century, it is clear that there are no easy solutions. Once again, China will have to adapt measures from different sources and apply them to its own unique situation. The studies in this volume strongly suggest that the Chinese people will rise to the challenge.

Appendix: Timeline

	Before 1900	1900s
Significant National, International Biomedical Events		
Nursing	1884: First missionary nurse arrives in China	1909: Nurses Association of China (NAC) established
Maternal and Child Health	1873: Lucinda Combs, first female medical missionary to China, arrives in Beijing 1896: Chinese Christians Shi Meiyu and Kang Cheng graduate from the University of Michigan's medical school and return to China	
Disease Prevention and Control	1890–1911: Anti–Juvenile Smoking Movement	1905: Schistosomiasis discovered in China
Chinese Medicine		
Health and Medical Delivery	1835 onwards: Missionary-run hospitals	1906: First govt. hospitals (*Minzhengbu yiyuan*) 1908: Railway hospitals
Relevant Policy "Era"		1900–1911: Qing dynasty, "New Policies"

	1910s	1920s
Significant National, International Biomedical Events		
Nursing	1915: NAC examinations introduced	1920: *Nursing Journal of China* 1921: PUMC School of Nursing
Maternal and Child Health	1913: Early government attempts to regulate midwives	
Disease Prevention and Control	1911–1912: North Manchurian Plague Prevention Service	
Chinese Medicine	1911–1948: National Medical Movement	
Health and Medical Delivery	1914: China Medical Board established	1921: Peking Union Medical College established 1925: Beijing, first PUMC-affiliated Health Station
Relevant Policy "Era"	1911: Republic of China 1916–1927: Warlordism	1923: Education and rural reconstruction movements 1928–1937: "Nanjing Decade" of Nationalists (Guomindang)

1930s	1940s	1950s
1935: Antimicrobial "sulfa drugs" mass produced	1945: Penicillin mass produced 1946: Streptomycin available for TB	
1935: Ministry of Health assumes responsibility for nurse registration	1940: First Chinese Dean of Nursing at PUMC, Neih Yuchan (Vera Neih)	Higher education of nurses replaced by secondary-level training
1929: The Ministries of Health and Education establish the National Midwifery Board and the First National Midwifery School	1949: PRC implements two-tiered system of midwifery training	1952: Promotion of Soviet "psychoprophylactic painless childbirth method"
New Life Movement targets smoking 1933: Chinese Anti-Tuberculosis Association established	1949: First anti-schistosomiasis campaign	1950: BCG vaccine promoted widely for TB 1957–1958: Shanghai, 17 TB prevention and treatment stations 1956: First Mao-sponsored anti-schistosomiasis mass campaign
		1954: Mao supports TCM
1929: Wusong, first rural Demonstration Station	GMD military hospitals, CCP field hospitals, and mass campaign strategies	Three-tier health system with hospitals at apex and "union clinics" in villages 1950–1952: Four "Principles of Health Work" training scheme 1951: Labour Medical Service (LIS) 1952: Government Medical Service 1955: Cooperative Medical Service (Rural)
New Life Movement 1937–1945: War of Resistance against Japan/Japanese Occupation 1939–1945: World War II	1945–1949: Civil war, Guomindang vs. China Communist Party	1949: People's Republic of China 1953–1958: Collectivization and work-unit system 1950–1953: Korean War

	1960s	1970s
Significant National, International Biomedical Events	1967–1970: Measles and epidemic cerebrospinal meningitis vaccines	
Nursing		
Maternal and Child Health		
Disease Prevention and Control		
Chinese Medicine	1966: "Simplification"	
Health and Medical Delivery	1968: Notion of barefoot doctors introduced; promoted widely from 1970	Medical and nursing schools closed
Relevant Policy "Era"	1958–1962: Great Leap Forward 1966–1976: Great Proletarian Cultural Revolution	1970: Cultural Revolution cont. 1978: Economic reform; decollectivization and rise of market economy; household responsibility system

1980s	1990s	After 2000
1980: Praziquantel for effective schistosomiasis treatment		
1983: First University medical school (Tianjin) reestablishes nursing degree	1998: Seven master's degree programs in place	2013: ICN accepts Chinese Nursing Association as a member
1980: The "one-child policy" officially codified 1982: New PRC Constitution identifies "family planning" as a state priority	1995: Promoting hospital-based births becomes governmental priority	
	1990: Chinese Association on Tobacco Control 1992: DOTS strategy for TB 1998: Shanghai Center for Disease Control established	
Post-Mao "Diversification"	"Integration"	
Collapse of medical insurance schemes; disintegration of barefoot doctors scheme.	1998: Basic medical insurance scheme (urban)	2003: New cooperative medical system (rural) 2009: Three-year health care reform initiated

Bibliography

The bibliography is organized into three sections: first English and other Western-language references, then Chinese- and Japanese-language sources, and finally archival sources.

English Sources

Achtenberg, Hannah. 1983. "Mental Health Care in China." *Journal of Psychiatric Treatment and Evaluation* 53: 371–375.

Adams, F. 1972. "Mental Care in Peking." *China Now,* January.

Andrews, Bridie J. 1996. "The Making of Modern Chinese Medicine, 1895–1937." PhD diss., University of Cambridge.

———. 2001. "From Bedpan to Revolution: Qiu Jin and Western Nursing in China." In *Women and Modern Medicine,* edited by Anne Hardy and Lawrence Conrad, 53–72. Amsterdam: Rodopi.

———. 2014. *The Making of Modern Chinese Medicine, 1850–1960.* Vancouver: University of British Columbia Press.

Arias, Elizabeth. 2010. "United States Life Tables, 2006." *National Vital Statistics Reports* 58 (21): 1–40.

Ash, Robert. 1981. "The Quest for Food Self-Sufficiency." In *Shanghai: Revolution and Development in an Asian Metropolis,* edited by Christopher Howe, 188–221. Cambridge: Cambridge University Press.

Ashton, Basil, Kenneth Hill, Alan Piazza, and Robin Zeitz. 1984. "Famine in China, 1958–61." *Population and Development Review* 10 (4): 613–645.

Balasegaram, Mangai, and Alan Schnur. 2006. "China: From Denial to Mass Mobilization." In *SARS: How a Global Epidemic Was Stopped,* edited by the World Health Organization, Western Pacific Region, 73–85. Geneva: World Health Organization Press.

Bangdiwala, Shrikant I., Joseph D. Tucker, Sanjay Zodpey, Sian M. Griffiths, Li-Ming Li, K. Srinath Reddy, Myron S. Cohen, Miriam Gross, Kayva Sharma, and Jin-Ling Tang. 2011. "Public Health Education in India and China: History, Opportunities, and Challenges." *Public Health Reviews* 33 (1): 204–224.

Banister, Judith. 1984. "An Analysis of Recent Data on the Population of China." *Population and Development Review* 10 (2): 241–271.

Barham, Peter. 1984. *Schizophrenia and Human Values.* Oxford: Basil Blackwell.

Barnes, Linda L. 2005. *Needles, Herbs, Gods, and Ghosts: China, Healing, and the West to 1848.* Cambridge, MA: Harvard University Press.

Barnes, Nicole Elizabeth. 2012a. "Disease in the Capital: Nationalist Health Services and the 'Sick (Wo)man of East Asia' in Wartime Chongqing." *European Journal of East Asian Studies* 11 (2): 283–303.

———. 2012b. "Protecting the National Body: Gender and Public Health in Southwest China during the War of Resistance against Japan, 1937–1945." PhD diss., University of California, Irvine.

Bartsch, Bernhard. 2005. "High-Tech Helps a Million Patients." *Pictures of the Future,* Fall, 81. http://www.siemens.com/innovation/pool/en/publikationen/publications_pof/pof _fall_2005/digital_health/suzhou_municipal_hospital/pof205_editorial_1334505.pdf.

Bashford, Alison, and Philippa Levine, eds. 2010. *The Oxford Handbook of the History of Eugenics.* Oxford: Oxford University Press.

"Basic Research Program for Chinese Medicine Formulae." 2001. *Medical China Update* 1 (1): 30.

Baum, Richard. 1982. "Science and Culture in Contemporary China: The Roots of Retarded Modernization." *Asian Survey* 22 (12): 1166–1186.

Benedict, Carol. 1996. *Bubonic Plague in Nineteeth-Century China.* Stanford, CA: Stanford University Press.

———. 2011. *Golden-Silk Smoke: A History of Tobacco in China, 1550–2010.* Berkeley: University of California Press.

Berry-Cabán, CS. 2007. "Return of the God of Plague: Schistosomiasis in China." *Journal of Rural and Tropical Public Health* 6: 45–53.

Bieler, Stacey. 2004. *"Patriots" or "Traitors"? A History of American Educated Chinese Students.* Armonk, NY: M. E. Sharpe.

Bloom, Gerald, and Tang Shenglan, eds. 2004. *Health Care Transition in Urban China.* Burlington, VT: Ashgate.

Blumenthal, David, and William Hsiao. 2005. "Privatization and Its Discontents—The Evolving Chinese Health Care System." *New England Journal of Medicine* 353 (11): 1165–1170.

Bolt, Richard A. 1913. "A Plea for More Systematic Medical Inspection and Physical Examination of Chinese Students." *China Medical Journal* 27 (4): 208–226.

Borowy, Iris. 2009a. "Thinking Big—League of Nations Efforts towards a Reformed National Health System in China." In *Uneasy Encounters: The Politics of Medicine and Health in China, 1900–1937,* edited by Iris Borowy, 205–228. New York: Peter Lang.

———. 2009b. *Coming to Terms with World Health: The League of Nations Health Organization, 1921–1946.* New York: Peter Lang.

Bowers, John Z. 1972. *Western Medicine in a Chinese Palace: Peking Union Medical College, 1917–1951.* Philadelphia: Josiah Macy Jr. Foundation.

Bramall, Chris. 2009. *Chinese Economic Development.* London: Routledge.

Brandtstädter, Susanne. 2000. "Elias in China?: 'Civilising Process,' Kinship and Customary Law in the Chinese Countryside." Max Planck Institute for Social Anthropology: Working Papers 6.

Breay, Margaret. 1937. "Professional Review." *British Journal of Nursing,* May: 136–137.

Bu, Liping. 2009a. "Public Health and Modernization: The First Campaigns in China, 1915–1916." *Social History of Medicine* 22 (2): 305–319.

———. 2009b. "Social Darwinism, Public Health and Modernization in China, 1895–1925." In *Uneasy Encounters: The Politics of Medicine and Health in China 1900–1937,* edited by Iris Borowy, 93–124. New York: Peter Lang.

———. 2011. "Cultural Communication in Picturing Health: W. W. Peter and the Public Health Campaigns in China, 1912–1926." In *Imagining Illness: Public Health and Visual Culture,* edited by David Serlin, 24–39. Minneapolis: University of Minnesota Press.

———. 2012a. "Beijing First Health Station: Innovative Public Health Education and Influence on China's Health Profession." In *Science, Public Health and the State in Modern Asia,* edited by Liping Bu, Darwin Stapleton, and Ka-che Yip. London: Routledge.

———. 2012b. "From Public Health to State Medicine: John B. Grant and China's Health Profession." *Asia Quarterly* 14 (4): 8–15.

Buck, Peter. 1980. *American Science and Modern China, 1876–1936.* Cambridge: Cambridge University Press.

Bueber, M. 1992. "Letter from China (No. 1)." *Archives of General Nursing* 6: 61–64.

———. 1993a. "Letter from China (No. 2)." *Archives of General Nursing* 7: 111–115.

———. 1993b. "Letter from China (No. 3)." *Archives of General Nursing* 7: 249–253.

Bullock, Mary Brown. 1980. *The American Transplant: The Rockefeller Foundation and Peking Union Medical College.* Berkeley: University of California Press, 1980.

———. 2011. "The Rockefeller Foundation and China Medical Board in Asia, 1913 to 1950." Unpublished paper.

Caldwell, John C. 1976. "Toward a Restatement of Demographic Transition Theory." *Population and Development Review* 2: 321–366.

———. 1990. "Introductory Thoughts on Health Transition." In *What We Know about Health Transition: The Cultural, Social and Behavioural Determinants of Health,* edited by John C. Caldwell, Salley Findley, Pat Caldwell, Gigi Santow, Wendy Cosford, Jennifer Braid, and Daphne Broers-Freeman, xi–xii. Canberra: Health Transition Center, Australian National University.

Campbell, Cameron. 1997. "Public Health Efforts in China before 1949 and Their Effects on Mortality: The Case of Beijing." *Social Science History* 21 (2): 179–218.

Cerny, J. 1965. "Chinese Psychiatry." *International Journal of Psychiatry* 1: 229–247.

Chan, Sally, and Frances Wong. 1999. "Development of Basic Nursing Education in China and Hong Kong." *Journal of Advanced Nursing* 29 (6): 1300–1307.

Chang Che-Chia. 1998. "The Therapeutic Tug of War: The Imperial Physician-Patient Relationship in the Era of Empress Dowager Cixi (1874–1908)." PhD diss., University of Pennsylvania.

Chang Chih-Tung. 1900. *China's Only Hope: An Appeal.* New York: Fleming H. Revel.

Chang, P. Y. 1993. *Record of Interviews with Chief Mei-Yu Chow.* Translated by Na Wu. Taipei: Institute of Modern History, Academia Sinica.

Chau, Adam Yuet. 2008. *Miraculous Response: Doing Popular Religion in Contemporary China.* Stanford, CA: Stanford University Press.

Checkland, Olive. 1994. *Humanitarianism and the Emperor's Japan, 1877–1977.* New York: St. Martin's.

Chen, C. C. 1989. *Medicine in Rural China: A Personal Account.* Berkeley: University of California Press.

Chen, Hanhui, Michael R. Phillips, Hui Cheng, Qiongqiong Chen, Xiaodong Chen, Drew Fralick, Yin'e Zhang, Meng Liu, Jia Huang, and Marlys Bueber. 2012. "Mental Health Law of the People's Republic of China (English Translation with Annotations)." *Shanghai Archives of Psychiatry* 24 (6): 305–321. doi: 10.3969/j.issn.1002-0829.2012.06.001.

Chen, Jiajian, Zhenming Xie, and Hongyan Liu. 2007. "Son Preference, Use of Maternal Health Care, and Infant Mortality in Rural China, 1989–2000." *Population Studies* 61 (2): 161–183.

Chen, K. K., and Carl F. Schmidt. 1930. "Ephedrine and Related Substances." *Medicine: Analytical Reviews of General Medicine, Neurology and Pediatrics* 9: 1–117.

Chen, Nancy N., ed. 2003. *Breathing Spaces.* New York: Columbia University Press.

Chen, William Y. 1961. "Medicine and Public Health." *China Quarterly* 6 (April–June): 153–169.

Chen Kaiyi. 1996a. "Missionaries and the Early Development of Nursing in China." *Nursing History Review* 4: 129–149.

———. 1996b. "Quality versus Quantity: The Rockefeller Foundation and Nurses Training in China." *Journal of American-East Asian Relations* 5 (1): 77–104.

Chen Pi-chao. 1985a. "Birth Control Methods and Organization in China." In *China's One-Child Family Policy,* edited by Elisabeth Croll, Delia Davin, and Penny Kane, 135–148. New York: St. Martin's.

Chen Xianyi, Wang Liying, Cai Jiming, Zhou Xiaonong, Zheng Jiang, Guo Jiagang, Wu Xiaohua, D. Engels, and Chen Minggang. 2005. "Schistosomiasis Control in China:

The Impact of a 10-Year World Bank Loan Project (1992–2001)." Bulletin of the World Health Organization 83: 1–80.

Chen Xueping. 1999. "An Attempt to Add Academic Nursing Knowledge in 4-Year System Clinical Class." *Secondary Medical Education* 17 (2): 24–25.

Chen Yunan. 2011a. "Health Information Use in Chronic Care Cycles." Paper presented at the 2011 Association of Computing Machinery Conference on Computer Supported Cooperative Work, Hangzhou, China, March 19–23.

———. 2011b. "Understanding and Designing for Patient-Centered Care in China." Paper presented at the Computer Supported Cooperative Work 2011 Workshop: Designing Social and Collaborative Systems for China, Hangzhou, China, July 15.

Chen Zhu, Shin Young-soo, and Robert Beaglehole. 2012. "Tobacco Control in China: Small Steps towards a Giant Leap." *Lancet* 379 (March 3): 779–780.

Cheng, K. F., and P. C. Leung. 2007. "What Happened in China during the 1918 Influenza Pandemic?" *International Journal of Infectious Diseases* 11: 360–365.

Cheng, M. Y. 1948. "Infant Mortality and Its Causes in China: Review and Discussion." *China Medical Journal* 34 (2): 53–63.

Cheng Tien-hsi. 1971. "Schistosomiasis in Mainland China: A Review of Research and Control Programs since 1949." *American Journal of Tropical Medicine and Hygiene* 20 (1): 26–53.

Cheng Yingqi. 2012. "First TCM Medicine OK'd for EU Market." *China Daily* (Beijing), April 19.

Cheung Ngai Fen, Rosemary Mander, and Linan Cheng. 2005. "The 'Doula-Midwives' in Shanghai." *Evidence-Based Midwifery* 3: 73–79.

Cheung Ngai Fen, Rosemary Mander, Xiaoli Wang, Wei Fu, Junghong Zhu. 2009. "Chinese Midwives' Views on a Proposed Midwife-Led Normal Birth Unit." *Midwifery* 25: 744–755.

Chiang Yung-chen. 2001. *Social Engineering and the Social Sciences in China, 1919–1949.* Cambridge: Cambridge University Press.

Chin, Robert, and Ai-Li S. Chin. 1969. *Psychological Research in Communist China 1949–1966.* Cambridge, MA: MIT Press.

China Centenary Missionary Conference. 1907. *China Centenary Missionary Conference Records: Report of the Great Conference Held at Shanghai, April 5th to May 8th, 1907.* New York: American Tract Society.

China Daily. 2011. "Free Hospital Delivery Improves Rural Women's Lives." August 22.

———. 2012a. "Birth Defects an Increasing Concern for Physicians." February 28.

———. 2012b. "Official Vows China Will Correct Gender Imbalance." May 24.

China Institute in America. *A Survey of Chinese Students in American Universities and Colleges in the Past One Hundred Years.* 1954. New York: National Tsing Hua University Research Fellowship Fund and China Institute in America.

China Medical Commission of the Rockefeller Foundation. 1914. *Medicine in China.* New York: China Medical Commission.

China National Health Economics Institute. 2005. "Assessing Government Health Expenditure in China." Background Paper, World Bank China Rural Health Study.

China Reconstructs (Peking). 1968. "First County to Wipe Out Schistosomiasis." July 17.

"China to Train 15,000 TCM Backbone Clinicians." 2012. Xinhua News Agency, May 30. http://news.xinhuanet.com/english/china/2012-05/30/c_131618924.htm.

Chinese People's Political Consultative Conference. 1949. *The Important Documents of the First Plenary Session of the Chinese People's Political Consultative Conference.* Peking: Foreign Languages Press.

Choa, Gerald H. 1990. *"Heal the Sick" Was Their Motto: The Protestant Medical Missionaries in China.* Hong Kong: Chinese University Press.

Chow Kai Wing. 1998. "Yin Yamei." In *Biographical Dictionary of Chinese Women: The Qing Period, 1644–1911,* Vol. 1, edited by Lily Xiao Hong Lee and translated by Stephanie Po-yin Chung, 94–96. Armonk, NY: M. E. Sharpe.

Chow Mei-Yu. 1945. *Nurses of China Fight On: The Story of China's Army Nursing School.* New York: American Bureau for Medical Aid to China.

Chun, J. W. H. 1923. "Pneumonic Plague in Harbin (Manchurian Epidemic, 1921)." *China Medical Journal* 37 (1): 7–17.

Clodfelter, M. 2001. *Warfare and Armed Conflict: A Statistical Reference to Casualty and Other Figures, 1500–2000.* Jefferson, NC: McFarland.

Cook, Harold, Sanjoy Battacharya, and Anne Hardy, eds. 2009. *History of the Social Determinants of Health: Global Histories and Contemporary Debates.* Hyderabad, India: Orient Blackswan.

Cormack, J. G. 1914. "Letter to the Editor." *Chinese Medical Journal* 28 (4): 237.

Cousland, Philip B. 1901. "The Medical School." *China Medical Missionary Journal* 15 (3): 199–200.

Cox, Howard. 2000. *The Global Cigarette: Origins and Evolution of British-American Tobacco, 1880–1945.* Oxford: Oxford University Press.

Croizier, Ralph. 1968. *Traditional Medicine in Modern China: Science, Nationalism, and the Tensions of Cultural Change.* Cambridge, MA: Harvard University Press.

———. 1975. "Medicine and Modernization in China: An Historical Overview." In *Medicine in Chinese Culture: Comparative Studies of Health Care in Chinese and Other Societies,* edited by Arthur Kleinman and Peter Kunstadter, 21–35. Bethesda, MD: National Institutes of Health.

Crosby, Alfred W. 2003. *America's Forgotten Pandemic: The Influenza of 1918.* Cambridge: Cambridge University Press.

Cui Weiyuan. 2010. "China Wrestles with Tobacco Control." *Bulletin of the World Health Organization* 88 (April): 251–252.

Cunningham, Andrew, and Ole Peter Grell. 2000. *The Four Horsemen of the Apocalypse: Religion, War, Famine and Death in Reformation Europe.* Cambridge: Cambridge University Press.

Davenport, Horace W. 1996. *Victor Vaughan: Statesman and Scientist.* Ann Arbor, MI: Historical Center for the Health Sciences.

Davies, A. Tegla. 1947. *Friends Ambulance Unit: The Story of the F.A.U. in the Second World War, 1939–1946.* London: George Allen and Unwin.

Davin, Delia. 1985. "The Single-Child Family Policy in the Countryside." In *China's One-Child Family Policy,* edited by Elisabeth Croll, Delia Davin, and Penny Kane, 37–82. New York: St. Martin's.

Davis, Andrew. 2003. "Schistosomiasis." In *Manson's Tropical Diseases,* edited by Gordon C. Cook and Alimuddin I. Zumla, 1425–1460. 21st ed. Philadelphia: Saunders-Elsevier Science.

Davis, Anne. 1983a. Unpublished interview with Vera Nieh. Beijing. Used by permission of Anne Davis.

———. 1983b. Unpublished interview with Lin Ju Ying. Beijing. Used by permission of Anne Davis.

———. 2001. "Interview with Madam Lin Ju Ying." *Nursing Ethics* 8 (4): 484–486.

Davis, Kingsley. 1963. "The Theory of Change and Response in Modern Demographic History." *Population Index* 29: 345–366.

Dikötter, Frank. 1998. *Imperfect Conceptions: Medical Knowledge, Birth Defects, and Eugenics in China*. London: Hurst.

———. 2010. *Mao's Great Famine: The History of China's Most Devastating Catastrophe, 1958–62*. London: Bloomsbury.

Ding, Qu Jian, and Therese Hesketh. 2006. "Family Size, Fertility Preferences, and Sex Ratio in China in the Era of the One Child Family Policy: Results from National Family Planning and Reproductive Health Survey." *British Medical Journal* 333: 371–373.

Dirlik, Arif. 1975. "The Ideological Foundations of the New Life Movement: A Study in Counterrevolution." *Journal of Asian Studies* 35 (4): 945–980.

Dower, John W. 1993. *War Without Mercy: Race and Power in the Pacific War*. New York: Pantheon Books.

Duckett, Jane. 2010. *The Chinese State's Retreat from Health: Policy and the Politics of Retrenchment*. Abingdon, UK: Routledge.

Duffy, John. 1992. *The Sanitarians: A History of American Public Health*. Urbana-Champaign: University of Illinois Press.

Dumoulin-Smith, Adrien. 2009. "Social Health Insurance in China: An Example of Nascent Social Security in China." Cornell University Center for the Study of Inequality. http://inequality.cornell.edu/people/PapersAbstracts/Dumoulin%20Smith_paper.pdf.

Dyckerhoff, Claudia Sussmuth, and Jin Wang. 2010. "China's Health Care Reform." *Health International* 10: 55–67.

Elling, Ray H. 1978. "Medical Systems as Changing Social Systems." *Social Science & Medicine* 12: 107–115.

Elman, Benjamin. 2006. *A Cultural History of Modern Science in China*. Cambridge, MA: Harvard University Press.

Eyler, John M. 1997. *Sir Arthur Newsholme and State Medicine, 1889–1935*. Cambridge: Cambridge University Press.

Faber, Knud Helge. 1931. *Report on Medical Schools in China*. Geneva: League of Nations Health Organization.

Fan, Kawai, and Honkei Lai. 2008. "Mao Zedong's Fight against Schistosomiasis." *Perspectives in Biology and Medicine* 51 (2): 176–187.

Fan Lizhu. 2003. "The Cult of the Silkworm Mother as a Core of Local Community Religion in a North China Village: Field Study in Zhiwuying, Boading, Hebei." *China Quarterly* 174 (June): 359–372.

Fang, Xiaoping. 2012. *Barefoot Doctors and Western Medicine in China*. New York: University of Rochester Press.

Farley, John. 1991. *Bilharzia: A History of Imperial Tropical Medicine*. Cambridge: Cambridge University Press.

———. 2004. *To Cast Out Disease: A History of the International Health Division of the Rockefeller Foundation, 1913–1951*. New York: Oxford University Press.

Farquhar, Judith. 1994a. "Multiplicity, Point of View, and Responsibility in Traditional Chinese Healing." In *Body, Subject and Power in China*, edited by Angela Zito and Tani E. Barlow, 78–99. Chicago: University of Chicago Press.

———. 1994b. *Knowing Practice: The Clinical Encounter in Chinese Medicine*. Boulder, CO: Westview.

———. 1995. "Re-Writing Traditional Medicine in Post-Maoist China." In *Knowledge and the Scholarly Medical Traditions*, edited by Don Bates, 251–276. Cambridge: Cambridge University Press.

———. 1996a. "'Medicine and the Changes are One': An Essay in Divination Healing." *Chinese Science* 16: 107–134.

———. 1996b. "Market Magic: Getting Rich and Getting Personal in Medicine after Mao." *American Ethnologist* 23 (2): 239–257.

Faust, Ernest Carroll, and Henry Edmund Meleney. 1924. *Studies on Schistosomiasis Japonica.* Baltimore, MD: American Journal of Hygiene.

Fee, Elizabeth. 1987. *Disease and Discovery: A History of the Johns Hopkins School of Hygiene and Public Health, 1919–1939.* Baltimore, MD: Johns Hopkins University Press.

Feng Wang, Xuejin Zuo, and Daching Ruan. 2002. "Rural Migrants in Shanghai: Living under the Shadow of Socialism." *International Migration Review* 36 (2): 520–545.

Ferguson, Mary. 1970. *China Medical Board and Peking Union Medical College: A Chronicle of Fruitful Collaboration, 1914–1951.* New York: China Medical Board.

First Affiliated Hospital of Soochow University. 2012. "Hospital Profile." http://fyy.sdfyy.cn.

Flohr, Carsten. 1996. "The Plague Fighter: Wu Lien-teh and the Beginning of the Chinese Public Health System." *Annals of Science* 53: 361–380.

Fogarty, John E. 1990. *A Barefoot Doctor's Manual.* Philadelphia: Running Press.

Frears, M. 1976. "Fighting for Freedom: Mental Health Care in China." *Rehabilitation World* 2: 21–22.

Frederiksen, H. 1969. "Feedbacks in Economic and Demographic Transition." *Science* 166: 837–847.

Frenk, Julio, José L. Bobadilla, Claudio Stern, Tomas Frejka, and Rafael Lozano. 1994. "Elements for a Theory of the Health Transition." In *Health and Social Change in International Perspective,* edited by Lincoln C. Chen, Arthur Kleinman, and Norma C. Ware, 25–49. Boston: Harvard School of Public Health.

Frenk, Julio, José L. Bobadilla, Jaime Sepulveda, and Malaquias López-Cervantes. 1989. "Health Transition in Middle Income Countries: New Challenges for Health Care." *Health Policy and Planning* 4: 29–39.

Fu Qing-zhu. 1995. *Fu Qing-zhu's Gynecology.* Translated by Yang Shou-zhong and Liu Da-wei. Boulder, CO: Blue Poppy.

Furth, Charlotte. 1999. *A Flourishing Yin: Gender in China's Medical History, 960–1665.* Berkeley: University of California Press.

Gamble, Sidney D. 1921. *Peking: A Social Survey.* New York: G. H. Doran.

———. 1968. *Ting Hsien: A North China Rural Community.* Stanford, CA: Stanford University Press.

Gan Quan, Kirk R. Smith, S. Katharine Hammond, and Teh-wei Hu. 2008. "Disease Burden from Smoking and Passive Smoking in China." In *Tobacco Control Policy Analysis in China: Economics and Health,* edited by Hu Teh-wei, 83–104. Singapore: World Scientific.

Gao, Xi. 2012. "Between the State and the Private Sphere: Chinese State Medicine Movement, 1930–1949." In *Science, Public Health and the State in Modern Asia,* edited by Liping Bu, Darwin Stapleton, and Ka-Che Yip, 145–148. New York: Routledge.

Gao Yu, Lesley Barclay, Sue Kildea, Min Hao, and Suzanne Belton. 2010. "Barriers to Increasing Hospital Birth Rates in Rural Shanxi Province, China." *Reproductive Health Matters* 18 (36): 35–45.

Gardner, John. 1969. "The Wu-fan Campaign in Shanghai." In *Chinese Communist Politics in Action,* edited by A. Doak Barnett, 477–539. Seattle: University of Washington Press.

"General Practitioner System to Take Shape in China by 2020." 2011. *Xinhua News,* July 7. http://news.xinhuanet.com/english2010/health/2011-07/07/c_13971885.htm.

Gillespie, Robert S. 2006. "The Train Doctors: A Detailed History of Railway Surgeons." http://railwaysurgery.org/HistoryLong.htm#_ednref68.

Glaziou, Philippe, Katherine Floyd, Eline L. Korenromp, Charalambos Sismanidis, Ana L. Bierrenbach, Brian G. Williams, Rifat Atun, and Mario Raviglione. 2011. "Lives Saved by Tuberculosis Control and Prospects for Achieving the 2015 Global Target for Reducing Tuberculosis Mortality." *Bulletin of the World Health Organization* 89: 573–582. http://www.who.int/bulletin/volumes/89/8/11-087510/en/.

Goffman, William, and Kenneth S. Warren. 1980. *Scientific Information Systems and the Principle of Selectivity.* New York: Praeger.

Goldschmidt, Asaf. 2009. *The Evolution of Chinese Medicine: Song Dynasty, 960–1200.* London: Routledge.

Goldstein, Joshua. 1998. "Scissors, Surveys, and Psycho-Prophylactics: Prenatal Health Care Campaigns and State Building in China, 1949–1954." *Journal of Historical Sociology* 11 (2): 153–183.

Golub, JE, CI Mohan, GW Comstock, and RE Chaisson. 2005. "Active Case Finding of Tuberculosis: Historical Perspective and Future Prospects." *International Journal of Tuberculosis and Lung Disease* 9 (11): 1183–1203.

Good, Mary-Jo Delvecchio, and Byron J. Good. 2012. "Significance of the 686 Program for China and for Global Mental Health." *Shanghai Archives of Psychiatry* 24 (3): 175–177.

Grant, John B. 1928. "State Medicine—A Logical Policy for China." *National Medical Journal of China* 14 (2): 65–80.

Grant, John B., and T. M. Peng. 1934. "Survey of Urban Public Health Practice in China." *Chinese Medical Journal* 48: 1074–1079.

Greene, Roger S. 1918. "Medical Needs of the Chinese." *Chinese Record,* April.

Greenhalgh, Susan. 2008. *Just One Child: Science and Policy in Deng's China.* Berkeley: University of California Press.

Greenhalgh, Susan, and Edwin A. Winckler. 2005. *Governing China's Population: From Leninist to Neoliberal Biopolitics.* Stanford, CA: Stanford University Press.

Grypma, Sonya. 2008. *Healing Henan: Canadian Nurses at the North China Mission, 1888–1947.* Vancouver: University of British Columbia Press.

———. 2011. "Missionary Nursing: Internationalizing Religious Ideals." In *Religion, Religious Ethics, and Nursing,* edited by Marsha D. M. Fowler, Sheryl Reimer-Kirkham, Richard Sawatzky, and Elizabeth Johnston Taylor, 129–150. New York: Springer.

Gu Dongfeng, Tanika N. Kelly, Xigui Wu, Jing Chen, Jonathan M. Sarnet, Jian-feng Huang, Manlu Zhu et al. 2009. "Mortality Attributable to Smoking in China." *New England Journal of Medicine* 360 (2): 150–159.

Gui Shixun, and Liu Shan. 1992. "Urban Migration in Shanghai, 1950–88: Trends and Characteristics." *Population and Development Review* 18 (3): 533–548.

Guo Jiagang. 2003. "Schistosomiasis Control in China: Strategy of Control and Rapid Assessment of Schistosomiasis Risk by Remote Sensing (RS) and Geographic Information System (GIS)." PhD diss., University of Basil. http://pages.unibas.ch/diss/2003/DabsB_7169.pdf.

Guo Sufang, Sabu S. Padmadas, Zhao Fengmin, James J. Brown, and R. William Stones. 2007. "Delivery Settings and Caesarean Section Rates in China." *Bulletin of the World Health Organization* 85 (10): 755–762.

Halpern, Fanny G. 1940. "Insulin Shock Treatment of Schizophrenia." *American Journal of Psychiatry* 96 (5): 1153–1165.

Hanson, Marta. 2008. "The Art of Medicine: Maoist Public-Health Campaigns, Chinese Medicine, and SARS." *Lancet* 372 (October 25): 1457–1458.

Harris, Amanda, Suzanne Belton, Lesley Barclay, and Jenny Fenwick. 2009. "Midwives in China: 'Jie sheng po' to 'zhu chan shi.'" *Midwifery* 25: 203–212.

Harris, Amanda, Yu Gao, Lesley Barclay, Suzanne Belton, Zweng Wei Yue, Hao Min, Xu Augun, Liao Hua, and Zhou Yun. 2007. "Consequences of Birth Policies and Practices in Post-Reform China." *Reproductive Health Matters* 15: 114–124.

Hayford, Charles W. 1990. *To the People: James Yen and Village China*. New York: Columbia University Press.

"Health Work in Kiangsi." 1934. *Chinese Medical Journal* 48 (11): 1173.

Henderson, Gail. 1989. "Issues in the Modernization of Medicine in China." In *Science and Technology in Post-Mao China*, edited by Denis Fred Simon and Merle Goldman, 199–221. Cambridge, MA: Council of East Asian Studies, Harvard University.

———. 1990. "Increased Inequality in Health Care." In *Chinese Society on the Eve of Tiananmen*, edited by Deborah Davis & Ezra F. Vogel, 263–282. Cambridge, MA: Harvard University Asia Center.

Henderson, Gail, and Myron Cohen. 1984. *The Chinese Hospital: A Socialist Work Unit*. New Haven, CT: Yale University Press.

Hermalin, Albert I., and Deborah Lowry. 2010. "The Age Prevalence of Smoking among Chinese Women: A Case of Arrested Diffusion?" Population Studies Center Research Report 10-718.

Henriot, Christian. 2006. "Shanghai and the Experience of War: The Fate of Refugees." *European Journal of East Asian Studies* 5 (2): 215–245.

Hershatter, Gail. 2008. "Birthing Stories: Rural Midwives in 1950s China." In *Dilemmas of Victory: The Early Years of the People's Republic of China*, edited by Jeremy Brown and Paul Pickowicz, 337–358. Cambridge, MA: Harvard University Press.

Hesketh, Therese, Li Lu, and Zhu Wei Xing. 2005. "The Effect of China's One-Child Family Policy after 25 Years." *New England Journal of Medicine* 353 (11): 1171–1176.

Hillier, Sheila M., and Tony Jewell. 1983. *Health Care and Traditional Medicine in China, 1800–1982*. London: Routledge and Kegan Paul.

Ho, David Y. F. 1974. "Prevention and Treatment of Mental Illness in the People's Republic of China." *American Journal of Orthopsychiatry* 44: 621–636.

Hoekman, Arie. 2012. "Op-ed on International Day of the Midwife: Investing in Midwifery Urgently Needed in China." United Nations in China, May 5. www.un.org.cn/cms/p /news/27/1946/contentl.html.

Honig, Emily. 1986. *Sisters and Strangers: Women in the Shanghai Cotton Mills, 1919–1949*. Stanford, CA: Stanford University Press.

Horn, Joshua. 1969. *Away with All Pests: An English Surgeon in People's China: 1954–1969*. New York: Monthly Review Press.

Hsiao, WC. 1984. "Transformation of Health Care in China." *New England Journal of Medicine* 310: 932–936.

———. 2004. "Disparity in Health: The Underbelly of China's Economic Development." *Harvard China Review* 5: 64–70.

Hsu H. F., and Li S. Y. Hsu. 1974. "Schistosomiasis in the Shanghai Area." In *China Medicine as We Saw It*, edited by Joseph R. Quinn, 345–363. DHEW Publication No. (NIH) 75, issue 684. Washington, DC: John E. Fogarty International Center, U.S. Department of Health, Education, and Welfare.

Hu Teh-wei, ed. 2008a. *Tobacco Control Policy Analysis in China: Economics and Health*. Singapore: World Scientific.

Hu Xing-Juan, and Bao-Juan Zhang. 1982. "Women's Health Care." *American Journal of Public Health* 72: 33–35.

Huang, Efen, and Simon Li. 2011. "China Healthcare & Wellness Consumer Survey Burson-Marsteller Asia-Pacific." Prepared by Burson-Masteller and Kantar Health. http://

www.slideshare.net/bursonmarstellerchina/china-healthcare-wellness-consumer
-survey.

Huang, Tsefang F. 1935. "Developing a Railway Health Service." *Chinese Medical Journal* 49 (9): 973–989.

Hui, Edwin C. 2007. "The Patient-Doctor Relationship in China." *Guanxi: The China Letter* 1 (11).

Hunter, Jane. 1984. *The Gospel of Gentility: American Women Missionaries in Turn-of-the-Century China.* New Haven, CT: Yale University Press.

Hyde, Sandra T. 2007. *Eating Spring Rice: The Cultural Politics of AIDS in Southwest China.* Berkeley: University of California Press.

Iijima, Wataru. 2008. "'Farewell to the God of Plague': Anti-Schistosoma Japonicum Campaign in China and Japanese Colonial Medicine." *Memoirs of the Research Department of the Toyo Bunko* 66: 45–79.

Ingram, J. H. 1918. "The Pitiable Condition of the Insane in North China." *China Medical Journal* 32: 134–135.

International Council of Nurses. 2012. "International Council of Nurses Members." http://www.icn.ch/members/.

———. 2013. "International Council of Nurses Expands Global Membership." http://www.icn.ch/images/stories/documents/news/press_releases/2013_PR_12_New_ICN_Members.pdf.

Jefferys, W. Hamilton, and James L. Maxwell. 1910. *The Diseases of China: Including Formosa and Korea.* Philadelphia: P. Blakiston's Son.

Jenkins, Rachel. 2012. "Meeting Population Needs for Mental Health—The Chinese Example." *Shanghai Archives of Psychiatry* 24 (3): 178–180.

Jia Huanguang. 1997. "Chinese Medicine in Post-Mao China: Standardization and the Context of Modern Science." PhD diss., University of North Carolina.

Jiang Jingmei, Boqi Liu, Freddy Sitas, Junyao Li, Xianjia Zeng, Wei Han, Xiaonong Zou, Yanping Wu, and Ping Zhao. 2010. "Smoking-Attributable Deaths and Potential Years Lost from a Large, Representative Study in China." *Tobacco Control* 19 (1): 7–12.

Johnson, Tina Phillips. 2011. *Childbirth in Republican China: Delivering Modernity.* Lanham, MD: Lexington Books.

Jun Lv, Meng Su, Zhiheng Hong, Ting Zhang, Xuemei Huang, Bo Wang, and Liming Li. 2011. "Implementation of the WHO Framework Convention on Tobacco Control in Mainland China." *Tobacco Control* 20: 309–314.

Kan Huai-chieh, and Kung Jen-chi. 1936. "Incidence of Schistosomiasis Japonica in an Endemic Area in Chekiang." Supplement, *China Medical Journal* 50: 449–456.

Kan Huai-chieh, and Yao Yung-tsung. 1934. "Some Notes on the Anti-Schistosomiasis Japonica Campaign in Chih-huai-pan, Kaihua, Chekiang." *China Medical Journal* 48 (4): 323–326.

Kane, Penny. 1984. "An Assessment of China's Health Care." *Australian Journal of Chinese Affairs* 11: 1–24.

Kao, John J. 1979. *Three Millennia of Chinese Psychiatry.* New York: Institute for Advanced Research in Asian Science and Medicine.

Karchmer, Eric. 2004. "Orientalizing the Body: Postcolonial Transformations in Chinese Medicine." PhD diss., University of North Carolina.

Kau, Michael, and John Leung, eds. 1986. *The Writings of Mao Zedong, 1949–1976.* Vol. 1. Armonk, NY: M. E. Sharpe.

———, eds. 1992. *The Writings of Mao Zedong, 1949–1976.* Vol. 2. Armonk, NY: M. E. Sharpe.

Kerr, John G. 1898. "The Refuge for the Insane, Canton." *China Medical Missionary Society* 12: 177–178.

Kety, Seymour S. 1976. "Psychiatric Concepts and Treatment in China." *China Quarterly* 66: 315–323.

King, P. Z. 1941. "China's Civilian Health." In *United China Relief Series, no. 6: Looking after China's Civilians.* Chungking: China Publishing Company.

Kleinman, Arthur. 1986. *Social Origins of Distress and Disease: Depression, Neurasthenia, and Pain in Modern China.* New Haven, CT: Yale University Press.

Klemetti, Reijia, Elena Regushevsklaya, Wei-Hong Zhang, Zhuochun Wu, Hong Yan, Yang Wang, and Elina Hemminki. 2011. "Unauthorised Pregnancies and Use of Maternity Care in Rural China." *European Journal of Contraception and Reproductive Health Care* 16: 359–368.

Klotzbucher, Sascha, Peter Lässig, Qin Jiangmei, and Susanne Weigelin-Schwiedrzik. 2010. "What's New in the 'New Rural Co-Operative Medical System?' An Assessment in One Kazak County of the Xinjiang Uyghur Autonomous Region." *China Quarterly* 201 (March): 38–57.

Knowledge@Wharton. 2011. "China's Hospitals: Is a Window of Opportunity Finally Opening for Investors?" Wharton School of Business, University of Pennsylvania. http://www.knowledgeatwharton.com.cn/index.cfm?fa=viewArticle&Articleid=2383&languageid=1.

Kohrman, Matthew. 2007. "Depoliticizing Tobacco's Exceptionality: Male Sociality, Death, and Memory-Making among Chinese Cigarette Smokers." *China Journal* 58: 85–109.

———. 2010. "New Steps for Tobacco Control in and outside of China." Supplement, *Asia-Pacific Journal of Public Health* 22 (3): 189S–196S.

Komiya, Y. 1957. "Recommendatory Note for the Control Problem of Schistosomiasis in China." *Japanese Journal of Medical Science and Biology* 10: 461–471.

Köster, Anne-Dorothee. 2009. "Das Gesundheitssystem der VR China: Gesundheitspolitik zwischen fragmentiertem Autoritarismus, Kaderkapitalismus und Familiarismus" [The health system of the People's Republic of China: Health policy between fragmented authoritarianism, cadre capitalism, and family policy]. WIP-Diskussionspapier, Wissenschaftliches Institut der PKV, Köln.

Kwok, D. W. Y. 1965. *Scientism in Chinese Thought, 1900–1950.* New Haven, CT: Yale University Press.

Lai, Daniel G. (Lai Douyan), and C. M. Chu (Zhu Jiming). 1940. "The Ku-tsung (Yunnan) Demonstration Health Centre—A Review for 1939–40." *Chinese Medical Journal* 59 (May): 468–475.

Lai, Lili. 2003. "Irresistable Scientization: Rhetoric of Science in Institutional Chinese Medicine." Master's thesis, University of North Carolina.

Lamberts, L. J. 1950. *The Life Story of Dr. Lee S. Huizenga.* Grand Rapids, MI: Eerdmans.

Lampton, David M. 1972. "Public Health and Politics in China's Past Two Decades." *Health Services Report* 87 (10): 895–904.

———. 1974. *Health, Conflict, and the Chinese Political System.* Michigan Papers in Chinese Studies, No. 18. Ann Arbor: University of Michigan.

———. 1977. *The Politics of Medicine in China: The Policy Process 1949–1977.* Folkestone: Dawson.

Lamson, Herbert Day. 1935. *Social Pathology in China.* Shanghai: Commercial Press.

Langwick, Stacey Ann. 2011. *Bodies, Politics, and African Healing: The Matter of Maladies in Tanzania.* Bloomington: Indiana University Press.

Lao She. 2005. *Camel Xiangzi.* Translated by Shi Xiangzi. Bilingual edition. Hong Kong: Chinese University Press.

Lapham, Robert J., and W. Parker Mauldin. 1984. "Family Planning Program Effort and Birthrate Decline in Developing Countries." *International Family Planning Perspectives* 10 (4): 109–118.

Law Pui-Lam. 2005. "The Revival of Folk Religion and Gender Relationships in Rural China: A Preliminary Observation." *Asian Folklore Studies* 64 (1): 89–109.

Lazure, Denis. 1964. "Politics and Mental Health in New China." *American Journal of Orthopsychiatry* 34: 925–933.

League of Nations Health Organization. 1937. *Intergovernmental Conference of Far Eastern Countries on Rural Hygiene: Report of China.* Geneva: League of Nations.

Lee, Anita H., and Yuan Jiang. 2008. "Tobacco Control Programs in China." In *Tobacco Control Policy Analysis in China: Economics and Health,* edited by Hu Teh-wei, 33–56. Singapore: World Scientific.

Lee, Leo Ou-fan. 2000. "The Cultural Construction of Modernity in Urban Shanghai: Some Preliminary Explorations." In *Becoming Chinese: Passages to Modernity and Beyond,* edited by Wen-hsin Yeh, 31–61. Berkeley: University of California Press.

Lee, Vincent. 2004. "Snail Scare." *Shanghai Star,* July 24.

Lee Hsien-wei. 1934. *The Tobacco in China.* Tientsin: Haute études; Shanghai: Université l'Aurore, Institut des hautes études industrielles et commerciales, Faculty of Commerce, Economic Studies.

Lei, Sean Hsiang-lin. 1999. "When Chinese Medicine Encountered the State: 1910–1949." PhD diss., University of Chicago.

——. 2002. "How Did Chinese Medicine Become Experiential? The Political Epistemology of Jingyan." *Positions: East Asia Cultures Critique* 10 (2): 33–64.

——. 2010. "Sovereignty and the Microscope: Constituting Notifiable Infectious Diseases and Containing the Manchurian Plague (1910–11)." In *Health and Hygiene in Chinese East Asia: Policies and Publics in the Long Twentieth Century,* edited by Angela Ki Che Leung and Charlotte Furth, 73–106. Durham, NC: Duke University Press.

Lennox, William G. 1932. "A Self Survey By Mission Hospitals in China." *Chinese Medical Journal* 46 (5): 484–534.

Lesch, John E. 2007. *The First Miracle Drugs: How the Sulfa Drugs Transformed Medicine.* New York: Oxford University Press.

Leung, Angela Ki Che. 2003. "Medical Learning from the Song to the Ming." In *The Song-Yuan-Ming Transition in Chinese History,* edited by Paul Jakov Smith, 374–400. Cambridge, MA: Harvard University Press.

——, ed. 2006. *Medicine for Women in Imperial China.* Leiden: Brill.

Levine, Aaron D. n.d. "Trends in the Movement of Scientists between China and the United States and Implications for Future Collaboration." Unpublished paper.

Li, K. H. 1928. *Report of the Soochow Hospital, Soochow China: 1928.* Shanghai: Shanghai Times.

Li Danke. 2010a. *Echoes of Chongqing: Women in Wartime China.* Urbana: University of Illinois Press.

Li Hongshan. 2008a. *U.S.–China Educational Exchange: State, Society, and Intercultural Relations, 1905–1950.* New Brunswick, NJ: Rutgers University Press.

Li Jingwu. 2008b. "Understanding the Nurse Management Regulations of PRC." *Chinese Nursing Management* 8 (3): 8–9.

Li Keqiang. 2010b. "Attendance and Speech." Paper presented at the National Schistosomiasis Treatment and Prevention Working Conference, Wuhan, Hubei Province, September 6.

Li Qiang, Jason Hsia, and Gonghuan Yang. 2011. "Prevalence of Smoking in China in 2010." *New England Journal of Medicine* 364 (25): 2469–2470.

Li Shang-jen. 2010c. "Eating Well in China: Diet and Hygiene in Nineteenth-Century Treaty Ports." In *Health and Hygiene in Chinese East Asia: Policies and Publics in the Long Twentieth Century,* edited by Angela Ki Che Leung and Charlotte Furth, 109–131. Durham, NC: Duke University Press.

Li Shuzhuo. 2007a. "Imbalanced Sex Ratio at Birth and Comprehensive Intervention in China." Paper presented at the Fourth Asia Pacific Conference on Reproductive and Sexual Health and Rights, Hyderabad, India, October 29–31.

Li Ting'an. 1934a. "Summary Report on Rural Public Health Practice in China." *Chinese Medical Journal* 48 (October): 1086–1090.

———. 1934b. "The Campaign against Tuberculosis." *Chinese Medical Journal* 48: 301–303.

Li Zhisui, and Anne Thurston. 1996. *The Private Life of Chairman Mao: The Memoirs of Mao's Personal Physician.* New York: Random House.

Liang Juan, Xiaohong Li, Li Dai, Weiyue Zeng, Qi Li, Mingrong Li, Rong Zhou, Chunhua He, Yanping Wang, and Jun Zhu. 2012. "The Changes in Maternal Mortality in 1000 Counties in Mid-Western China by a Government-Initiated Intervention." *PLOS ONE* 7 (5). doi:10.1371/journal.pone.0037458.

Lim, Khati (Lin Qiaozhi). 1959. "Obstetrics and Gynecology in the Past Ten Years." *Chinese Medical Journal* 79 (5): 375–383.

Lin, Evelyn. 1938. "Nursing in China." *American Journal of Nursing* 38 (1): 1–8.

Lin, Justin Yifu, and Dennis Tao Yang. 1998. "On the Causes of China's Agricultural Crisis and the Great Leap Famine." *China Economic Review* 9 (2): 125–140.

Lin, Tsung Yi 1985. "The Shaping of Chinese Psychiatry." In *Mental Health Planning for One Billion People: A Chinese Perspective,* edited by Tsung Yi Lin and Leon Eisenberg, 3–37. Vancouver: University of British Columbia Press.

Litsios, Socrates. 2005. "Selskar Gunn and China: The Rockefeller Foundation's 'Other' Approach to Public Health." *Bulletin of the History of Medicine* 79 (2): 295–318.

———. 2011. "John Black Grant: A 20th-Century Public Health Giant." *Perspectives in Biology and Medicine* 54 (4): 532–549.

Liu, J. H., and J. T. Jia. 1994. "Medicine and the Law in the People's Republic of China." Paper presented at the Taniguchi Foundation Nineteenth International Symposium, Division of Medical History, Fuji Institute of Education and Training, Shizuoka, Japan, September 4–10.

Liu, J. Heng. 1929. "The Chinese Ministry of Health." *National Medical Journal of China* 15: 135–148.

Liu, Xiehe. 1980. "Mental Health Work in Sichuan." *British Journal of Psychiatry* 137: 371–376.

Liu Bo-Qi, Richard Peto, Zheng-Ming Chen, Jillian Boreham, Ya-Ping Wu, Jun-Yao Li, T. Colin Campbell, and Jun-Shi Chen. 1998. "Emerging Tobacco Hazards in China: 1. Retrospective Proportional Mortality Study of One Million Deaths." *British Medical Journal* 317 (November 21): 1411–1422.

Liu Chung-tung. 1991. "From San Guiliupo to 'Caring Scholar:' The Chinese Nurse in Perspective." *International Journal of Nursing Studies* 28 (4): 315–324.

Liu Jin, Hong Ma, Yanling He, Bin Xie, Yifeng Xu, Hongyu Tang, Ming Li et al. 2011a. "Mental Health System in China: History, Recent Service Reform and Future Challenges." *World Psychiatry* 10: 210–216.

Liu Wennan. 2009a. "'No-Smoking' for the Nation: Anti-Cigarette Campaigns in Modern China, 1910–1935." PhD diss., University of California, Berkeley.

Liu Xiaoning, Hong Yan, and Dulao Wang. 2010. "The Evaluation of 'Safe Motherhood' Program on Maternal Care Utilization in Rural Western China: A Difference in Difference Approach." *BMC Public Health* 10: 566.

———. 1981. "Psychiatry in Traditional Chinese Medicine." *British Journal of Psychiatry* 138: 429–433.

Liu Xingzhu, and Wang Junle. 1991. "An Introduction to China's Health Care System." *Journal of Public Health Policy* 12 (1): 104–116.

Liu Yuanli. 2002. "Reforming China's Urban Health Insurance System." *Health Policy* 60: 133–150.

Liu Yuanli, and Lincoln Chen. 2011. "New Medical Data and Leadership on Tobacco Control in China." *Lancet* 377 (April 9): 1218–1220.

Lo Chiu-jing. 2003. "Chou Mei-yu." In *Biographical Dictionary of Chinese Women*, Vol. 2, edited by Lily Xiao Hong Lee and Clara Wing-Chung and translated by Barbara Law, 114–116. Armonk, NY: M. E. Sharpe.

Logan, O. T. 1905. "A Case of Dysentery in Hunan Province Caused by the Trematode, *Schistosoma Japonicum*." *China Medical Journal* 19: 243–245.

Lora-Wainwright, Anna. 2006. "Perceptions of Health, Illness and Healing in a Sichuan Village, China." PhD diss., University of Oxford.

Lou, Vivian W. Q., Veronica Pearson, and Yu Cheung Wong. "Humanitarian Welfare Values in a Changing Social Environment: A Survey of Social Work Undergraduate Students in Beijing and Shanghai." *Journal of Social Work* 12: 65–83.

Lu, Yi-Chuang. 1978. "The Collective Approach to Psychiatric Practice in the People's Republic of China." *Social Problems* 26: 2–14.

Lu Hanchao. 1999. *Beyond the Neon Lights: Everyday Shanghai in the Early Twentieth Century*. Berkeley: University of California Press.

Lucas, AnElissa. 1980. "Changing Medical Models in China: Organizational Options or Obstacles?" *China Quarterly* 83 (September): 461–489.

———. 1982. *Chinese Medical Modernization: Comparative Policy Continuities, 1930s–1980s*. New York: Praeger.

Luk, J, P Gross, and WW Thompson. 2001. "Observations on Mortality during the 1918 Influenza Pandemic." *Clinical Infectious Diseases* 33: 1375–1378.

Lumbiganon, Pisake, Malinee Laopaiboon, A. Metin Gülmezoglu, João Paulo Souza, Surasak Taneepanichskul, Pang Ruyan, Deepika Eranjanie Attygalle et al. 2010. "Method of Delivery and Pregnancy Outcomes in Asia: The WHO Global Survey on Maternal and Perinatal Health, 2007–08." *Lancet* 375 (February 6): 490–499.

Lyman, Robert S. 1937. "Psychiatry in China." *Archives of Neurology and Psychiatry* 37 (4): 765–771.

Lyman, R. S., V. Maeker, and P. Liang, eds. 1939. *Social and Psychological Studies in Neuropsychiatry in China*. Beijing: Henri Vetch.

Ma, Hong. 2012. "Integration of Hospital and Community Services—the '686 Project'—Is a Crucial Component in the Reform of China's Mental Health Services." *Shanghai Archives of Psychiatry* 24: 172–174.

MacPherson, Kerrie L. 1987. *A Wilderness of Marshes: The Origins of Public Health in Shanghai, 1843–1893*. Hong Kong: Oxford University Press.

Mander, Rosemary, Cheung Ngai Fen, Wang Xiaoli, Fu Wei, and Zhu Junghong. 2010. "Beginning an Action Research Project to Investigate the Feasibility of a Midwife-Led Normal Birthing Unit in China." *Journal of Clinical Nursing* 19: 517–526.

Manning, Kimberley Ens. 2006. "The Gendered Politics of Woman-Work: Rethinking Radicalism in the Great Leap Forward." *Modern China* 32 (3): 349–384.

Mao Shou-Pai. 1983. "Parasitological Research in Institutes in China." In *Parasitology: A Global Perspective,* edited by Kenneth S. Warren and John Z. Bowers, 117–126. New York: Springer-Verlag.

Markel, Howard. 2000. "Victor C. Vaughan." *Journal of the American Medical Association* 283 (7): 848.

Marr, Kendra, and Ariana Eunjung Cha. 2008. "Shaking Up China's Medical System." *Washington Post,* June 23.

Mathers, Colin, Ties Boerma, and Doris Ma Fat. 2008. *The Global Burden of Disease: 2004 Update.* Geneva: World Health Organization.

McBain, Alan. 1945. "Letter from Tengcheng, Yunnan, Free China." January 28. Private collection (family letters).

McCartney, J. Lincoln. 1926. "Neuropsychiatry in China: A Preliminary Observation." *Chinese Medical Journal* 40: 616–626.

McIsaac, Mary Lee. 1994. "The Limits of Chinese Nationalism: Workers in Wartime Chongqing, 1937–1945." PhD diss., Yale University.

McKeown, Thomas. 1976. *The Modern Rise of Population.* London: Edward Arnold.

Meng Qingyue, Clas Rehnberg, Zhuang Ning, Bian Ying, Goran Tomson, and Tang Shenglan. 2004a. "The Impact of Urban Health Insurance Reform on Hospital Charges: A Case Study from Two Cities in China." *Health Policy* 68: 197–209.

Meng Qingyue, Clas Rehnberg, Zhuang Ning, Bian Ying, and Tang Shenglan. 2004b. "Public Hospitals: Policy Reform, Productivity and Cost." In *Health Care Transition in Urban China,* edited by Gerald Bloom and Tang Shenglan, 143–162. Burlington, VT: Ashgate.

Minden, Karen. 1979. "The Development of Early Chinese Communist Health Policy: Health Care in the Border Region, 1936–1949." *American Journal of Chinese Medicine* 7 (4): 299–315.

Ministry of Finance. 2012. *Report on the Implementation of Central and Local Budgets for 2011 and on Draft Central and Local Budgets for 2012: Fifth Session of the Eleventh National People's Congress.* March 5. http://online.wsj.com/public/resources /documents/2012NPC_FinanceWorkReport_English.pdf.

Ministry of Health. 2011a. *Report on Women and Children's Health Development in China.* www.moh.gov.cn/publicfiles/business/cmsresources/mohfybjysqwss/cmsrsdocument/ doc12910.pdf.

———. 2011b. *2011 Annual of Statistics of Health in China.* Beijing: Peking Union Medical College.

Ministry of Health, UNICEF, World Health Organization, and United Nations Fund for Population Activities. 2006. *Joint Review of the Maternal and Child Survival Strategy in China.* Beijing: Ministry of Health.

Ministry of Information. 1943. *China Handbook 1937–1943: A Comprehensive Survey of Major Developments in China in Six Years of War.* American ed. New York: Macmillan.

Ministry of the Interior. 2011. *Abridged Life Table of the Taiwan Area, Republic of China.* Taipei: Ministry of the Interior.

Mo, Ganming 1959. "The Achievements of the Guanghou City Mental Hospital over Ten Years." *Chinese Journal of Neurology and Psychiatry* 5: 310–311.

Mosley, W. Henry, and Lincoln C. Chen. 1984. "An Analytical Framework for the Study of Child Survival in Developing Countries." In "Child Survival: Strategies for Research," edited by W. Henry Mosley and Lincoln C. Chen, supplement, *Population and Development Review* 10: 25–45.

Mullowney, John J. 1912. "Modern Hospitals for Chinese by Chinese." *Chinese Medical Journal* 26 (1): 34–43.

Nagajima, Chieko. 2008. "Health and Hygiene in Mass Mobilization: Hygiene Campaigns in Shanghai, 1920–1945." *Twentieth Century China* 34 (1): 43.

Nathan, Carl F. 1967. *Plague Prevention and Politics in Manchuria, 1910–1931.* Cambridge, MA: Harvard University Press.

National People's Congress of the People's Republic of China. 2011. *Debates over Proposals to Improve Family Planning Policy during the "Two Sessions."* Special report, March 10. http://www.npc.gov.cn/englishnpc/Special_11_4/2011-03/10/content_1640208.htm.

Needham, Joseph. 1970. *Clerks and Craftsmen in China and the West.* Cambridge: Cambridge University Press.

"News about Nursing." 1940. *American Journal of Nursing* 40 (11): 1280.

Ng, Vivien W. 1980. "Ching Laws concerning the Insane: An Historical Survey." *Ch'ing-shih wen-t'i* 4: 55–89.

———. 1990. *Madness in Late Imperial China: From Illness to Deviance.* Norman: University of Oklahoma Press.

Ngok Kinglun, and Dian Li. 2010. "Tobacco Control in China: Process, Actors, and Policy Initiatives." *Journal of Asian Public Policy* 3 (1): 100–110.

NHACFHS (National Health Administration and Central Field Health Station). 1934. *National Epidemic Prevention Bureau, a Report, Being a Review of Its Activities from Its Foundation in March 1919 to June 1934.* Peiping: NHACFHS.

Ni, J. 1986. "Life Expectancy of China: Past, Current and Future Trend." *Statistical Research* 2: 21–27.

Niu Shiru, Gonghuan Yang, Zhengming Chen, Junling Wang, Gonghao Wang, Xingzhou He, Helen Schoepff, Jillian Boreham, Hongchao Pan, and Richard Peto. 1998. "Emerging Tobacco Hazards in China: Early Mortality Results from a Prospective Study." *British Medical Journal* 317 (November 21): 1423–1424.

"Nursing Doctoral Program Partnership with Peking Union Medical College." 2012. Johns Hopkins Bloomberg School of Public Health Global Research. http://www.jhsph.edu/faculty/research/map/CN/1376.

Omran, Abdel R. 1971. "The Epidemiological Transition: A Theory of the Epidemiology of Population Change." *Milbank Memorial Fund Quarterly* 49: 509–538.

Ong Aihwa. 1995. "Anthropology, China and Modernities." In *The Future of Anthropological Knowledge,* edited by Henrietta L. Moore, 60–92. London: Routledge.

Pan Yueh. 1957. "Ending the Scourge of Schistosomiasis." *China Reconstructs* 6 (8): 8–10.

Pang, S. C., and L. M. Kao. 1995. *China Health Care Management.* Jilin: Jilin Science and Technology.

Parry-Jones, William Llewellyn. 1986. "Psychiatry in the People's Republic of China." *British Journal of Psychiatry* 148: 632–641.

Patterson, David, and Gerald Pyle. 1991. "The Geography and Mortality of the 1918 Influenza Pandemic." *Bulletin of the History of Medicine* 65 (1): 4–21.

Pearson, Veronica. 1991. "The Development of Modern Psychiatric Services in China, 1890–1949." *History of Psychiatry* 2: 133–147.

———. 1992. "Community and Culture: A Chinese Model of Care for the Mentally Ill." *International Journal of Social Psychiatry* 38 (3): 163–178.

———. 1993. "Families in China: An Undervalued Resource in Mental Health." *Journal of Family Therapy* 15 (2): 163–185.

———. 1995. *Mental Health Care in China: State Policies, Professional Services and Family Responsibilities.* London: Gaskell.

———. 1996. "The Chinese Equation in Mental Health Policy and Practice: Order Plus Control Equal Stability." *International Journal of Law and Psychiatry* 19 (3–4): 437–458.

———. 2007. "Psychiatric Services in China—Guangzhou." In *Culture and Mental Health: A Comprehensive Textbook,* edited by Kamaldeep Bhui and Dinesh Bhugra, 294–298. London: Hodder Arnold.

———. 2008. "A Plague upon Our Houses: The Consequences of Underfunding the Health Sector." In *A Sense of Place: Hong Kong West of Pottinger Street,* edited by Veronica Pearson and Tim Keung Ko, 242–261. Hong Kong: Joint Publishing.

Pearson, Veronica, and Paul C. W. Lam. 2001. "On Their Own: Caregivers in Guangzhou." In *Family Interventions in Mental Illness: International Perspectives,* edited by Harriet P. Lefley and Dale L. Johnson, 174–181. London: Praeger.

Pearson, Veronica, and Michael R. Phillips. 1994. "The Social Context of Psychiatric Rehabilitation in China." In "Models for Change in a Changing Society: Psychiatric Rehabilitation in China," edited by Michael R. Phillips, Veronica Pearson, and Ruiwen Wang, supplement 24, *British Journal of Psychiatry* 165: 11–18.

Peng Jing, Shengnian Zhang, Wei Lu, and Andrew T. L. Chen. 2003. "Public Health in China: the Shanghai CDC Perspective." *American Journal of Public Health* 93 (12): 1991–1993.

Peng, X. 1987. "Demographic Consequences of the Great Leap Forward in China's Provinces." *Population and Development Review* 13 (4): 639–670.

People's Daily. 2001. "Tianjin Takes the Lead in Bidding Farewell to Midwives." April 26.

———. 2002. "Midwifery Phased Out in China's Rural Areas." September 30.

Peto, Richard, Zheng-Ming Chen, and Jillian Boreham. 2009. "Tobacco: The Growing Epidemic in China." *CVD Prevention and Control* 4 (1): 61–70.

Pfeiffer, Stefani. 2005. "'Still Arguing Over Cost': Bargaining, Etiquette and the Modern Patient in Republican Beijing." *Asian Medicine* 1 (2): 355–386.

Phillips, Michael R. 1993. "Strategies Used by Chinese Families Coping with Schizophrenia." In *Chinese Families in the Post-Mao Era,* edited by Deborah Davis and Steven Harrell, 277–306. Berkeley: University of California Press.

Phillips, Michael R., Jingxuan Zhang, Qichang Song, Zhijie Ding, Shutao Pang, Yuli Zhang, and Zhiqing Wang. 2009. "Prevalence, Treatment, and Associated Disability of Mental Disorders in Four Provinces in China during 2001–05: An Epidemiological Survey." *Lancet* 373 (June 13): 2041–2053.

Phillips, Michael R., and Veronica Pearson. 1994a. "Future Opportunities and Challenges for Psychiatric Rehabilitation in China." In "Models for Change in a Changing Society: Psychiatric Rehabilitation in China," edited by Michael R. Phillips, Veronica Pearson, and Ruiwen Wang, supplement 24, *British Journal of Psychiatry* 165: 128–142.

———. 1994b. "Rehabilitation Interventions in Urban Communities." In "Models for Change in a Changing Society: Psychiatric Rehabilitation in China," edited by Michael R. Phillips, Veronica Pearson, and Ruiwen Wang, supplement 24, *British Journal of Psychiatry* 165: 66–69.

Phillips, Michael R., Veronica Pearson, Feifei Li, Minjie Xu, and Lawrence Yang. 2002. "Stigma and Expressed Emotion: A Study of People with Schizophrenia and Their Family Members in China." *British Journal of Psychiatry* 181: 488–493.

Phillips, Michael R., Xiong Wei, and Xiong H. 1993. "The Economic Benefits of Family-Based Intervention for Urban Schizophrenic Patients in China: A Randomized Controlled Trial." Paper presented at the Sixth Scientific Meeting of the Pacific Rim College of Psychiatrists, Shanghai, China, April.

Porter, Edgar. 1997. *The People's Doctor: George Hatem and China's Revolution.* Honolulu: University of Hawai'i Press.

Poston, Dudley L., and Baochang Gu. 1987. "Socioeconomic Development, Family Planning, and Fertility in China." *Demography* 24 (4): 531–551.

Priemus-Noach, Mieke. 1988. "Mental Health in China: Notes and Impressions." *China Information* 3: 55–63.

Proctor, Robert N. 2011. *Golden Holocaust: Origins of the Cigarette Catastrophe and the Case for Abolition.* Berkeley: University of California Press.

Qian Juncheng, Min Cai, Jun Gao, Shenglan Tang, Ling Xu, and Julia Alison Critchley. 2010. "Trends in Smoking and Quitting in China from 1993 to 2003: National Health Service Survey Data." *Bulletin of the World Health Organization* 88 (10): 769–776.

Qiu, Fugen, and Shouqing Lu. 1994. "Guardianship Networks for Rural Psychiatric Patients: A Non-Professional Support System in Jinshan County, Shanghai." In "Psychiatric Rehabilitation in China: Models for Change in a Changing Society," edited by Michael R. Phillips, Veronica Pearson, and Ruiwen Wang, supplement 24, *British Journal of Psychiatry* 165: 114–120.

Rao, K., and Y. Chen. 1995. "An Analysis of Population Data of Beijing City during 1910s–1940s." *Chinese Journal of Health Statistics* 12 (6): 27–33.

Records of China Centenary Missionary Conference, Held at Shanghai April 25 to May 8, 1907. 1907. Shanghai: Centenary Conference Committee.

Reed, John Harland. 1979. "Brass Butterflies of the Thoughts of Mao Tsetung: The Sociology of Schistosomiasis Control in China." PhD diss., Cornell University.

"Registration of Schools of Nursing in China." 1923. *American Journal of Nursing* 23 (5): 410.

Reinhardt, Anne. 2002. "Navigating Imperialism in China: Steamship, Semicolony, and Nation, 1860–1937." PhD diss., Princeton University.

Remington, Gary, Ofer Agid, George Foussiasis, Magie Hahn, N. Rao, and Mark Sinyor. 2013. "Clozapine's Role in the Treatment of First Episode Schizophrenia." *American Journal of Psychiatry* 170: 146–151.

Renshaw, Michelle. 2005. *Accommodating the Chinese: The American Hospital in China, 1880–1920.* New York: Routledge.

"Report of the American Schistosomiasis Delegation to the People's Republic of China." 1977. *American Journal of Tropical Medicine and Hygiene* 26 (3): 427–462.

Report of the Soochow Hospital, Soochow, Ku. 1940. Suzhou: China Conference of the Methodist Episcopal Church.

Rese, Andrey, Dina Balabanova, Kirill Danishevski, Martin McKee, and Rod Sheaff. 2005. "Implementing General Practice in Russia: Getting Beyond the First Steps." *British Medical Journal* 331 (July 23): 204–207.

Ristaino, Marcia R. 2008. *The Jacquinot Safe Zone: Wartime Refugees in Shanghai.* Stanford, CA: Stanford University Press.

Robb, Isabel Hampton. 1901. *Nursing Ethics: For Hospital and Private Use.* Cleveland, OH: JB Savage.

Rogaski, Ruth. 2004. *Hygienic Modernity: Meanings of Health and Disease in Treaty Port China.* Berkeley: University of California Press.

Rosenberg, Charles E. 1974. "Social Class and Medical Care in Nineteenth-Century America: The Rise and Fall of the Dispensary." *Journal of the History of Medicine and Allied Science* 29 (1): 32–54.

Rudan, Igor, Kit Yee Chan, Jian S. F. Zheng, Evropi Theodoratou, Xing Lin Feng, Joshua A. Salomon, Joy E. Lawn et al. 2010. "Causes of Death in Children Younger Than 5 Years in China in 2008." *Lancet* 375 (March 27): 1083–1089.

Sainsbury, MJ. 1974. "Psychiatry in the People's Republic of China." *Medical Journal of Australia* 1: 669–675.

Sandbach, FR. 1977. "Farewell to the God of Plague—The Control of Schistosomiasis in China." *Social Science and Medicine* 11: 27–33.

Scheid, Volker. 2002. *Chinese Medicine in Contemporary China: Plurality and Synthesis.* Durham, NC: Duke University Press.

———. 2007. *Currents of Tradition in Chinese Medicine, 1626–2006.* Seattle: Eastland.

Schoenhals, Michael. 1996. *China's Cultural Revolution, 1966–1969: Not a Dinner Party.* Armonk, NY: M. E. Sharpe.

Scull, A. 1985. "Deinstitutionalization and Public Policy." *Social Science and Medicine* 20 (5): 545–552.

Seifert, Harry E. 1935. "Life Tables for Chinese Farmers." *Milbank Memorial Fund Quarterly* 13 (3): 223–236.

Seipp, Conrad. 1963. Introduction to *Health Care for the Community: Selected Papers of Dr. John B. Grant,* by John B. Grant, xiii–xiv. Edited by Conrad Seipp. Baltimore, MD: Johns Hopkins University Press.

Selden, Charles 1905. "Work amongst the Chinese Insane and Some of Its Results." *Chinese Medical Missionary Journal* 19: 1–17.

———. 1937. "The Story of the John G. Kerr Hospital for the Insane." *China Medical Journal* 22: 82–91.

Sen, Amartya. 1982. *Poverty and Famines: An Essay on Entitlement and Deprivation.* New York: Oxford University Press.

———. 1987. *Food and Freedom.* Cambridge, MA: Harvard Institute of Economic Research.

Sha, Wei, Yu Cheung Wong, Vivian W. Q. Lou, Veronica Pearson, and Dong Hui Gu. 2012. "Career Preferences of Social Work Students in China: The Case of Beijing and Shanghai." *Social Work Education* 31 (1): 4–21.

Shemo, Connie A. 2011. *The Chinese Medical Ministries of Kang Cheng and Shi Meiyu, 1872–1937: On a Cross-Cultural Frontier of Gender, Race, and Nation.* Bethlehem, PA: Lehigh University Press.

Shen Ch'i-chen. 1961. "Report on Prevention of Schistosomiasis." In *Speeches Given at the Second Session of the Second National People's Congress, Communist China.* Washington, DC: U.S. Joint Publications Research Service.

Shen, RG., HJ Yang, H Li, F He, H Ding, XH Deng, X Xiao, and G Liu. 2006. "Study on the Maternal Mortality Rate from 1995 to 2004 among Residential and Migrant Women in Beijing." *Chinese Journal of Epidemiology* 27: 223–225.

Shen, Yu-Cun. 1983. "Community Mental Health Care within Primary Care in the People's Republic of China: The Home Care Program in the Beijing Countryside." *International Journal of Mental Health* 12: 123–131.

"Shi Meiyu." n.d. Biographical Dictionary of Chinese Christianity. Accessed February 25, 2014. http://www.bdcconline.net/en/stories/s/shi-meiyu.php.

Sidel, Ruth. 1973. "The Role of Revolutionary Optimism in the Treatment of Mental Illness in the People's Republic of China." *American Journal of Orthopsychiatry* 43: 732–736.

Sidel, Victor W. 1972. "The Barefoot Doctors of the People's Republic of China." *New England Journal of Medicine* 286 (24): 1292–1300.

Sidel, Victor W., and Ruth Sidel. 1973. *Serve the People: Observations on Medicine in the People's Republic of China.* New York: Josiah Macey Foundation.

———. 1977. "Health Care Services." *Social Scientist* 5: 114–130.

Simpson, Cora. 1922. *A Joy Ride through China for the NAC.* Shanghai: KwangHsuek.

Smedley, Agnes. 1939. "Hospitals in China: A Contrast; Progress of the Fourth Army Scientific Methods." *Manchester Guardian,* January 17.

Snell, John A. 1919. *Report of the Soochow Hospital, Soochow China: 1919.* Shanghai: Oriental Press.

———. 1924. *Report of the Soochow Hospital, Soochow China: 1924.* Shanghai: Oriental Press.

Song Shige, and Sarah A. Burgard. 2011. "Dynamics of Inequality: Mother's Education and Infant Mortality in China, 1970–2001." *Journal of Health and Social Behavior* 52 (3): 349–364.

Song Yi, Jun Ma, Bing Zhang, Chengye Ji, and Jiali Duan. 2008. "Analyses of the Prevalence Changes of Overweight and Obesity in Han Students in Beijing, 1995–2005." *Chinese Journal of Reproductive Health* 19 (3): 149–153.

"Specialist Online." 2012. Suzhou Municipal Hospital. http://www.smh.cc.

Spence, Jonathan. 1980. *To Change China: Western Advisers in China, 1620–1960*. New York: Penguin.

Splane, Richard, and Verna Huffman Splane. 1994. *Chief Nursing Officer Positions in National Ministries of Health: Focal Points for Nursing Leadership*. San Francisco: University of San Francisco.

Stanley, John R. 2010. "Establishing a Female Medical Elite: The Early History of the Nursing Profession in China." In *Pioneer Chinese Christian Women: Gender, Christianity, and Social Mobility,* edited by Jessie G. Lutz, 274–291. Bethlehem, PA: Lehigh University Press.

Stapleton, Kristin. 2000. *Civilizing Chengdu: Chinese Urban Reform, 1895–1937.* Cambridge, MA: Harvard University Press.

Stein, Gunther. 1945. *The Challenge of Red China*. London: Pilot Press.

Szto, Peter P. 2002. "The Accomodation of Insanity in Canton, China: 1857–1935." PhD diss., University of Pennsylvania.

Tang, YL, PX Mao, F Jiang, Q Chen, CY Wang, ZJ Cai, and PB Mitchell. 2008. "Clozapine in China." *Pharmacopsychiatry* 41 (1): 1–9.

"Tasly Pharmaceuticals Selects ICON as It Seeks First FDA Approval of a Traditional Chinese Medicine." 2012. http://www.iconplc.com/news-events/news/tasly-pharmaceuticals -sel/.

Taubenberger, Jeffery K., and David M. Morens. 2006. "1918 Influenza: The Mother of All Pandemics." *Emerging Infectious Diseases* 12 (1):15–22.

Taylor, Kim. 1999. "Paving the Way for TCM Textbooks: The Chinese Medical Improvement Schools." Paper presented at the Ninth International Conference on the History of Science in East Asia, East Asian Institute, National University of Singapore, Singapore, August 23–27.

———. 2005. *Chinese Medicine in Early Communist China, 1945–63: A Medicine of Revolution.* London: Routledge Curzon.

"Tenth Medical Care Dedication Prize: Awarded to 93 Year Old General Chou Mei-yu." 2000. *TWNNA News: Nursing in Taiwan* 7: 3.

Teow, See Heng. 1999. *Japan's Cultural Policy toward China, 1918–1931: A Comparative Perspective*. Cambridge, MA: Harvard University Asia Center.

Thompson, R. K., W. C. MacKenzie, and A. F. Peart. 1967. "A Visit to the People's Republic of China." *Canadian Medical Association Journal* 97: 349–360.

Thornicroft, Graham. 1987. "Contemporary Psychiatry in China." *International Journal of Mental Health* 16: 86–94.

Thoroughman, J. C. 1938. *Report of the Soochow Hospital, Soochow, China: 1937–1938*. Suzhou: China Conference of the Methodist Episcopal Church, South.

Thurston, Anne. 1987. *Enemies of the People*. New York: Knopf.

Tian, Weicai, Veronica Pearson, Ruiwen Wang, and Michael R. Phillips. 1994. "A Brief History of the Development of Rehabilitative Services in China." In "Models for Change in a Changing Society: Psychiatric Rehabilitation in China," edited by Michael R. Phillips, Veronica Pearson, and Ruiwen Wang, supplement 24, *British Journal of Psychiatry* 165: 19–27.

Tiedemann, R. G. 2010. "Medical Missions." In *Handbook of Christianity in China*, Vol. 2, *1800 to the Present*, edited by R. G. Tiedemann, 436–446. Leiden: Brill.

Tien Hung-Mao. 1972. *Government and Politics in Kuomintang China 1927–1937.* Stanford, CA: Stanford University Press.

Tien, Ju K'ang. 1985. "Traditional Chinese Beliefs and Attitudes towards Mental Illness." In *Chinese Culture and Mental Health*, edited by Wen Shing Tseng and David Wu, 67–82. New York: Academic Press.

Toman, K. 1979. *Tuberculosis Case-Finding and Chemotherapy: Questions and Answers.* Geneva: World Health Organization.

Tousley, Martha M. 1985. "China: Psychiatric Nursing in the People's Republic." *Journal of Psychosocial Nursing and Mental Health Services* 23: 569–577.

Tow, Edna. Forthcoming. "Life under Fire: State and Society in Wartime Chongqing, 1937–1945." PhD diss., University of California, Berkeley.

Tseng, Wen Shing. 1983. "The Development of Traditional Psychiatric Concepts in Traditional Chinese Medicine." *Archives of General Psychiatry* 29: 569–577.

"Tsung Sing SZE." 1997. Citations, Honorary Degrees Congregation, University of Hong Kong. http://www4.hku.hk/hongrads/index.php/archive/citation_detail/247.

Tucker, Sarah. 1983. "The Canton Hospital and Medicine in 19th Century China (1835–1900)." PhD diss., Indiana University.

U, Eddy. 2007. *Disorganizing China: Counter-Bureaucracy and the Decline of Socialism.* Stanford, CA: Stanford University Press.

United Nations. 2011. *Millennium Development Goals Report 2011.* New York: United Nations.

Unschuld, Paul. 1979. *Medical Ethics in Imperial China: A Study in Historical Anthropology.* Berkeley: University of California Press.

U.S. CDC (Centers for Disease Control and Prevention). 2009. "Consumption Data." In *Smoking and Tobacco Use*, 1–4. Atlanta, GA: U.S. Centers for Disease Control and Prevention.

Utzinger, Jürg, Zhou Xiao-Nong, Chen Ming-Gang, and Robert Bergquist. 2005. "Conquering Schistosomiasis in China: The Long March." *Acta Tropica* 96 (2–3): 69–96.

Vaughan, Victor C. 1926. *A Doctor's Memories.* Indianapolis: Bobbs-Merrill.

Vigarello, Georges. 1988. *Concepts of Cleanliness: Changing Attitudes in France since the Middle Ages.* Translated by Jean Birrell. Cambridge: Cambridge University Press.

Visher, John S., and Emily B. Visher. 1979. "Impressions of Psychiatric Problems and Their Management in China." *American Journal of Psychiatry* 136: 28–32.

Walls, PD, LH Walls, and DG Langsley. 1975. "Psychiatric Training and Practice in the People's Republic of China." *American Journal of Psychiatry* 132: 121–128.

Wang, Chuanyue, and Lijun Li. 2012. "Proper Use of Clozapine: Experiences in China." *Shanghai Archives of Psychiatry* 24 (2): 108–109.

Wang, Qingtong, Yuzhu Gong, and Kezhen Niu. 1994. "The Yantai Model of Community Care for Psychiatric Patients." In "Models for Change in a Changing Society: Psychiatric Rehabilitation in China," edited by Michael R. Phillips, Veronica Pearson, and Ruiwen Wang, supplement 24, *British Journal of Psychiatry* 165: 107–113.

Wang, Xishi. 1994. "An Integrated System of Community Services for the Rehabilitation of Chronic Psychiatric Patients in Shenyang, China." In "Models for Change in a Changing Society: Psychiatric Rehabilitation in China," edited by Michael R. Phillips, Veronica Pearson, and Ruiwen Wang, supplement 24, *British Journal of Psychiatry* 165: 80–88.

Wang, Y. C. 1966. *Chinese Intellectuals and the West, 1872–1949.* Chapel Hill: University of North Carolina.

Wang Bing-shun, Li-feng Zhou, David Coulter, Hong Liang, Ye Zhong, Yu-na Guo, Li-ping Zhu, Xiao-ling Gao, Wei Yuan, and Er-sheng Gao. 2010. "Effects of Caesarean Section on Maternal Health in Low Risk Nulliparous Women: A Prospective Matched Cohort Study in Shanghai, China." *BMC Pregnancy Childbirth* 10: 78.

Wang Jian-Bing, Yong Jiang, Wen-Qiang Wei, Gong-Huan Yuan, You-Lin Qiao, and Paolo Bofetta. 2010. "Estimation of Cancer Incidence and Mortality Attributable to Smoking in China." *Cancer Causes Control* 21 (6): 959–965.

Wang Jing. 1996a. *High Culture Fever: Politics, Aesthetics, and Ideology in Deng's China.* Berkeley: University of California Press.

Wang Jun. 2003. "A Life History of Ren Yingqiu: Historical Problems, Mythology, Continuity and Difference in Chinese Medical Modernity." PhD diss., University of North Carolina.

Wang Longde, Jiajun Liu, and Daniel P. Chin. 2007. "Progress in TB Control and the Evolving Public-Health System in China." *Lancet* 369 (February 24): 691–695.

Warren, Kenneth. 1988. "Farewell to the Plague Spirit: Chairman Mao's Crusade against Schistosomiasis." In *Science and Medicine in Twentieth-Century China: Research and Education,* edited by John Bowers, J. Hess, and Nathan Sivin, 123–140. Ann Arbor: Center for Chinese Studies, University of Michigan.

Warrick, Susan. 2005–2012. "Lucinda L. Coombs, 1849–1919." Biographical Dictionary of Chinese Christianity. http://www.bdcconline.net/en/stories/c/coombs-lucinda-l.php.

Watt, John R. 2004. "Breaking into Public Service: The Development of Nursing in Modern China, 1870–1949." *Nursing History Review* 12: 62–91.

———. 1914. *Saving Lives in Wartime China.* Leiden: E. J. Brill.

Way, E. Leong. 1961. "Pharmacology." In *Sciences in Communist China,* edited by Sidney H. Gould, 363–382. Washington, DC: American Association for the Advancement of Science.

Wei Xiaolin, Jing Chen, Ping Chen, James N. Newell, Hongdi Li, Chenguang Sun, Jian Mei, and John D. Walley. 2009. "Barriers to TB Care for Rural-to-Urban Migrant TB Patients in Shanghai: A Qualitative Study." *Tropical Medicine & International Health* 14 (7): 754–760.

White, Sidney D. 1998. "From 'Barefoot Doctor' to 'Village Doctor': A Case Study of Health Care Transformation in Socialist China." *Human Organization* 57 (4): 480–490.

Whitney, H. T. 1901a. "Chinese Medical Education." *China Medical Missionary Journal* 15 (3): 195–199.

———. 2001b. "Medical Education for the Chinese." *China Medical Missionary Journal* 15 (3): 217.

Whyte, Martin King, and William L. Parish. 1984. *Urban Life in Contemporary China.* Chicago: University of Chicago Press.

Wilms, Sabine. 2007. *Sun Simiao, Bei Ji Qian Jin Yao Fang: Essential Prescriptions Worth A Thousand Gold for Every Emergency, Volumes 2–4 on Gynecology.* Portland, OR: Chinese Medicine Database.

Wilson, H. S., and S. A. Hutchison. 1983. "Nursing in China: Three perspectives—Psychiatric Diagnoses Range from Depression and Violence to Social and Sexual Non-conformity." *American Journal of Nursing* 83: 393–395.

Winfield, Gerald F. 1948. *China: The Land and the People.* New York: William Sloane.

Witte, E. B., George J. Kunz, Walter E. Peters, and H. M. Randall. 1900. *Does China Need an American Hospital?* Los Angeles: Missionary Department of the National Holiness Association.

Wong, K. Chimin. 1950. "A Short History of Psychiatry and Mental Health in China." *Chinese Medical Journal* 68: 44–48.

Wong, K. Chimin, and Wu Lien-teh. 1936. *History of Chinese Medicine: Being a Chronicle of Medical Happenings in China from Ancient Times to the Present Period.* 2nd ed. Shanghai: National Quarantine Service.

Woods, Andrew H. 1929. "The Nervous Diseases of the Chinese." *Archives of Neurology and Psychiatry* 21: 546–570.

World Bank. 1992. *China: Long-Term Issues and Options in the Health Transition.* Washington, DC: World Bank.

World Health Organization. 2013. *Global Tuberculosis Report 2013.* Geneva: World Health Organization.

World Health Organization (WHO) Department of Mental Health and Substance Abuse. 2005. *Mental Health Atlas: 2005.* Geneva: World Health Organization.

World Population Prospects: The 2010 Revision. 2011. New York: United Nations, Department of Economic and Social Affairs, Population Division.

Worsley, Peter. 1982. "Non-Western Medical Systems." *Annual Review of Anthropology* 11: 349–375.

Wright, Pearce. 2004. "Obituary: Yingkai Wu." *Lancet* 363 (February 14): 575.

Wu, Yi-Li. 2010. *Reproducing Women: Medicine, Metaphor, and Childbirth in Late Imperial China.* Berkeley: University of California Press.

Wu Jibo. 1936. "On the Force of Health Movement." *Popular Health* 5 (2).

Wu Lien-teh. 1913. "First Report of the North Manchurian Plague Prevention Service." *Journal of Hygiene (Lond)* 13 (3): 237–290.

———. 1920. "Medical Progress in China since the Republic." *Lancet* 195 (5048): 1203–1204.

Wu Tai-Yin, Azeem Majeed, and Ken N. Kuo. 2010. "An Overview of the Healthcare System in Taiwan." *London Journal of Primary Care* 3: 115–119.

Wu Zhuochun, Kirsi Viisainen, Ying Wang, and Elina Hemminki. 2003. "Perinatal Mortality in Rural China: Retrospective Cohort Study." *British Medical Journal* 327 (December 6): 1–4.

Xia, Zhenyi, Heqin Yan, and C. H. Wang. 1987. "Mental Health Care in Shanghai." *International Journal of Mental Health* 16 (3): 81–85.

Xia, Zhenyi, and Mingyuan Zhang. 1981. "History and Present Status of Modern Psychiatry in China." *Chinese Medical Journal* 94: 277–282.

Xiao Lin, Yan Yang, Qiang Li, Cong-Xiao Wang, and Gong-Huan Yang. 2010. "Population-Based Survey of Secondhand Smoke Exposure in China." *Biomedical and Environmental Sciences* 23 (6): 430–436.

Xu Xiaoqun. 2001. *Chinese Professionals and the Republican State: The Rise of Professional Associations in Shanghai 1912–1937.* Cambridge: Cambridge University Press.

Yan, SM, DZ Xiang, YZ Chao, DY Chen, DQ Zhang, and MA Taylor. 1984. "The Frequency of Major Psychiatric Disorder in Chinese Inpatients." *American Journal of Psychiatry* 141: 690–692.

Yang, Lawrence, Graciete Lo, Ahtoy J. WonPat-Borja, Daisy R. Singla, Bruce G. Link, and Michael R. Phillips. 2012. "Effects of Labeling and Interpersonal Contact upon Attitudes towards Schizophrenia: Implications for Reducing Mental Illness Stigma in Urban China." *Social Psychiatry and Psychiatric Epidemiology* 47: 1459–1473.

Yang, Lawrence, and Veronica Pearson. 2002. "Understanding Families in their Own Context; Schizophrenia and Structural Family Therapy in Beijing." *Journal of Family Therapy* 24: 233–257.

Yang, Marion. 1928a. "Midwifery Training in China." *China Medical Journal* 42: 768–775.

Yang Gonghuan. 2008. "Prevalence of Smoking in China." In *Tobacco Control Policy Analysis in China: Economics and Health,* edited by Hu Teh-wei, 13–32. Singapore: World Scientific.

———. 2010. "Monitoring Epidemic of Tobacco Use, Promote Tobacco Control." *Biomedical and Environmental Sciences* 23 (6): 420–421.

Yang Gonghuan, Lixin Fan, Jian Tan, Cuoming Qi, Yifang Zhang, Jonathan M. Samet, Carl E. Taylor, Karen Becker, and Jing Xu. 1999. "Smoking in China: Findings of the 1996 National Prevalence Survey." *Journal of the American Medical Association* 282 (13): 1247–1253.

Yang Lian, Hai-Yen Sung, Zhengzhong Mao, Teh-wei Hu, and Keqin Rao. 2011. "Economic Costs Attributable to Smoking in China: Update and an 8-Year Comparison, 2000–2008." *Tobacco Control* 20 (4): 266–272.

Yang Yan, Ji-Jiang Wang, Cong-Xiao Wang, Qiang Li, and Gong-Huan Yang. 2010. "Awareness of Tobacco-Related Health Hazards among Adults in China." *Biomedical and Environmental Sciences* 23 (6): 437–444.

Ye Weili. 1994. "'Nu Liuxuesheng': The Story of American-Educated Chinese Women, 1880s–1920s." *Modern China* 20 (3): 315–346.

———. 2001. *Seeking Modernity in China's Name: Chinese Students in the United States, 1900–1927.* Stanford, CA: Stanford University Press.

Yen, F. C. 1915. "An Example of Cooperation with the Chinese in Medical Education." *Journal of the American Medical Association* 64 (17): 1385.

———. 1927. "A Plan Suggested for Public Health Administration in the Central Government of China." *National Medical Journal of China* 13 (1): 1.

Yip, Ka-che. 1992. "Health and Nationalist Reconstruction: Rural Health in Nationalist China, 1928–1937." *Modern Asian Studies* 26 (2): 395–415.

———. 1095. *Health and National Reconstruction in Nationalist China: The Development of Modern Health Services, 1928–1937.* Ann Arbor, MI: Association of Asian Studies.

———. 2001. "Disease and the Fighting Men: Nationalist Anti-Epidemic Efforts in Wartime China, 1937–1945." In *China in the Anti-Japanese War, 1937–1945: Politics, Culture, and Society,* edited by David P. Barrett and Larry N. Shyu, 171–188. New York: Peter Lang.

Yip, Winnie, and William C. Hsiao. 2008. "The Chinese Health System at a Crossroads." *Health Affairs* 27 (2): 460–468.

Yip, Winnie Chi-Man, William C. Hsiao, Wen Chen, Shanlian Hu, Jin Ma, and Alan Maynard. 2012. "Early Appraisal of China's Huge and Complex Health-Care Reforms." *Lancet* 379 (March 3): 833–842.

You, J., H. Quan, and J. Xu. 1991. "Re-analysis of Life Data of Guangxi Population Before 1949." *Chinese Journal of Health Statistics* 8 (6): 5–8.

Yung, W. W. 1936. "Child Health Work in Peiping First Health Area." *Chinese Medical Journal* 50: 562–572.

Zaslawaski, Christopher, and Myeong Soo Lee. 2011. "International Standardization of East Asian Medicine: The Quest for Modernization." In *Integrating East Asian Medicines into Modern Health Care,* edited by Volker Scheid and Hugh MacPherson, 89–104. London: Elsevier.

Zenoff, Alexandra. 2010. "The Role of Johns Hopkins in Promoting Professionalized Medical Education at Peking Union Medical College: 1915–1947." Bachelor's thesis, Johns Hopkins University.

Zhan Mei. 2009. *Other-Worldly: Making Chinese Medicine through Transnational Frames.* Durham, NC: Duke University Press.

Zhang, Daqing, and Paul U. Unschuld. 2008. "China's Barefoot Doctor: Past, Present, and Future." *Lancet* 372 (9653): 1865–1867.

Zhang, Minglian, Mingtao Wang, Jianjun Li, and Michael R. Phillips. 1994. "Randomised-Control Trial of Family Intervention for 78 First-Episode Male Schizophrenic Patients:

An 18-month Study in Suzhou, Jiangsu." In "Models for Change in a Changing Society: Psychiatric Rehabilitation in China," edited by Michael R. Phillips, Veronica Pearson, and Ruiwen Wang, supplement 24, *British Journal of Psychiatry* 165: 96–102.

Zhang, Mingyuan, Heqin Yan, and Michael R. Phillips. 1994. "Community-Based Psychiatric Rehabilitation in Shanghai: Facilities, Services, Outcome and Culture Specific Characteristics." In "Models for Change in a Changing Society: Psychiatric Rehabilitation in China," edited by Michael R. Phillips, Veronica Pearson, and Ruiwen Wang, supplement 24, *British Journal of Psychiatry* 165: 70–79.

Zhang Dewen. 2009a. "Rockefeller Foundation and China's Wartime Nursing, 1937–1945." Research Reports, Rockefeller Archive Center. http://www.rockarch.org/publications /resrep/zhang.pdf.

Zhang Dongying. 1997. "Current Situation and Reform for Chinese Secondary Nursing Education." *Chinese Health Service Management* 12: 652–654.

Zhang Hong and Cai Baiqiang. 2003. "The Impact of Tobacco on Lung Health in China." *Respirology* 8 (1): 17–21.

Zhang Yixia, and Mark Elvin. 1998. "Environment and Tuberculosis in Modern China." In *Sediments of Time: Environment and Society in Chinese History*, edited by Mark Elvin and Liu Ts'ui-jing, 520–544. New York: Cambridge University Press.

Zhao, J. 1990. "Analysis of Mortality and Causes of Death of Population in Northeastern China in 1907–1938." *Chinese Journal of Population Science* 6: 47–53.

Zheng, Jiang, Gu Xueguang, Xu Yonglong, Ge Jihua, Yang Xianxiang, He Changhao, Tang Chao et al. 2002. "Relationship between the Transmission of Schistosomiasis Japonica and the Construction of the Three Gorge Reservoir." *Acta Tropica* 82: 147–156.

Zhou Jingnan. 2012. "China Imposes Regulation to Fight Antibiotics Abuses." *China Radio International,* August 1. http://english.cri.cn/7146/2012/07/31/2702s714530.htm.

Zhou XN, JB Malone, TK Kristensen, and NR Bergquist. 2001. "Application of Geographic Information Systems and Remote Sensing to Schistosomiasis Control in China." *Acta Tropica* 79 (1): 97–106.

Zhu Yu. 2008. "The Resurgence of Shanghai and Its Demographic and Employment Changes in the 1990s." In *Mega-Urban Regions in Pacific Asia: Urban Dynamics in a Global Era*, edited by Gavin Jone and Mike Douglass, 251–283. Singapore: National University of Singapore Press.

Chinese Sources

An Yansheng 安燕生. 2003. "Beijing shi shishi DOTS25 nian: Jiehebing chuanbing lv, siwang lv ji fabing qushi xiaoguo fenxi yanjiu" 北京市实施 DOTS25 年: 结核病患病率、死亡率及发病趋势效果分析研究 [Beijing city implements the year of DOTS25: Research and analysis of the rate of tuberculosis infection, rate of death, and the results of morbidity trends]. Supplement, *Zhonguo fanglao zazhi* 中国防痨杂志 25: 19–20.

Anhui sheng weishengzhi bianzuan weiyuanhui 安徽省卫生志编纂委员会. 1990. *Anhui xuexichong bing fangzhizhi* 安徽血吸虫病防治志 [Record of the prevention and history of schistosomiasis in Anhui Province]. Hefei: Huangshan shushe.

"Beijing shi weisheng ju" 北京市衛生局 [Beijing city department of health]. 1928. *Weisheng gongbao* 衞生公報, no. 1.

BJSWJ (Beijing shi weisheng ju) 北京市卫生局. 2012. "2011 nian Beijing shi weisheng fazhan maishang xin taijie" 2011 年北京市卫生发展迈上新台阶 [In 2011, the development of hygiene in the city of Beijing ascended new heights]. June 1. http://www.bjhb.gov.cn /wsxw/201206/t20120601_50439.htm.

Boerdeliefu 波尔德列夫 [Tikhon E. Boldyrev]. 1956. "Guanyu xiaomie xue xi chongbing cuoshi de jidian yijian" 关于消灭血吸虫病措施的几点意见 [Several suggestions on schistosomiasis elimination]. *Jiankangbao* 健康报 425 (February 17).

———. 1959. "Guanyu lingdao gongzuo de jixiang zong de yuanze ji qi zai baojian bumen-zhong de yingxiang" 关于领导工作的几项总的原则及其在保健部门中的应用 [Concerning several principles of leadership work and their influence on the department of public health]. In *Sulian zhuanjia fuyou gongzuo jiangyan ji* 苏联专家妇幼工作讲演集 [Collections of lectures by Soviet experts on maternal and child work], edited by Weisheng bu fuyou weisheng si 卫生部妇幼卫生司编, 1–26. Beijing: People's Health Press.

BSDZBW (Beijing shi difang zhi bianzhuan weiyuanhui) 北京市地方志编撰委员会, ed. 2000. *Beijing zhi, shizheng juan, huanjing weisheng zhi* 北京志·市政卷·环境卫生志 [Beijing gazetteer, city administration, environmental health]. Beijing: Beijing chubanshe.

BSWC (Beiping shi weisheng chu) 北平市衛生處. 1934. *Di er weisheng qu shiwu suo di yi niandu nianbao* 第二衛生區事務所第一年度年報 [Report of the first year of work in the Second Hygiene Area], no. 1.

BSWJ (Beiping shi weisheng ju) 北平市衛生局. 1928a. "Beiping tebie shi weisheng weiyuanhui zhangcheng" 北平特別市衛生委員會章程 [Beiping special city public health committee regulations]. *Weisheng gongbao* 衛生公報 1: 13.

———. 1928b. "Beiping shi weisheng shiye gangyao" 北平市衛生事業綱要 [Essentials of Beiping city public health service]. *Weisheng gongbao* 衛生公報 1: 257–262.

BWNW (Beijing shi weisheng ju "Beijing weisheng nianjian" bianji weiyuanhui) 北京市卫生局《北京卫生年鉴》编辑委员会. 1992–1999. Beijing weisheng nianjian 北京卫生年鉴 [Health annals of Beijing].

BWZBW (Beijing weisheng zhi bianzuan weiyuanhui) 北京卫生志编纂委员会. 2001. *Beijing weisheng zhi* 北京卫生志 [Beijing health record]. Beijing: Beijing kexue jishu chubanshe.

BYYXBZ (Beijing yixueyuan yishi xue baojian zuzhi xue jiaoyan shi) 北京医学院医史保健组织学教研室, ed. 1964. *Beijing yiyao weisheng shiliao* 北京医药卫生史料 [Beijing historical records of medicine and hygiene]. Beijing: Beijing chubanshe.

Cai Jingfeng 蔡景峰, Li Qinghua 李庆华, and Zhang Binghuan 张冰皖, eds. 1999. *Zhongguo yixue tongshi: Xiandai juan* 中国医学通史: 现代卷 [A comprehensive history of medicine in China: Modern volume]. Beijing: Renmin weisheng chubanshe.

Cao Jingxing 曹景行, ed. 2008. *Qinli—Shanghai gaige kaifang sanshi nian* 亲历—上海改革开放三十年 [Personal experiences: Thirty years of reform and opening in Shanghai]. Shanghai: Shanghai cishu chubanshe.

Cao Shuji 曹树基 and Li Yushang 李玉尚. 2006. *Shuyi: Zhanzheng yu heping—zhongguo de huanjing yu shehui bianqian (1230–1960)* 鼠疫: 战争与和平—中国的环境与社会变迁 (1230–1960年) [Plague: War and peace—China's environmental and societal changes, 1230–1960]. Ji'nan: Shandong huabao chubanshe.

Chen Cunren 陈存仁. 2000. *Yinyuan shidai de shenghuo shi* 银元时代的生活史 [History of life in the era of the silver dollar]. Shanghai: Shanghai renmin chubanshe.

Chen Fangzhi 陳方之. 1929a. "Kaocha Riben yishi yu weisheng yanjiu qingkuang" 考察日本醫事與衛生研究情況 [Survey of medical issues and the situation of public health research in Japan]. *Weisheng gongbao* 衛生公報 1 (8): 91–103.

Chen Jianmin 陈健民. 1990. "Lu Yuanlei xiansheng de xueshusixiang" 陆渊雷先生的学术思想 [Mr. Lu Yuanlei's scholarly thoughts]. *Zhonghua yishi zazhi* 中华医史杂志 20 (2): 91–95.

Chen Minzhang 陈敏章. 1985b. "Chen Minzhang tongzhi zai yijiubawunian quanguo weishengtingjuzhang huiyi shang de zongjie jianghua" 陈敏章同志在一九八五年全国卫生厅局长会议上的总结讲话 [Minister of Health Comrade Chen Minzhang's summary speech at the National Health Department director meeting in 1985]. Cited in *Zhongguo gaige quanshu: yiliao weisheng tizhi gaigejuan* 中国改革全书: 医疗卫生体制改革卷 [China reform: Medical and health system reform], edited by Ma Hong 马洪, 137. Dalian: Dalian chubanshe.

Chen Wanqing 陈万青, Zhang Siwei 张思维, Zou Xiaonong 邹小农, and Zhao Ping 赵平. 2010. "2004–2005 nian Zhongguo fei'ai siwang qingkuang fenxi 2004–2005" 年中国肺癌死亡情况分析 [An analysis of lung cancer mortality in China, 2004–2005]. *Zhonghua yufang yixue zazhi* 中华预防医学杂志 44 (5): 378–382.

Chen Zhiqian 陈志潜. 1929b. "Wu guo quan yi jianshe wenti" 吾國全醫建設問題 [Problems in our nation's medical system]. *Yixue zhoukan ji* 醫學周刊集 2: 89–110.

"Chen Zhongyang zhixing weiyuanhui zhengzhi huiyi chenfu yixue hui zhang Lin Kesheng duiyu yi xiao liang jizhi zhi jianyi yi an, yi zhuan zi jiao bu he ban wen" 稱中央執行委員會症治會議臣服醫學會長林克生對於醫校兩機制之建議議案,已轉自教部??? [The central executive committee's feedback to Chinese medical association president Lin Kesheng's suggestion for a two-tiered medical education system has been sent to the Ministry of Education to be implemented]. 1929. *Weisheng gongbao* 衛生公報 1 (9): 70–71.

Chongqing shi tongji ju 重庆市统计局, ed. 2010. *Chongqing tongji nianjian* 重庆统计年鉴 [Chongqing statistical yearbook, 2010]. Beijing: Zhongguo tongji chubanshe.

Chongqingshi tongji tiyao 重慶市統計提要 [A summary of Chongqing statistics]. 1942. Chongqing: Chongqing shi zhengfu.

"Cong 'chijiao yisheng' de chengzhang kan yixue jiaoyu geming de fangxiang: Shanghaishi de diaocha baogao" 从'赤脚医生'的成长看医学教育革命的方向: 上海市的调查报告 [Fostering a revolution in medical education through the growth of the barefoot doctors: An investigative report from Shanghai municipality]. 1968. *Renmin ribao* 人民日报, September 14.

Cui Yueli 崔月梨, ed. 1997. *Zhongyi chensï lu* 中医沉思录 [Record of meditations on Chinese medicine]. Beijing: Zhongyi guji chubanshe.

Cui Yueli 崔月犁 and Wei Gonghao 韦功浩, eds. 1987. *Zhongguo dangdai yixuejia huicui* 中国当代医学家荟萃 [A distinguished assembly of contemporary medical experts in China]. Changchun: Jilin kexue jishu chubanshe.

Dai Zhicheng 戴志澄, ed. 1993. *Zhongguo weisheng fangyi gongzuo huigu yu zhanwang—jinian quanguo weisheng fangyi zhan chengli sishi zhou nian* 中国卫生防疫工作回顾与展望—纪念全国卫生防疫站成立四十周年 [The past and future of public health and disease prevention work in China—Remembering the disease prevention hygiene stations that have been established across the nation over forty years]. Beijing: Weishengbu weisheng fangyi si.

Dan Li 单丽. 2008. "1902 nian huoluan zai Zhongguo de liuxing" 年霍乱在中国的流行 [The spread of cholera in China in 1902]. Master's thesis, Qingdao University.

"Dazongtong jiejian boyihui waiguo yishi daci" 大總統接見博醫會外國醫士答辞 [Reply to the president receiving Medical Missionary Association foreign physicians' assistants]. 1913. *Zhonghua yixue zazhi* 中華醫學雜誌 27 (1): 91.

Deng Tietao 邓铁涛. 1999. *Zhongyi jindai shi* 中医近代史 [A modern history of Chinese medicine]. Guangzhou: Guangdong gaodeng jiaoyu chubanshe.

———, ed. 2006. *Zhongguo fangyi shi* 中国防疫史 [A history of epidemic prevention in China]. Nanning: Guangxi keji chubanshe.

Deng Tietao 邓铁涛 and Cheng Zhifan 程之范, eds. 2000. *Zhongguo yixue tongshi: Jindai juan* 中国医学通史·近代卷 [A comprehensive history of medicine in China: Modern volume]. Beijing: Renmin weisheng chubanshe.

Di Ruide 狄瑞德. 1934. "Yixue jiaoyu yu Beiping xiehe yixueyuan zhi kecheng" 醫學教育與北平協和醫學院之課程 [Medical education and the curriculum of Beiping Union Medical College]. *Zhonghua yixue zazhi* 中華醫學雜誌 20 (12): 1544.

"Di san jie quanguo weisheng xingzheng huiyi jueyi" 第三屆全国卫生行政会议决议 [Resolutions of the third national health administration conference]. 1954. *Jiangxi zhengbao* 江西政报, no. 14, 17.

Di si ye zhan jun hou qin weisheng bu 第四野戰軍後勤衛生部. 1949. *Huoluan chili nueji xiao tui xie kuiyang riben xuexichong bing* 霍亂赤痢瘧疾小腿潰瘍日本血吸蟲病 [Cholera, Bacillian dysentery, malaria, Ulcus cruris and Schistosomiasis japonica].

"Di yi qian yi bai wu shi qi hao, zhezou lei" 第一千一百五十七号, 折奏类 [Memorial submitted to the emperor, no. 1157]. 2006 [1911]. *Zhengzhi guanbao* 政治官報, January 12, 7–8. Quoted in Pan Maoyuan 潘懋元, and Liu Haifeng 刘海峰, eds. *Zhongguo jindai jiaoyushi ziliao huibian: Gaodeng jiaoyu* 中国近代教育史资料汇编 高等教育 [Collected materials on the history of modern education in China: higher education]. Shanghai: Shanghai jiaoyu chubanshe, 307.

Ding Fubao 丁福保. 1903. *Weishengxue wenda* 衛生學問答 [Questions and answers on hygiene]. Shanghai: Wenming shuju jiaoyin.

———. 1910. Riben yixue ji 日本醫學記 [Record of Japanese medicine]. *Zhongxi yixue bao* 中西醫學報, no. 1, 5–9.

———. 1949. *Chouyin jushi xueshu shi* 疇隱居士學術史 [An academic history of past scholars living in seclusion]. Shanghai: Shanghai gulin jingshe chubanshe.

Ding Youhe 丁有和. 1993. *20 shiji wenyi: Aizibing* 20世纪瘟疫: 艾滋病 [20th century epidemics: AIDS]. Chengdu: Sichuan renmin chubanshe.

Ding Zhongying 丁仲英. 1936. "Zhongyiyao zhi qianzhan" 中醫藥之前瞻 [Prospects of Chinese drugs]. *Guanghua yiyao zazhi* 光華醫藥雜誌 4 (9): 8.

Dong Jianhua 董建华, Hou Dianyuan 侯点元, and Zhang Xijun 张锡君, eds. 1990. *Dangdai zhongyi* 当代中医 [Contemporary Chinese medicine]. Chongqing: Chongqing chubanshe.

"Fagui: Daxue yixueyuan ji yike zanxing ke mubiao" 《法規》大學醫學院及醫科暫行課目表 [Law: University, medical school, and temporary medical catalogue]. 1935. *Yishi huikan* 醫事匯刊 24: 329–332.

Fan Xingzhun 范行准. 1953. *Zhongguo yufang yixue sixiang shi* 中国预防医学思想史 [An intellectual history of preventive medicine in China]. Shanghai: Huadong yiwu shenghuoshe.

———. 1954. "You guan riben zhuxuexichong bing de zhongyi wenxian de chubu tantao" 有關日本住血吸蟲病的中醫文獻的初步探討 [A preliminary investigation of the Chinese medical literature relating to schistosomiasis]. *Zhonghua yixue zazhi* 中華醫學雜誌 11: 862–864.

Fang Shishan 方石珊, ed. 1928. Zhongguo weisheng xingzheng yange 中國衛生行政沿革 [The development of hygiene administration in China]. *Weisheng gongbao* 卫生公报, no. 1: 223.

Feng Depei 冯德培 and Pan Shu 潘菽. 1949. "Sulian zenyang jinian Bafuluofu 苏联怎样纪念巴夫洛夫 [How the Soviet Union remembers Pavlov]. *Kexue tongxun* 科学通讯, no. 6: 6.

Feng Qiuji 冯秋季. 2010. "Jindai yubei Jianada chuan jiao shi cuo yi chuan jiao yu fuyou weisheng guannian biange yanjiu" 近代豫北加拿大传教士借医传教与妇幼卫生观

念变革研究 [Research on Canadian missionary work through medical service and changes of ideas on women and children's health in modern northern Henan]. *Henan daxue xuebao (shehui kexue ban)* 河南大学学报 (社会科学版) 1: 105–110.

Fu Hui 傅惠 and Deng Zongyu 邓宗禹. 1989. "Jiu Weishengbu zuzhi de bianqian" 旧卫生部组织的变迁 [Changes in the organization of the old Ministry of Health]. In *Wenshi Ziliao Xuanbian* 文史资料选编 [Anthology of literary and historical materials], no. 37, 275–276. Beijing: Beijing chubanshe.

Fu Jihua 傅继华 and Yu Guofang 于国防, eds. 2000. *Aizibing yufang yu kongzhi* 艾滋病预防与控制 [Prevention and control of AIDS]. Ji'nan: Shandong keji chubanshe.

Fu Lianzhang 傅连暲. 1952. "Xuexi Sulian de xianjin yixue" 学习苏联的先进医学 [Studying the advances in Soviet medicine]. *Renmin ribao* 人民日报, November 5.

———. 1954. "Di san jie quanguo weisheng xingzheng huiyi jueyi" 第三届全国卫生行政会议决议 [Resolutions of the third national health administration conference]. *Jiankang bao* 健康报, August 6.

———. 1957. "Jianding bu yi de xuexi Sulian xianjin yixue" 坚定不移地学习苏联先进医学 [We must unswervingly continue to study advanced Soviet medicine]. *Renmin ribao* 人民日报, October 19.

Gan Houci 甘厚慈. 1907. *Beiyang gongdu leicuan* 北洋公牍类纂 [Official documents of the type seized from the coastal provinces of Liaoning, Hebei, and Shandong]. Weisheng 衛生 [Hygiene]. Vol. 25. Beijing: Yi sen yinshua youxian gongsi.

"Ganwu lishi digou weilai: jinian 'Zhongguo shiyong huli zazhi' chuangkan 20 zhou nian" 感悟历史缔构未来—纪念《中国实用护理杂志》创刊20周年 [A History of Comprehension and the Construction to Come: 20 Year Anniversary for Chinese Journal of Practical Nursing]. 2005. *Zhongguo shiyong huli zazhi* 中国实用护理杂志 21 (1): 1–2.

Gao Yaojie 高耀洁, ed. 2005. *Zhongguo aizibing diaocha* 中国艾滋病调查 [Survey of AIDS in China]. Guilin: Guangxi shifan da xue chubanshe.

Gao Zonglu 高宗鲁, trans. 1982. *Zhongguo youtong liu mei shi* 中國幼童留美史 [A history of Chinese children studying in America]. Taipei: Huaxin wenhua shiye zhongxin chuban.

Ge Shaolong 戈绍龙. 1952. "Sulian de yiliao yu baojian" 苏联的医疗与保健 [Soviet medicine and health]. *Zhongsu youhao* 中苏友好, no. 6: 24.

Gong Naiquan 宫乃泉. 1950. Introduction to *Sulian de yixue he baojian* 苏联的医学和保健 [Soviet medicine and health], by Xigelisi [Henry S. Sigerist] 西格里斯. Translated by Gong Naiquan 宫乃泉. Shanghai: Huadong yiwu shenghuo chubanshe.

Guangdong sheng zhengfu jingchating 廣東省政府警察廳 [Guangdong Provincial Government Police Department]. 1913. "Jingchating gongbu shixing suo ni xiyisheng chankesheng yaojishi tiaoji yaofang xiyiyuan shihongzihui ge li'an zhangcheng wen" 警察廳公布試行所拟西醫生產科生藥劑師調劑藥方西醫院十紅字會各立案章程聞 [Police Department announcement of draft regulations for registered Western doctors, obstetrists, pharmacists, prescriptions, Western hospitals and the Red Cross]. *Guangdong Bulletin,* January 23: 14–25.

"Guangdongsheng Qujiangxian Qunxing dadui jianchi hezuo yiliao zhidu shiyinian de qingkuang diaocha" 广东省曲江县群星大队坚持合作医疗制度十一年的情况调查 [Investigative report of Qunxing production brigade, Qujiang county, Guangdong Province, persisting in implementing cooperative medical services for 11 years]. 1969. *Renmin ribao* 人民日报, January 11.

"Guangxu ershijiu nian guanxue dachen zhang (bai xi) zunzhi yi qinhuguang zongdu zhang (zhidong) deng qin cidi xingban xuetang zhe" 光绪二十九年管学大臣张 (百熙) 遵旨议秦湖广总督张 (之洞) 等秦次第兴办学堂折 [Guangxu year 29 report of the consultation between Minister of Education Zhang (Baixi) and Governor-General of Shaanxi and Huguang Zhang (Zhidong) on the progress of establishing schools in Shaanxi]. 1903. In *Zhengyi congshu zhengshu tongji, juan er* 政艺丛书 政书通辑, 卷二 [Collection on the administrative arts, series of political records, Vol. 2], cited in Zhu (1987), 67.

Guo Jianyao 郭建堯. 1990. *Lin Qiaozhi: Zhongguo jiechu fuchanke nu yisheng* 林巧稚: 中國傑出婦產科女醫生 [Lin Qiaozhi: China's outstanding female obstetrician-gynecologist]. Hong Kong: Xin ya wenhua shiye youxian gongsi.

Guo Moruo 郭沫若. 1950. "Zai di yi jie quanguo weisheng huiyi shang de jianghua" 在第一届全国卫生会议上的讲话 [Discussion of the First National Health Conference]. *Dongbei weisheng* 东北卫生 2 (6): 3.

Guo Rugui 郭汝瑰. 2005. *Zhongguo kangri zhanzheng zhengmian zhanchang zuozhan ji* 中国抗日战争正面战场作战记 [China's Anti-Japanese War combat operations]. Nanjing: Jiangsu renmin chubanshe.

"Guoli Beijing yixue zhuanmen xuexiao zhangcheng" 國立北京醫學專門學校章程 [National Beijing Medicine Technical School regulations]. 1920. *Jiaoyu gongbao* 教育公報, no. 7 (September): 14–22.

Guomin zhengfu weishengbu 國民政府衛生部, ed. 1928. "Wuwu saochu tiaoli" 污物掃除條例 [Regulations for cleaning up sewage]. In *Weisheng fagui* 衛生法規 [Hygiene laws]. Nanjing: Guomin zhengfu weishengbu.

Guowu yuan yanjiu shi keti zu 国务院研究室课题组. 1993. *Jingti aizibing: Weile Zhonghua minzu de shengcun* 警惕艾滋病: 为了中华民族的生存 [On guard against AIDS: For the survival of the Chinese nation]. Beijing: Xinhua chubanshe.

Gu Yunyu 谷韫玉. 1936. "Sulian fuying zhi weisheng" 苏联妇婴之卫生 [Soviet women's and infants' health]. *Zhonghua yixue zazhi* 中华医学杂志 22 (7): 455–468.

"Han guoji lianmeng hui weisheng bu Laximan boshi qing yi guwen zi ge lai hua zhidao bing zhuan qing zhi pai zhuan zhang ren yuan xiang ban hai gang jian yi shiyi wen" 函國際聯盟會衛生部拉西曼博士請以顧問資格來華指導並轉請指派專長人員襄辦海港檢疫事宜文 [Letter to the League of Nations Health Organization's Dr. Rajchman to invite him to come to China as a senior advisor to provide guidance, and also to pass on an invitation to select and send specialist staff to act as assistants in managing matters concerning seaport quarantines]. 1929. *Weisheng gongbao* 衛生公報 1 (8): 80.

Hangzhou shi weisheng fangyizhan 杭州市卫生防疫站, ed. 1982. *Yiqing ziliao huibian, 1950–1979* 疫情资料汇编, 1950–1979 [Compiled data of epidemic disease prevention, 1950–1979]. Hangzhou: Hangzhoushi fangyizhan.

Hao Xianzhong 郝先中. 2005. "Riben feichu hanyi yu Zhongguo jindai yixue" 日本废除汉医与中国近代医学 [Japan's abolishment of Han medicine and modern medicine in China]. *Wan xi xueyuan xuebao* 皖西学院学报 21 (6): 69–76.

He Shixi 何時希. 1997. *Jindai yilin yishi* 近代医林佚事 [Anecdotes of modern medical circles]. Shanghai: Shanghai zhongyiyao daxue chubanshe.

Hou Yuwen 侯毓汶. 1939. "Fa kan ci" 發刊詞 [Inaugural introduction to this periodical]. *Weisheng yuebao* 衛生月報 1: 1.

Hsiung Ping-chen 熊秉真. 1995. *Youyou: Chuantong zhongguo de qiangbao zhi dao* 幼幼: 傳統中國的襁褓之道 [To care for the young: The way of the swaddling cloth in traditional China]. Taipei: Lianjing.

———. 1999. *An yang: Jindai zhongguo ertong de jibing yu jiankang* 安恙: 近世中國兒童的疾病與健康 [To preserve from worry: Children's diseases and health in late imperial China]. Taipei: Lianjing.

Hu Cheng 胡成. 2008b. "Dongbei diqu fei shuyi manyan qijian de zhuquan zhi zheng (1910.11–1911.4)" 东北地区肺鼠疫蔓延期间的主权之争 (1910.11–1911.4) [The competition over sovereign rights during the course of the spreading of pneumonic plague in Manchuria (November 1910–April 1911)]. In *Zhongguo shehui lishi pinglun, di jiu juan* 中国社会历史评论, 第九卷 [Discussion of the social history of China, Vol. 9], edited by Chang Jianhua 常建华, 214–232. Tianjin: Tianjin guji chubanshe.

Hu Dingan 胡定安. 1934. Zhongguo yishi qiantu jidai jiejue zhi ji ge genben wenti 中國醫事前途急待解決之幾個根本問題 [The prompt settlement of some fundamental problems of the future of Chinese medical matters]. *Yishi gonglun* 醫事公論, no. 6: 17.

Hu Juanjuan 胡娟娟. 2009. "Jianguo hou gaodeng jiao chong xuexi sulian moshi de huigu he lishi jiaoxun" 建国后高等教充学习苏联模式的回顾和历史教训 [Memories and historical lessons of studying the Soviet model in higher education after the establishment of the nation]. *Gaige yu kaifang* 改革与开放, December.

Hu Shih 胡适. 1938. Foreword to *Ren yu yixue* 人與醫學 [Man and medicine], by Xigelisi [Henry S. Sigerist] 西格里斯. Translated by Gu Qianji 顾谦吉. Shanghai: Shangwu chubanshe.

Hu Shijie 胡世杰, ed. 1990. *Xin'an yiji congkan* 新安医集丛刊 [A collection of medical records from Xin'an]. Anhui: Anhui kexue jishu chubanshe.

Hu Ting'an 胡廷安. 1928. *Zhongguo weisheng xingzheng sheshi jihua* 中國衛生行政設施計劃 [Planning and carrying out public health administration in China]. Shanghai: Shangwu yinshuguan.

Hu Xiansu 胡先骕. 1925. "Liuxue wenti yu wu guo gaodeng jiaoyu zhi fangzhen" 留學問題與吾國高等教育之方針 [The problem of studying abroad and our nation's higher education policy]. *Dongfang zazhi* 東方雜誌 22 (9): 15.

Huang Fuqing 黃福庆. 1988. "Jindai Zhongguo jideng jiaoyu yanjiu guoli zhongshan daxue (1924–1937)" 近代中国记等教育研究国立中山大学 (1924–1937) [Modern China remembers education and research at National Sun Yat-sen University]. *Zhongyang yanjiuyuan jindaishi yanjiusuo zhuankan* 中央研究院近代史研究所专刊, no. 56: 141.

Huang Qijing 黃其晶 and Luo Zhuliu 罗柱流. 1989. "Tongxin xieli song wenshen-qing puxiang xue xi chongbing yiqing ji fangzhi chengguo" 同心协力送瘟神—青浦县血吸虫病疫情及防治成果 [Unite together to say farewell to the God of Plague—Achievements of prevention and treatment of epidemic of schistosomiasis in Qingpu county]. In *Qingpu wenshi, di si qi* 青浦文史, 第四期 [Qingpu culture and history, Vol. 4]. Qingpu, Shanghai: Zhongguo renmin zhengzhi xieshang huiyi Qingpu xian weiyuanhui wenshi ziliao weiyuanhui.

Huang Shi 黃石. 1930. "Shenme shi taijiao" 甚麼是胎教 [What is "fetal education"?]. *Funü zazhi* 婦女雜誌 17 (1): 19–28.

Huang Yongqiu 黃永秋. 2007. "Xin Zhongguo chengli chuqi sulian dui wo guo gaodeng jiaoyu de yingxiang" 新中国成立初期苏联对我国高等教育的影响 [The influence of the Soviet Union upon our nation's higher education during the early years of the newly established China]. *Zhongguo gaodeng yixue jiaoyu* 中国高等医学教育, no. 9: 26–28.

Huang Zifang (Tsefang) 黃子方. 1927. "Zhongguo weisheng chuyi" 中國衛生芻議 [My humble opinion of hygiene in China]. *Shehuixue jie* 社會學界 1: 193.

Hunt, Mary H., and John Fryer. 1893. *Haitong weisheng bian* 孩童衛生編 [Health for little folks]. Shanghai: Gezhi shushi.

HYSBW (Hangzhou yiyao shangyezhi bianzuan weiyuanhui) 杭州医药商业志编纂委员会, ed. 1990. *Hangzhou yiyao shangyezhi* 杭州医药商业志 [Hangzhou pharmaceutical commerce gazetteer]. Beijing: Zhongguo qingnian chubanshe.

Iijima, Wataru 飯島涉. 2000. *Pesuto to kindai Chūgoku: Eisei no 'seido-ka' to shakai hen'yō* ペストと近代中国: 衛生の「制度化」と社会変容 [Bubonic plague and modern China: Hygiene's "systematization" and social change]. Tokyo: Ken bunshuppan.

———. 2008. "Riben xueshu zhenxing hui kexue yanjiufei yanjiu" 日本学術振興会 科学研究費研究 [A brief history of Japanese colonial medicine]. Working paper, Aoyama Gakuin University, Tokyo.

Ji Chengye 季成叶. n.d. "Shao nian ertong wuda jiankang wenti" 少年儿童五大健康问题 [Five big health questions for young children]. Accessed March 4, 2014. http://www.govedu.com.cn/news_detailed.asp?param1=%D3%AA%D1%F8&param2=%C9%D9%C4%EA%B6%F9%CD%AF%CE%E5%B4%F3%BD%A1%BF%B5%CE%CA%CC%E2&param3=12186.

Jia Hongwei 佳宏伟. 2012. "20 shiji 30 niandai chengshi jumin de jibing yu siwang—Yi Nanjing, Beiping he Guangzhou wei li" 20世纪30年代城市居民的疾病与死亡—以南京、北平和广州为例 [20th century 1930s city dwellers' morbidity and mortality: Using Nanjing, Beiping, and Guangzhou as examples]. Paper presented at the fourteenth annual meeting of the Chinese Social History Association, Shanxi University, Taiyuan, Shanxi, China, May.

"Jianashi de Qing guo jiaoyu tan" 嘉纳氏的清国教育谈 [Gardner's discussion of education in the Qing dynasty]. 1902. *Jiaoyushilun* 教育時論, no. 633: 38

Jiang Anli 姜安丽. 2004. "21 shiji huli jiaoyu fazhan xianzhuang ji wo guo huli jiaoyu mianlin de tiaozhan he fazhan celve" 21世纪护理教育发展现状及我国护理教育面临的挑战和发展策略 [The development status of Chinese nursing education in the 21st century and the challenges and development strategies that our nation's nursing education faces]. *Jiefang jun huli zazhi* 解放军护理杂志 21 (12): 1–3.

Jiang Jieshi (Chiang Kai-shek) 蔣介石. 1975 [1934]. "Xinshenghuo yundong zhi yaoyi" 新生活運動之要義 [The essential meaning of the New Life Movement]. In *Xinshenghuo yundong shiliao* 新生活運動史料 [Historical documents of the New Life Movement], edited by Xiao Jizong 萧继宗, 13–23. Taipei: Zhongyang wenwu gongyingshe.

Jiangsu sheng tongji ju 江苏省统计局. 2011. *Jiangsu tongji nianjian* 江苏统计年鉴 [Jiangsu statistical yearbook]. Beijing: Zhongguo tongji chubanshe.

Jiangsu xinyi xueyuan 江苏新医学院. 1979. *Zhongyao dacidian* 中药大辞典 [Dictionary of Chinese drugs]. Shanghai: Shanghai kexue jishu chubanshe.

"Jiaoyu bu pin ding yixue jiaoyu weiyuan" 教育部聘定醫學教育委員 [The Ministry of Education intends to establish a committee of medical education]. 1929. *Yiyao pinglun* 醫藥評論, no. 24: 28.

Jin Zizhi 金子直. 1922. "Beiguan yu xiwang" 悲觀與希望 [Regrets and hopes]. *Weisheng yuekan* 衛生月刊, no. 2: 58. Beijing: Shenghuo, dushu, xinzhi sanlian shudian.

Kellogg, John Harvey, and John Fryer. 1896. *Chuxue weisheng bian* 初學衛生編 [Hygiene for young children]. Shanghai: Gezhi shushi.

King, P. Z. (Jin Baoshan) 金宝善. 1984. "Banfengjian banzhimindi shiqi de weisheng" 半封建半殖民地时期的卫生 [Public health in the semi-feudal, semi-colonial age]. In *Zhongguo yixue baike quanshu: Shehui yixue yu weisheng guanlixue* 中国医学百科全书.社会医学与卫生管理学 [A comprehensive encyclopedia of medicine in China: Social medicine and public health administration], edited by Qian Xinzhong 钱信忠, 9. Shanghai: Shanghai kexue jishu chubanshe.

———. 1985. "Jiu Zhongguo de xiyi paibie yu weisheng shiye de yanbian" 旧中国的西医派别与卫生事业的演变 [Schools of Western medicine in old China and the evolution of public health service]. In *Wenshi ziliao xuanji* 文史资料选辑 [Selection of cultural and historical materials], Vol. 1, edited by Zhongguo renmin zhengzhi xieshang huiyi, quan guo weiyuanhui, wenshi ziliao weiyuanhui 中国人民政治协商会议全国委员会文史资料研究委员会, 125–138. Beijing: Wenshi ziliao chubanshe.

King, P. Z. (Jin Baoshan) 金宝善 and Xu Shijin 许世瑾. 1991. "Ge sheng shi xian you gong-gong weisheng sheshi zhi gaikuang" 各省市现有公共卫生设施之概况 [A survey of the public health facilities that province and city now have]. In *Jin Baoshan Wenji: Yang ben* 金宝善文集:样本 [Jin Baoshan's collected works], edited by Beijing yike daxue gonggong weisheng xueyuan 北京医科大学公共卫生学院, 170–180. Beijing: Beijing yike daxue gonggong weisheng xueyuan.

Kolbanovskii, V. N. 柯尔潘诺夫斯基, B. H. (в. н. колбановский). 1953. *Ba fu luo fu de xueshuo yu jiaoyu xue shang de jige wenti* 巴甫洛夫的学说与教育学上的几个问题 [Pavlov's theory and pedagogy on several issues]. Nanjing: Zhengfeng chubanshe.

Kōseishō imukyoku 厚生省医务局. 1974. *Isei hyakunenshi* 医制百年史 [One hundred years' history of the medical system]. Tokyo: Gyōsei.

Lee, Jen-Der 李貞德. 2008. *Nüren de zhongguo yiliao shi: Hantang zhi jian de jiankang zhaogu yu xingbie* 女人的中國醫療史—漢唐之間的健康照顧與性別 [A women's history of Chinese medicine—Health care and gender from the Han to the Tang dynasties]. Taipei: Sanmin shuju.

Lei, Sean Hsiang-lin (Lei Xianglin) 雷祥麟. 2011. "Xiguan cheng si wei: Xin shenghuo yundong yu feijiehe fangzhi zhong de lunli, jiating yu shenti" 習慣成四維: 新生活運動與肺結核防治中的倫理, 家庭與身體 [Custom becomes morality: The New Life Movement and ethics, families and health in the prevention and cure of pulmonary tuberculosis]. *Zhongyang yanjiu yuan jindai shi yanjiu suo jikan* 中央研究院近代史研究所集刊, no. 74 (December): 133–177.

Lei Zhifang 雷芝芳. 1990. "Wo guo jihua shengyu de tuohuangzhe" 我国计划生育的拓荒者 [Our country's family planning pioneer]. In *Yang Chongrui boshi: Danchen bai nian ji nian* 杨崇瑞博士: 诞辰百年纪念 [Dr. Yang Chongrui: Centennial commemoration], edited by Yan Renying 严仁英, 15–19. Beijing: Beijing yike daxue, zhongguo xiehe yike daxue lianhe chubanshe.

Leung, Angelia Ki Che (Liang Qizi) 梁其姿. 1987. "Ming-Qing yufang tianhua cuoshi zhi yanbian" 明清預防天花措施之演變 [The development of measures to prevent smallpox in the Ming and Qing]. In *Guoshi shilun* 國史釋論 [Explanatory discussion of national history], chief editor Yang Liansheng 楊聯陞, 239–253. Taipei: Shihuo chubanshe.

———. 2007. "Yiliaoshi yu zhongguo 'xiandaixing' wenti" 醫療史與中國"現代性"問題 [Medical history and the issue of Chinese "modernity"]. *Zhongguo shehui lishi pinglun* 中國社會歷史評論 8: 1–18.

Li Dequan 李德全. 1950. "Zai di yi jie quanguo weisheng huiyi shang de baogao" 在第一届全国卫生会议上的报告 [Report from the First National Health Conference]. *Dongbei weisheng* 东北卫生 2 (6): 6.

———. 1957a. "Ganxie Sulian wu si de bangzhu—Wei Beijing sulian hongshizi yiyuan wuchang de yijiao Zhongguo er xie" 感谢苏联无私的帮助—为北京苏联红十字医院无偿地移交中国而写 [Thanks to the selfless aid of the Soviet Union: Written in response to the Beijing Soviet Red Cross Hospital given to China free of charge]. *Renmin ribao* 人民日报, March 22.

———. 1957b. "Xuexi sulian de xianjin gongzuo jingyan genghao de jianshe woguo weisheng shiye" 学习苏联的先进工作经验 更好地建设我国卫生事业 [Studying Soviet advanced work experience in order to better establish public health work in our nation]. *Zhongyi zazhi* 中医杂志, no. 11: 562.

Li Dongzhen 李揀珍. 1935a. "Yunfu Yingyoude Changshi" 孕婦應有的常識 [General knowledge that pregnant women need]. *Dazhong Weisheng* 大眾衛生 1 (4): 12–15.

Li Fujing 李賦京. 1935b. "Pinglun Nanjing yixue jiaoyu weiyuanhui ji qi ni yixueyuan kecheng dagang" 評論南京醫學教育委員會及其擬醫學院課程大綱 [A discussion of the Nanjing medical education committee and a summary of the curriculum for its planned medical school]. *Yiyao pinglun* 醫藥評論, no. 2: 2–10.

Li Honghe 李洪河. 2007b. *Xin Zhongguo de yibing liuxing yu shehui yingdui, 1949–1959* 新中国的疫病流行与社会应对 (1949–1959) [Epidemic spread and social responses in the new China, 1949–1959]. Beijing: Zhonggongdangshi chubanshe.

Li Jingwei 李经纬. 1987. *Zhongguo yixue baike quanshu yixue shi* 中国医学百科全书医学史 [Encyclopedia of medicine in China: Medical history]. Shanghai: Kexue jishu chubanshe.

Li Junjiu 李俊九. 1992a. "Diyi mian hongqi shi zenyang chashang de" 第一面红旗是怎样插上的 [How the first red flag was put in place]. In *Songwenshen jishi* 送瘟神纪实 [Record of bidding farewell to the God of Plague], edited by Liu Yurui 刘玉瑞 and Wan Guohe 万国和, 94–101. Jiangxi wenshi ziliao 江西文史资料 [Literary and historical materials of Jiangxi Province] 43. Nanchang: Jiangxi Sheng zhengxie wenshi ziliao yanjiu weiyuanhui.

Li Tieying 李铁映. 1992c. "Gaige kaifang xingshi xia geng yao jiaqiang fangbing gongzuo" 改革开放形势下更要加强防病工作 [It is more important to strengthen disease prevention work under the circumstances of the reform and opening]. In *Zhongguo gaige quanshu (1978–1991): Yiliao weisheng tizhi gaige juan* 中国改革全书 (1978–1991): 医疗卫生体制改革卷 [A comprehensive volume of China's reform (1978–1991): Volume on medicine and health system reform], edited by Peng Ruicong 彭瑞聰, Cai Renhua 蔡仁华, and Zhou Caiming 周采铭, 94. Dalian: Dalian chubanshe.

Li Ting'an 李廷安. 1935c. *Zhongguo xiangcun weisheng wenti* 中國鄉村衛生問題 [China's rural health care problems]. Shanghai: Shangwu yinshuguan.

Li Wenbo 李文波. 2004. *Zhongguo chuanranbing shiliao* 中国传染病史料 [Historical materials relating to infectious disease in China]. Beijing: Huaxue gongye chubanshe.

Li Xiaojiang 李小江. 2003. *Rang nuren ziji shuohua* 让女人自己说话 [Let women speak for themselves]. Beijing: Shenghuo, dushu, xinzhi san lian shudian.

Li Yousong 李友松. 2006. "Wo guo xuexichongbing ruogan shiliao yu kaozheng" 我国血吸虫病若干史料与考证 [Research and historical materials on China's schistosomiasis]. In *Zhongguo xuexichongbing fangzhi licheng yu zhanwang* 中国血吸虫病防治历程与展望 [The retrospection and prospect of schistosomiasis prevention in China], edited by Wang Longde 王陇德, 16–23. Beijing: Renmin weisheng chubanshe.

Li Zhenglan 李正兰. 1992b. "Wo canjia xuefang kepu gongzuo" 我参加血防科普工作 [I participated in the work to popularize the science of prevention]. Compiled by Ning Haisheng 宁海生. In *Songwenshen jishi* 送瘟神纪实 [Record of bidding farewell to the God of Plague], edited by Liu Yurui 刘玉瑞 and Wan Guohe 万国和, 132–134. Jiangxi wenshi ziliao 江西文史资料 [Literary and historical materials of Jiangxi Province] 43. Nanchang: Jiangxi Sheng zhengxie wenshi ziliao yanjiu weiyuanhui.

Li Zhonglai 李仲来. 2002. "Zhongguo 1901–2000 nian ren jian shuyi dongtai guilv" 中国1901–2000 年人间鼠疫动态规律 [Laws and trends governing human plague in China between 1901 and 2000]. *Zhongguo difang bingxue zazhi* 中国地方病学杂志, no. 4, 294.

Liang Shuming 梁漱溟. 2002 [1921]. *Dongxi wenhua ji qi zhexue* 東西文化及其哲學 [Eastern and Western cultures and their philosophies]. Taibei: Taiwan shangwu.

Lin Juying 林菊英. 2004. "*Zhonghua huli zazhi* yu huli xueke gongjin" 《中华护理杂志》与护理学科共进 [*Chinese Journal of Nursing* and the advance of the discipline of nursing]. *Zhonghua huli zazhi* 中华护理杂志 39 (5): 321.

Lin Kesheng 林可胜. 1937. "Sulian de yixue jiaoyu" 素連的醫學教育 [Soviet medical education]. *Yiyu* 醫育 2 (8): 1–9.

Lin Peng 林鹏, He Qun 何群, and Wan Zhuoye 万卓越. 2004. *Aizibing yufang yu kongzhi* 艾滋病预防与控制 [Prevention and control of AIDS]. Guangzhou: Guangzhou keji chubanshe.

"Linshi jiaoyu weiyuanhui jishi" 臨時教育委員會紀事 [Temporary education committee record]. 1912. *Minlibao* 民立報, July 26.

Liu (J. Heng) Ruiheng 刘瑞恒. 1996 [1937]. "Shi nian lai de Zhongguo yiyao weisheng" 十年来的中国医药卫生 [Ten years of medicine and hygiene in China]. In *Shi nian lai de Zhongguo* 十年来的中国 [The last ten years in China], edited by Zhongguo wenhua jianshe xiehui 中国文化建设协会, 434–459. Minguo congshu 民国丛书, vol. 5, no. 69. Shanghai: Shanghai shudian.

Liu Bingfan 劉炳凡 and Zhou Shaoming 周紹明, eds. 1999. *Huxiang mingyi dianji jinghua* 湖湘名医典籍精华 [The essence of canonical writings of famous doctors of Hunan]. Changsha: Hunan kexue jishu chubanshe.

Liu Bingtao 刘炳涛. 2007. "1932 nian Shanxi sheng de huoluan yiqing ji qi shehui yingdui" 1932 年陕西省的霍乱疫情及其社会应对 [The cholera situation and its social reactions in Shanxi Province in 1932]. *Zhongguo lishi dili luncong* 中国历史地理论丛, no. 3: 113–124.

Liu Jianjun 刘剑君, Wang Lixia 王黎霞, Yao Hongyan 么鸿雁, Wang Ping 王萍, and Zheng Wenjing 郑文静. 2011b. "1984–2008 nian Zhongguo jiehebing siwang shuju gaikuang fenxi" 1984–2008 年中国结核病死亡数据概况分析 [Profile analysis of China TB mortality information from 1984 to 2008]. Zhongguo fanglao zazhi 中国防痨杂志 33 (7): 438–441.

Liu Lihong 刘力红. 2006. *Sikao zhongyi* 思考中医 [Contemplating Chinese medicine]. 3rd ed. Guilin: Guanxi shifan daxue chubanshe.

Liu Yanping. 刘燕萍. 2009b. "Waixiang hushi dui Zhongguo jindai huli de zuoyong yu yingxiang" 外籍护士对中国近代护理的作用与影响 [Foreign nurses' roles and influences on Chinese modern nursing]. Translated by Na Wu. *Zhongguo huli shi* 中国护理史 3: 34–35.

Liu Zhemin 劉振民 and Cui Wenzhi 崔文志. 1990. *Shixian yu tansuo: Zhongguo gaodeng zhonyiyao jiaoyu shi* 实践与探索: 中国高等中医药教育四十年史 [Practice and exploration: The history of forty years of higher education in Chinese medicine]. Beijing: Zhongguo zhongyiyao chubanshe.

Liu Zhiqin 刘志琴, ed. 1998. *Jindai Zhongguo shehui wenhua bianqian lu* 近代中國社會文化變遷錄 [A Record of social and cultural change in modern China]. Vol. 2. Hangzhou: Zhejiang renmin chubanshe.

Lü Ci 吕慈, Yu Yingli 于英丽, Wang Zhandong 王占东, and Han Yukai 韩雨凯. 1997. "1950 nian yilai wo guo chuanranbing tongji ziliao liuxingbingxue fenxi" 1950 年以来我国传染病统计资料流行病学分析 [Epidemiological analysis of our nation's statistical materials on contagious diseases since 1950]. *Zhongguo weisheng tongji* 中国卫生统计, no. 4: 38–39.

Lu Fenyao 陆焚尧, chief ed. 1999. *Lu Shouyan xueshu jingyan ji* 陆瘦燕学术经验集 [Collected scholarly experiences of Lu Shouyan]. Shanghai: Shanghai zhongyiya daxue chubanshe.

Lu Yongchun 卢永春. 1930. "Beiping xuexiao weisheng wenti" 北平學校衛生問題 [Issues in Beiping school public health]. *Yixue zhoukan ji* 醫學周刊集 4: 15.

———. 1937. *Laobing lun* 癆病論 [Discussion of tuberculosis]. Beiping: Zhonghua yixue hui fan lao ji jin she.

Lu Zonghan 盧崇漢. 2006. *Fu yang jiangji* 扶陽講記 [Notes on supporting yang]. Beijing: Zhongguo zhongyiyao chubanshe.

Lufei Kui 陆费逵. 2007. "Lun ge guo jiaokeshu" 论各国教科书 [Discussion of each nation's textbooks]. In *Zhongguo jindai jiaoyushi ziliao huibian: Jiaoyu sixiang* 中国近代教育史资料汇编·教育思想 [Collected historical materials of education in modern China:

Educational philosophy], edited by Qu Xingui 璩鑫圭 and Tong Fuyong 童富勇, 875–881. Shanghai: Shanghai jiaoyu chubanshe.

LWBW (Lin'anxian weishengzhi bianzhuan weiyuanhui) 临安县卫生志编撰委员会, ed. 1992. *Lin'anxian weishengzhi* 临安县卫生志 [Lin'an county health gazetteer]. Lin'an, Hangzhou, Zhejiang: Lin'an xian weishengju.

Ma Boying 马伯英. 1993. *Zhongguo yixue wenhua shi* 中国医学文化史 [A cultural history of Chinese medicine]. Shanghai: Shanghai People's Publishing House.

Ma Huanyun 马焕云, Wei Fang 魏芳, Li Yaozhen 李尧振, and Ma Lianshun 马连顺. 2001. "Guanyu dui sinian zhi huli zhuanye jiaoxue jihua ji dagang de ji dian yijian" 关于对四年制护理专业教学计划及大纲的几点意见 [On the 4-year nursing education and curriculum]. *Zhongdeng yixue jiaoyu* 中等医学教育 19 (S1): 4.

Mao Zhixiao 毛志霄. 1992. "Wo canjia songwenshen de licheng (Guangfeng)" 我参加送瘟神的历程 (广丰) [The process of my participation in bidding farewell to the God of Plague (Guangfeng county)]. In *Songwenshen jishi* 送瘟神纪实 [Record of bidding farewell to the God of Plague], edited by Liu Yurui 刘玉瑞 and Wan Guohe 万国和, 31–41. Jiangxi wenshi ziliao 江西文史资料 [Literary and historical materials of Jiangxi Province] 43. Nanchang: Jiangxi Sheng zhengxie wenshi ziliao yanjiu weiyuanhui.

Mei Renlang 梅人郎. 1993. *Zhongwai yixue jiaoyu shi* 中外医学教育比较 [A comparison of Chinese and foreign medical education]. Shanghai: Shanghai yike daxue chubanshe.

Mei Yulin 梅玉麟, Zhong Zhesheng 衷浙生, and Wang Wenzhen 王文珍, eds. 1991. "Xuhui qu jiehebing fei bu zhongliu fangzhi suo suo zhi" 徐汇区结核病肺部肿瘤防治所所志 [Chronicle of the Xuhui district TB and lung tumor prevention and treatment station]. Unpublished manuscript.

Meng Qingyun 孟庆云, ed. 1999. *Zhongguo zhongyiyao fazhan wushi nian* 中国中医药发展五十年 [Fifty years of development of Chinese medicine and drugs in China]. Zhengzhou: Henan yike daxue chubanshe.

Min Dahong 闵大洪. 1986. "'Su shang' shidai chubanshe yu 'Shidai' zhoukan, 'Shidai Ribao'" '苏商'时代出版社与<时代>周刊、<时代日报> [*The Soviet Union Times Press* and the *Times* magazine and *Times Daily*]. Xinwen yanjiu ziliao 新闻研究资料, no. 2, 134–144.

Min Zeng 敏增. 1952. "Yongyuan wei Zhongguo renmin huainian de Sulian yixue jiaoyu zhuanjia Bikuofu" 永远为中国人民怀念的苏联医学教育专家比阔夫 [The Soviet medical education expert whom the Chinese people will forever remember: Bykov]. *Renmin ribao* 人民日报, November 13.

Ministry of Health. 2010. *Zhongguo weisheng tongji nianjian* 中国卫生统计年鉴 [China public health statistical yearbook]. Beijing: Peking Union Medical College.

National Bureau of Statistics of China. 2011. *Zhongguo tongji nianjian* 中国统计年鉴 [China statistical yearbook]. Beijing: China Statistics Press.

Neizhengbu nianjian bianzuan weiyuanhui 內政部年鑒編纂委員會. 1936. *Neizheng nianjian* 內政年鑒 [Yearbook of internal affairs]. Vol. 4. Shanghai: Shangwu yinshuguan.

Niu Yahua 牛亚华. 2004. "Ding Fubao yu jindai zhongri yixue jiaoliu" 丁福保与近代中日医学交流 [Ding Fubao and modern Chinese and Japanese medical exchange]. *Zhongguo keji shiliao* 中国科技史料 25 (4): 315–329.

Ono Tokuichirō 小野得一郎. 1935. *Zhonghua minguo yishi zonglan* 中华民国医事综览 [A survey of medicine in the Republic of China]. Tokyo: Tongren hui.

Ono Yoshirō 小野芳朗. 1997. *Seiketsu no kindai: Eisei shōka kara kōkin gutsuzuhe* 清潔の近代: 衞生唱歌から抗菌グツズへ [The modernization of hygiene: From "the songs of hygiene" to "antibiotic substances"]. Tokyo: Kōdansha.

Pan Suiming 潘绥铭, Huang Yingying 黄盈盈, and Li Shun 李楯. 2006. "Zhongguo aizibing 'wenti' jiexi" 中国艾滋病"问题"解析 [An analysis of the "problem" of AIDS in China]. *Zhongguo shehui kexue* 中国社会科学, no. 1: 85–95.

Petrushevskii, S. A. 1953. *Bafuluofu weiwu zhuyi xueshuo* 巴甫洛夫唯物主义学说 [Pavlov's materialist doctrine]. Beijing: Zhongguo kexueyuan.

Pipunyrov, P. N. 1956. *Bafuluofu guanyu liang zhong xin hao xitong de xueshuo yu makesi zhuyi* 巴甫洛夫关于两种信号系统的学说与马克思主义 [Pavlov's theory on two kinds of signaling systems and Marxism]. Beijing: Kexue chubanshe.

Qian Jinyang 錢今陽, ed. 1950. *Shanghai mingyi zhi* 上海名醫誌 [Record of famous doctors in Shanghai]. Shanghai: Zhongguo yixue chubanshe.

Qin Bowei 秦伯未. 1929. "Jiaowu baogao" 教務報告 [Report on educational service]. *Zhongguo yixueyuan kan* 中國醫學院刊 1 (1): Appendix 6-7.

Qu Limei 曲黎梅. 2007. *Huangdi neijing yangsheng zhihui* 黃帝內經養生智慧 [The wisdom of the Huangdi neijing for nourishing life]. Xiamen: Lujiang chubanshe.

Ren Yingqiu 任應秋. 1980. *Zhongyi gejia xueshuo* 中醫各家學說 [Theories of each expert in Chinese medicine] Rev. ed. Shanghai: Shanghai kexue jishu chubanshe.

———. 1981. "Yixue liupai suhui lun" 医学流派溯洄论 [Discussion of medical sects going upstream]. *Beijing zhongyi xueyuan xuebao* 北京中医学院学报 1: 1-6.

Ren Yunlan 任云兰. 2009. "Dutong yamen shiqi Tianjin gonggong huanjing weisheng guanli chutan" 都统衙门时期天津公共环境卫生管理初探 [A first exploration of environmental public health administration in Tianjin by the yamen and military governor]. *Tianjin shehui kexue* 天津社会科学, no. 6: 127-131.

"Report of the Technical Agent of the Council on His Mission in China from the Date of Appointment until April 1, 1934." n.d. *Guo wen bao* 国闻报 11: 20-23.

Sanetō Keishū さねとう・けいしゅう (实藤惠秀). 1983. *Zhongguoren liuxue riben shi* 中国人留学日本史 [A history of Chinese studying in Japan]. Translated by Tan Ruqian 谭汝谦 and Lin Qiyan 林启彦.

Shanghai fanglao xiehui 上海防癆協會. 1953a. *Shanghai fanglao xiehui yi jiu wu er nian nianbao* 上海防癆協會一九五二年年報 上海防痨协会一九五二年年报 [Shanghai Anti-Tuberculosis Association 1952 annual report]. Shanghai: Shanghai fanglao xiehui.

———. 1953b. "Shanghai fanglao xiehui yi jiu wu er nian gongzuo zongjie" 上海防癆協會一九五二年工作總結 [SATA's 1952 work summary]. *Fanglao tongxun* 防痨通讯 6 (3): 1-5.

Shanghai tongjig nianjian 上海统计年鉴 [Shanghai statistical yearbooks]. 1992-2008. Shanghai: Shanghai kexue jishu wenxian chubanshe.

Shanghai zhongyi xueyuan 上海中醫學院, ed. 1962. *Jindai zhongyi liupai jingyan xuanji* 近代中醫流派經驗選集 [Selected experiences of Chinese medical currents of the modern era]. Shanghai: Shanghai kexue jishu chubanshe.

Shao Huaze 邵华泽, ed. 1993. *Guoqing zonglan* 国情总揽 [Assume responsibility for the state of the country]. Jinan: Shandong jiaoyu chubanshe.

Shao Jing 邵京. 2010. *Jilu yu sixiang: Nongcun you chang xian xue yu HIV ganran* 记录与思考: 农村有偿献血与HIV感染 [Record and consider: The countryside experiences the effects of payment for drawing blood and HIV]. In *Renming guantian* 人命关天 [A matter of life and death], edited by Xu Jiexun 徐杰舜 and Qing Hongzeng 秦红增, 228-239. Harbin: Heilongjian renmin chubanshe.

Shen Zhihua 沈志华. 2003. *Sulian zhuanjia zai Zhongguo 1948-1960* 苏联专家在中国 1948-1960 [Soviet experts in China, 1948-1960]. Beijing: Zhongguo guoji guangbo chubanshe.

"Shenshou pinxia zhongnong huanying de hezuo yiliao" 深受贫下中农欢迎的合作医疗 [Cooperative medical service warmly welcomed by poor and lower-middle peasants]. 1968. *Renmin ribao* 人民日报, December 5.

Shi Yali 施亚利. 2010. "Minguo shiqi Jiangsu sheng de xuefang gongzuo" 民国时期江苏省的血防工作 [The work of schistosomiasis prevention in Jiangsu Province during China's Republican period]. *Lishi jiaoxue* 历史教学 599 (10): 24-29.

Shidai gongbao 時代公報 [Times Bulletin]. 1933. No. 28.

Song Guobin 宋国宾. 1935. "Tan yi pai gao fa bi pai yijia" 谈医派, 告法比派医家 [Essay on the medical profession and talking to the French-Belgian Medical School]. *Yiyao pinglun* 医药评论 7 (3): 3.

Song Jiazhao 宋嘉钊. 1936. *Taijiao, Nuxue Congshu Zhiyi* 胎教, 女學叢書之一 [Fetal education, one of a series on women's studies]. 19th ed. Shanghai: Zhonghua shuje yinxing.

Song Yandong. 1953. "Xia chang fanglao de yi ge zhongdian shiyan: Shanghai guo mian wu chang tuixing fanglao gongzuo chubu zongjie" 下厂防痨的一个重点试验：上海国棉五厂推行防痨工作初步总结 [First anti-TB focal point testing: Initial results of TB prevention work at the Fifth National Cotton Factory]. *Shanghai fanglao* 上海防痨 3 (6): 6–10.

"Sulian gonggong weisheng shizhi" 苏联公共卫生实质 [The essence of Soviet public health]. 1934. *Zhonghua yixue zazhi* 中华医学杂志 20: 11–12.

Sun Baigang 孙百刚, ed. 1934. *Geguo jiaoyu zhidu ji gaikuang* 各国教育制度及概况 [Each nation's educational system and situation]. Shanghai: Xin Zhongguo jianshe xuehui chubanke.

Sun Qi 孙琦. 2007. "Shenti de zhengduo: 1950 niandai houqi de jiangnan xuexichongbing fangzhi—Yi Qingpu xian wei zhongxin" 身体的争夺：1950年代后期的江南血吸虫病防治—以青浦县为中心 [A contest of the body: Prevention and treatment of schistosomiasis in the Jiangnan region in the later 1950s—In which Qingpu county serves as the center]. *Lishi renleixue xuekan* 历史人类学学刊 5 (2): 105–112.

Sun Yanchang 孫延昌, ed. 2000. *Jingcheng guoyi pu* 京城國醫譜 [Guide to national medicine in the capital]. Beijing: Zhongguo zhongyiyao keji chubanshe.

Sun Zhongliang 孙忠亮. 1981. "Shanghai jiehebing fangzhi jinkuang yu jidian yijian" 上海结核病防治近况与几点意见 [Shanghai's prevention and treatment situation with suggestions]. *Shanghai fanglao tongxun* 上海防痨通讯 3 (1): 4–7.

Suzhou tongji ju 苏州统计局. 2010. *Suzhou tongji nianjian* 苏州统计年鉴－2010 [Suzhou statistical yearbook—2010]. Beijing: Zhongguo tongji chubanshe.

Suzhou xuefang shi zhi bianzuan weiyuanhui 蘇州血防史志編纂委員會. 1997. *Suzhou xuefang shi zhi* 蘇州血防史志 [Record of the prevention of schistosomiasis in Suzhou]. Shanghai: Shanghai kexue jishu chubanshe.

Tan Ruqian 谭汝谦. 1980. *Zhongguo yi Riben shu zhonghe mulu* 中国译日本书综合目录 [A comprehensive catalog of books translated from Chinese into Japanese]. Hong Kong: Xianggang zhongwen daxue chubanshe.

Tan Shouren 譚守仁. 1929. "Kaocha Ouzhou shehui weisheng jishi" 考察歐洲社會衛生紀事 [Chronicle of surveys of European social hygiene]. *Yiyao pinglun* 醫藥瓶論, no. 20: 12–15.

Tian Tao 田涛 and Guo Chengwei 郭成伟, eds. 1996. *Qing mo Beijing chengshi guanli fagui (1906–1910)* 清末北京城市管理法规 (1906–1910) [The administration and laws of the city of Beijing at the end of the Qing, 1906–1910]. Beijing: Beijing yanshan chubanshe.

———. 2004. "Zhongguo chengshi guanli zouxiang jindaihua de lichengbei: Xin faxian de Qing mo Beijing chengshi guanli fagui yanjiu" 中国城市管理走向近代化的里程碑—新发现的清末北京城市管理法规研究 [Milestones in the progress of China's urban administration toward modernization: Newly discovered legal research into the urban administration of Beijing at the end of the Qing]. In *Di'er fa men* 第二法门 [The second method of law], edited by Tian Tao 田涛, 14–27. Beijing: Falv chubanshe.

Tian Zhengping 田正平 and Yu Qian 于谦. 2010. "Jiaoyu juece minzhuhua de zuichu changshi" 教育决策民主化的最初尝试 [The first attempt to democratize educational policy]. *Gaodeng jiaoyu yanjiu* 高等教育研究 31 (1): 77–82.

12DQJ (12 di qu jingshen jibing liuxing xue diaocha xiezuo zu) 12地区精神疾病流行学调查协作组. 1986. "Ge lei jingshenbing, yaowu yilai, jiu yilai ji ren ge zhang'ai de diaocha ziliao fenxi" 各类精神病, 药物依赖, 酒依赖及人格障碍的调查资料分析 [Analysis of survey results of all types of psychiatric illnesses, drug and alcohol dependence and personality disorders]. *Zhonghua shenjing jingshen ke zazhi* 19 (2): 70–72.

"Waijiaobu pinqing Laximan deng san xi yuan wei benbu guwen" 外交部聘請拉西曼等三西員為本部顧問 [The foreign ministry has invited Rajchman and two other Western officials to serve as advisors]. 1929. *Weisheng gongbao* 衛生公報, no. 3: 62.

Wang Chongren 王忠仁. 2004. "Zhuiyi woguo jiehe bing fangzhi shiye de xian qu qiu zu yuan jiaoshou" 追忆我国结核病防治事业的先驱裘祖源教授 [Recalling the pioneer of our nation's tuberculosis prevention and treatment work, Professor Qiu Zuyuan]. *Zhonghua jiehe he huxi zazhi* 中华结核和呼吸杂志 27 (12): 794–796.

Wang Huobian 王火编. 1952. "Zhongyang weisheng bu gongkuang fanglao ban kaixue le" 中央卫生部工矿防痨班开学了 [Central Ministry of Health class for miners to prevent tuberculosis opened]. *Zhongguo fanglao zazhi* 中国防痨杂志, no. 6: 15.

Wang Kangjiu 王康久, ed. 1996b. *Beijing weisheng dashi ji (di yi juan)* 北京卫生大事记 (第一卷) [Chronicle of events related to hygiene in Beijing, Vol. 1]. Beijing: Beijing kexue jishu chubanshe.

———, ed. 2001. *Beijing weisheng zhi* (北京卫生志) [Health chronology of Beijing]. Beijing: Beijing Science and Technology Press.

Wang Ping 王平. 2011. "Kang zhan qian Nanjing guomin zhengfu weisheng yundong yanjiu" 抗战前南京国民政府卫生运动研究 [Research on hygiene movements conducted by the national government at Nanjing before the War of Resistance]. Master's thesis, Hunan Normal University.

Wang Qi 王琦. 1995a. "Ershiyi shiji—zhongyiyao de shiji" 二十一世紀—中醫藥的世紀 [21st century: The era of Chinese medicine]. *Chuantong wenhua yu xiandaihua* 传统文化与现代化 2: 64–67.

Wang Qiaochu 王翹楚. 1998. *Yilin chunqiu—Shanghai zhongyi zhongxiyi jiehe fazhan shi* 医林春秋: 上海中医中西医结合发展史 [The annals of medical circles—The history of Chinese medicine in Shanghai and the combination of traditional and Chinese medicine]. Shanghai: Wenhui chubanshe.

Wang Saite 王赛特. 2007. "Zhongyi xianzhuang diaocha" 中医现状调查 [A survey of the present conditions of Chinese medicine]. *Zhongguo xinwen zhoukan* 中国新闻周刊. http://www.chinanews.com.cn/other/news/2007/01-22/858935.shtml.

Wang Xiaojing 王小京. 2010. "Guanyu Taigang xuezhe dui 20 shiji 50–60 niandai Zhongguo dalu jiaoyu yanjiu wenti de pingxi" 关于台港学者对20世纪50–60年代中国大陆教育研究问题的评析 [On Taiwanese and Hong Kong scholars' critique of research questions relating to Chinese mainland education during the 1950s and 1960s]. *Xuelilun* 学理论, no. 3: 97–99.

Wang Ximeng 王希孟. 1988. *Shanghai xiaomie xuexichongbing de huigu* 上海消灭血吸虫病的回顾 [Review of elimination of schistosomiasis in Shanghai]. Shanghai: Shanghai kexue jishu chubanshe.

Wang Xiuying 王琇瑛. 1986. "Relie zhuhe 'Hushi jinxiu zazhi' chuangkan" 热烈祝贺《护士进修杂志》创刊 [Warm congratulations to founding of *Journal of Nurses Training*]. *Hushi jinxiu zazhi* 护士进修杂志 1: 4.

Wang Xuede 王学德, ed. 1995b. *Nanjing xuefang zhi* 南京血防志 [Record of the prevention of schistosomiasis in Nanjing]. Nanjing: Jiangsu kexue jishu chubanshe.

Wang Yiqiang 王益锵. 2000. *Zhongguo huli fazhan shi* 中国护理发展史 [A history of Chinese nursing]. Beijing: Zhongguo yiyao keji chubanshe.

Wang Yongyan 王永炎 and Wang Yaoting 王耀廷, eds. 2000. *Jinri zhongyi fuke* 今日中医妇科 [Today's traditional Chinese gynecology]. Beijing: Renmin weisheng chubanshe.

Wang Zhipu 王致谱 and Cai Jingfeng 蔡景峰, eds. 1999. *Zhongguo zhongyiyao 50 nian* 中国中医药50年 [Fifty years of Chinese medicine in China]. Fuzhou: Fujian kexue jishu chubanshe.

"Wei Zhongguo renmin fuwu de Beijing Sulian hongshizi yiyuan" 为中国人民服务的北京苏联红十字医院 [The Beijing-Soviet Red Cross Hospital for the service of the Chinese people]. 1954. *Renmin ribao* 人民日报, March 31.

"Weida lingxiu maozhuxi shenqie guanhuai guangda geming renmin zai quanguo fanwei nei shixian yaopin quanmian dafudu jiangjia" 伟大领袖毛主席深切关怀广大革命人民在全国范围内实现药品全面大幅度降价 [Great leader Chairman Mao takes care of the vast masses of revolutionary people and implements complete and large-scale price reduction]. 1969. *Renmin ribao* 人民日报, September 25.

"Weisheng yundong dahui shixing dagang" 衛生運動大會施行大綱 [Outline for implementation of hygiene movement rally]. 1928. *Shizheng yuekan* 市政月刊 (Hangzhou) 1 (9): 16–17.

"Weishengbu guwen laximan yijianshu zhaiyao" 衛生部顧問拉西曼意見書摘要 [Summary of the opinion of Department of Public Health consultant Laximan (Ludwik Rajchman)]. 1930. *Yiyao pinglun* 医药评论, no. 25: 45–47.

Weishengshu 衛生署. 1937. *Jiuzhong fading chuanranbing qianshuo* 九種法定傳染病淺說 [A brief introduction to the nine notifiable infectious diseases]. Nanjing: Weishengshu.

Weng Naiqun 翁乃群. 2001. "Aizibing de shehui wenhua jiangou" 艾滋病的社会文化建构 [The social and cultural construction of AIDS]. *Qinghua shehuixue pinglun* 清华社会学评论, no. 1: 17–37.

Woyi 我一 [pseud.]. 1912. "Linshi jiaoyu huiyi riji" 臨時教育會議日記 [Diary of the temporary education conference]. *Jiaoyu zazhi* 教育雜誌, no. 6: 1–16.

Wu Dui 吳兌. 1907. *Weisheng xin lun* 衛生新論 [New discussion of hygiene]. Shanghai: Zhongguo tushu gongsi.

Wu Lien-teh (Wu Liande) 伍连德. 1915a. *Lun Zhongguo dang chou fangbing zhi fang shixing weisheng zhi fa* 論中國當籌防病之方施行衛生之法 [Discussion of the ways in which China must plan to prevent disease and implement hygiene]. *Dongfang zazhi* 東方雜誌 12 (2): 6–10.

——. 1915b. "Zhongguo ji yi moujin yixue jiaoyu" 中國急宜謀進醫學教育 [China should anxiously plan to improve medical education]. *Dongfang zazhi* 東方雜誌, no. 1: 4.

——. 1929. Zhongguo gonggong weisheng zhi jingfei wenti 中國公共衛生之經費問題 [Financial problems of public health in China]. *Zhonghua yixue zazhi* 中華醫學雜誌 15 (4): 351–354.

——. 1934a. "Guanyu Zhongguo yixue zhi guanjian" 關於中國醫學之管見 [My humble opinion of Chinese medicine]. *Zhonghua yixue zazhi* 中華醫學雜誌 20 (1): 3–4.

——. 1934b. "Zhiliao feilao xinfa" 治療肺癆新法 [New methods of tuberculosis treatment]. *Fanglao zazhi* 防癆杂志 1 (4): 205–206.

Wu Qian 吳谦, ed. 2002 [1742]. *Yuzuan yizong jinjian* 御纂醫宗金鑒 [Imperially commissioned Golden Mirror of the Medical Lineage]. Beijing: Wuying dian. Reprint, Wenyuan ge Siku quanshu 文淵閣四庫全書, 1782. Modern facsimile edition Hong Kong: Dizhi wenhua chuban youxian gongsi.

Wu Shaoqing 吳紹青. 1952. "Shanghai ruhe fanglao" 上海如何防癆 [How does Shanghai prevent tuberculosis?]. *Shanghai weisheng* 上海卫生 2 (1): 34–36.

Wu Shenglin 吳生林, chief ed. 1955. "Translators' Note." In *Bafuluofu xuanji* 巴甫洛夫选集 [Selected works of Pavlov], edited by Zhongguo kexue xinli yanjiu shi 中国科学心理研究室编辑. Beijing: Kexue chubanshe.

Wu Zhongdao 吳忠道, Lu Zhiyue 呂志躍, Zhang Shuangmin張雙民, Wang Li 王麗, Hu Fei 胡斐, and Florian Rubelt. 2006. "1933–1949 nian Zhongguo xuexichong bing yanjiu qingkuang" 1933–1949 年中国血吸虫病研究情况 [Schistosomiasis research in China from 1933 to 1949]. In *Zhongguo Xuexichongbing fangzhi licheng yu zhanwang* 中国血吸虫病防治历程与展望, edited by Wang Longde 王隴德, 42–49. Beijing: Renmin weisheng chubanshe.

Wu Zunyou 吳尊友, Qi Guoming 祁国明, and Zhang Jiapeng 张家鹏, eds. 1999. *Aizibing liuxing yu kongzhi* 艾滋病流行与控制 [The spread and control of AIDS]. Beijing: Kexue chubanshe.

Wuzhong yiji bianxiezu 吳中医集编写组, ed. 1993. *Wuzhong yiji* 吳中医集 [Volume on Chinese medicine in the Wu region]. Changzhou: Jiangsu kexue jishu chubanshe.

Xian Weixun 冼维逊. 1988. *Shuyi liuxing shi* 鼠疫流行史 [History of the spread of plague]. Guangzhou: Guangdong sheng weisheng fangyi zhan.

Xiao Aishu 肖爱树. 2003. "1949–1959 nian aiguo weisheng yundong shulun" 1949–1959 年爱国卫生运动述论 [A narration and discussion of the Patriotic Hygiene Movement from 1949 to 1959]. *Dangdai zhongguo shi yanjiu* 当代中国史研究, no. 1: 498–514.

"Xijing yishi gonghui guoyixue jiaoyu dui Nanjing yixue jiaoyu weiyuanhui suo ni yix-ueyuan kecheng dagang pingyi dian dayao" 西京醫師公會國醫學教育對南京醫學教育委員會所擬醫學院課程大綱評議點大要 [Main points of the discussion that the Xijing (Xi'an) Medical Association for State Medical Education held on the medical school curriculum outline that the Committee on Medical Education in Nanjing has planned]. 1935. *Yishi huikan* 醫事匯刊 23: 165.

Xin Zhike 辛智科. 2002. "1956 nian Sulian zhuanjia zai Shaanxi diaocha difangbing de qing-kuang" 1956年苏联专家在陕西调查地方病的情况 [The 1956 survey by Soviet experts of the local disease situation in Shaanxi]. *Zhonghua yishi zazhi* 中华医史杂志, no. 4: 247.

Xin Zhongguo yufang yixue lishi jingyan weiyuanhui 新中国预防医学历史经验委员会, ed. 1988–1991. *Xin Zhongguo yufang yixue lishi jingyan* 新中国预防医学历史经验 [History and experiences of preventive medicine in the new China]. 5 vols. Beijing: Renmin weisheng chubanshe.

Xu Shijin 許世瑾. 1933. "Quanguo dengji yishi tongji" 全國登記醫師統計 [Statistics on doctors that the nation has registered]. *Zhonghua yixue zazhi* 中華醫學雜誌 19 (4): 677–678.

Xu Youjun 许友君. 2005. "Meiguo huli jiaoyu sixiang ji qi dui woguo de qishi" 美国护理教育思想及其对我国的启示 [American nursing education thought and inspiration for China]. *Dalian daxue xuebao* 大连大学学报 26 (6): 26–28.

Xu Yuangen 徐元根, ed. 1991. *Fuyangxian weishengzhi* 富阳县卫生志 [Fuyang county health gazetteer]. Beijing: Zhongguo yiyao keji chubanshe.

"Xunjingbu nipin weisheng guwenguan" 巡警部拟聘卫生顾问官 [Department of Police plan to engage health advisors]. 1906. *Shibao* 时报, January 3.

Yan Dakui 殷大奎. 2006. "Guanyu jianli Beiping gaoxiao de weisheng yiliao fuwu tixi" 关于建立公平高效的卫生医疗服务体系 [On establishing a highly efficient hygiene and healing service system in the city of Beiping]. September 20. http://finance.sina.com.cn/hy/20060920/15262932019.shtml.

Yan Fuqing 颜福庆. 1914. "Yixue gailun" 醫學概論 [General discussion of medicine]. In *Zhonghua jidujiao hui nianjian* 中華基督教會年鑒 [Yearbook of Chinese Christian missionaries], 124.

———. 1935. "Zhongguo yishi zhi qiantu" 中國醫事之前途 [Future of medical matters in China]. *Zhonghua yixue zazhi* 中華醫學雜誌 21 (11): 1187–1189.

Yan Renying 严仁英, ed. 1990. *Yang Chongrui boshi: Danchen bai nian ji nian* 杨崇瑞博士: 诞辰百年纪念 [Dr. Yang Chongrui: Centennial commemoration]. Beijing: Beijing yike daxue, zhongguo xiehe yike daxue lianhe chubanshe.

Yan S. M., D. Z. Xiang, Y. Z. Chao, D. Y. Chen, D. Q. Zhang, and M. A. Taylor. 1984. "The frequency of major psychiatric disorder in Chinese inpatients." *American Journal of Psychiatry* 139, 1150–1153.

Yan Weiran 严渭然. 1986. "Wei fazhan huli xueke er nuli—Zhuhe *Huli xue zazhi* chuangkan" 为发展护理学科而努力—祝贺《护理学杂志》创刊 [Work hard for nursing—Congratulation on the founding of the *Journal of Nursing Science*]. *Huli xue zazhi* 护理学杂志 1: 2.

Yan Youxiang 严有祥, ed. 1985. *Jiandexian yiyao weishengzhi* 建德县医药卫生志 [Jiande county health and pharmaceutical gazetteer]. Jiande: Jiandexian weishengju.

Yang Daozheng 杨道正. 1992. "Qumo you dang yizhi jian yin chu pikai xin tiandi (Fengxin)" 驱魔有党意志坚银锄劈开新天地 (奉新) [The party has unwavering determination to expel demons, a silver hoe can cleave open a new universe (Fengxin county)]. In *Songwenshen jishi* 送瘟神纪实 [Record of bidding farewell to the God of Plague], edited by Liu Yurui 刘玉瑞 and Wan Guohe 万国和, 16–22. Jiangxi wenshi ziliao 江西文史资料 [Literary and historical materials of Jiangxi Province] 43. Nanchang: Jiangxi Sheng zhengxie wenshi ziliao yanjiu weiyuanhui.

Yang Guo'an 杨国安, ed. 2002. *Zhongguo yanyeshi huidian* 中国烟业史汇典 [Documents on the history of Chinese tobacco]. Beijing: Guangming ribao chubanshe.

Yang, Marion (Yang Chongrui) 杨崇瑞. 1928b. "Chanke jiaoyu jihua" 産科教育計劃 [Plan for maternal health education]. *Zhonghua yixue zazhi* 中華醫學雜誌 14 (5): 61–68.

———. 1990. "Wode zizhuan" 我的自传 [My autobiography]. In *Yang Chongrui boshi: Danchen bai nian ji nian* 博士: 诞辰百年纪念 [Dr. Yang Chongrui: Centennial commemoration], edited by Yan Renying 严仁英, 143–153. Beijing: Beijing yike daxue, zhongguo xiehe yike daxue lianhe chubanshe.

Yang Nianqun 杨念群. 2006. *Zaizao "bingren": Zhongxiyi chongtuxia de zhengzhi kongjian, 1832–1985* 再造"病人": 中西医冲突下的空间政治 (1832–1985) [Remaking "patients": Spatial politics in the conflicts between Chinese and Western medicine, 1832–1985]. Beijing: Zhongguo renmin daxue chubanshe.

Yangpu qu jiehebing fangzhi suo. 杨浦区结核病防治所. 1992. "Shanghai shi Yangpu qu jiehebing fangzhi suo suozhi" 上海市杨浦区结核病防治所所志 [Chronicle of the Yangpu district tuberculosis prevention and treatment station]. Unpublished manuscript.

Yao 垚. 1929a. "Wasuo weisheng xueyuan zhi kecheng" 瓦梭衛生學院之課程 [The curriculum of Wasuo Hygiene School]. *Weisheng gongbao* 衛生公報 1 (3): 83–88.

———. 1929b. "Guoji lianmeng weishenghui yu Xila zhengfu hezuo jihua Xila weisheng zhi gaijin" 國際聯盟衛生會與希臘政府合作計劃希臘衛生之改進 [The League of Nations Health Organization and the Greek government's cooperative plan to improve Greek hygiene]. *Weisheng gongbao* 衛生公報 1 (8): 91–103.

"Yihu bili daozhi xianxiang dedao niuzhuan" 医护比例倒置现象得到扭转 [Optimizing the ratio of doctors to nurses]. 2011. *Huli guanli zazhi* 护理管理杂志 11 (6): 392.

"Yike daxue zhangcheng shangque" 醫科大學章程商榷 [Discussion of medical school regulations]. 1905. *Shibao* 時報, August.

Yin Lei 殷磊. 2006. "Zhongguo huli lilun yanjiu xianzhuang fenxi ji sikao" 中国护理理论研究现状分析及思考 [An analysis and suggestions on applying nursing theories in China]. *Zhongguo huli guanli* 中国护理管理 6 (6): 6–28.

Yiyao xuehui 醫藥學會. 1907. "Liuxuesheng riben yiyao xuexuai tongren xingming diaochabiao" 留學生日本醫藥學校同人姓名調查表 [Chart: Survey of names of foreign student classmates at Japanese schools of medicine and pharmacy]. *Yiyao Xuebao* 醫藥學報 6 (November): 1–4.

Yoshino Sakuzō 吉野作造. 1910. "Zai Qingguo fuwu zhi riben jiaoshi" 清国勤日本人教师 [Japanese educators in the service of the Qing]. *Guojia xuehui zazhi* 国家学会杂志 23 (5): 769–794.

Yu, Xinzhong 余新忠. 2003. *Qing dai jiangnan de wenyi yu shehui: Yi xiang yiliao shehui shi de yanjiu* 清代江南的瘟疫与社会——项医疗社会史的研究 [Plagues and society in the Jiangnan region during the Qing dynasty—Research on the social history of medical treatment]. Beijing: Zhongguo renmin daxue chubanshe.

———. 2008. "Cong biyi dao fangyi: Wan Qing yin ying yibing guannian de yanbian" 从避疫到防疫:晚清因应疫病观念的演变 [From escaping epidemics to preventing them: The evolution of concepts of coping with disease in late Qing]. *Huazhong Shifan Daxue xuebao* 华中师范大学学报, no. 2: 57–58.

———. 2009. *Fangyi, weisheng, shenti kongzhi: Wan Qing qingjie guannian he xingwei de yanbian* 防疫.卫生.身体控制—晚清清洁观念和行为的演变 [Preventing disease, hygiene, and controlling the body: The development of sanitary concepts and practices at the end of the Qing]. Beijing: Zhonghua shuju.

———. 2011a. "Lishi qingjing yu xianshi guanhuai: Wo yu Zhongguo jinshi weisheng shi yanjiu" 历史情境与现实关怀—我与中国近世卫生史研究 [Historical circumstance and practical concerns: Myself and research into China's contemporary history of hygiene]. *Anhui shi xue* 安徽史学, no. 4.

———. 2011b. "Wan Qing de weisheng xingzheng yu jindai shenti de xingcheng: Yi weisheng fangyi wei zhongxin 晚清的卫生行政与近代身体的形成—以卫生防疫为中心 [Hygiene administration at the end of the Qing and the formation of the modern body: Placing hygiene and disease prevention at the center]. *Qing shi yanjiu* 清史研究, no. 3: 48–68.

———. 2012. "Fuzaxing yu xiandaixing: Wan Qing jianyi ji zhi yin jian zhong de shehui fanying" 复杂性与现代性—晚清检疫机制引建中的社会反应 [Complexity and modernity: Social reactions to quarantine measures imposed in the late Qing]. *Jindai shi yanjiu* 近代史研究, no. 2: 47–64.

Yu, Xinzhong 余新忠, Zhao Xianhai 赵献海, Zhang Xiaochuan 张笑川, Hui Qinglou 惠清楼, Wuyungerile 乌云格日勒, and Zhao Qi 赵琦. 2004. *Wenyi xia de shehui zhengjiu: Zhongguo jin shi zhongda yiqing ji shehui yingdui yanjiu* 瘟疫下的社会拯救: 中国近世重大疫情及社会应对研究 [Saving a society gripped by pestilence: Research on China's great modern epidemics and society's response]. Beijing: Zhongguo shudian.

Yu Fengbin 俞鳳賓. 1930. *Weisheng conghua* 衛生叢話 [Chats on hygiene]. Shanghai: Shangwu yinshuguan.

Yu Guangyan 余光炎, ed. 1998. *Chun'anxian weishengzhi* 淳安县卫生志 [Chun'an county health gazetteer]. Chun'an: Chun'anxian renmin zhengfu jiguang yinshuachang.

Yu Laixi 余来喜. 1992. "Yujiang renmin fangzhi xuexichongbing de weida douzheng" 余江人民防治血吸虫病的伟大斗争 [The people of Yujiang's mighty battle to treat and prevent schistosomiasis]. In *Songwenshen jishi* 送瘟神纪实 [Record of bidding farewell to the God of Plague], edited by Liu Yurui 刘玉瑞 and Wan Guohe 万国和, 1–6. Jiangxi wenshi ziliao 江西文史资料 [Literary and historical materials of Jiangxi Province] 43. Nanchang: Jiangxi Sheng zhengxie wenshi ziliao yanjiu weiyuanhui.

Yu Qinglian 于清涟. 2001. "Zhishi jingji shidai yu woguo de gaodeng jiaoyu" 知识经济时代与我国的高等教育 [The era of the knowledge economy and Chinese higher education]. *Jiaoyu yu jingji* 教育与经济 1: 16–18.

Yu Yunxiu 余云岫 and Zu Shuxian 祖述宪. 2006. *Yu Yunxiu zhongyi yanjiu yu pipan* 余云岫中医研究与批判 [Yu Yunxiu's research and criticism of Chinese medicine]. Hefei: Anhui daxue chubanshe.

"Yuanqi" 缘起 [Origins]. 1929. *Yiyao pinglun* 医药评论 1 (1): 11.

Zhang, Daqing 张大庆. 2006a. *Zhongguo jindai jibing shehui shi (1912–1937)* 中国近代疾病社会史 (1912–1937) [A social history of disease in modern China, 1912–1937]. Jinan: Shandong jiaoyu chubanshe, 2006.

Zhang Feicheng 章斐成. 1934. "Wo guo fuying weisheng zhi gaikuang" 我國婦嬰衛生之概況 [The state of maternal and infant health in our nation]. *Yixue zhoukan ji* 醫學周刊集 6 (4): 85–88.

Zhang Gongyao 张功耀. 2006b. *Gao bie zhongyi zhongyao* 告别中医中药 [Farewell to Chinese medicine and Chinese herbs]. *Yixue yu zhexue (renwen shehui yixue ban)* 医学与哲学 人文社会医学版 27: 14–17.

Zhang Guojun 张国军, Sun Baoqing 孙宝清, and Zeng Haiqing 曾海清. 2004. "Yixue jiaoxue moshi qianxi" 医学教学模式浅析 [Medical education models and simple analysis]. *Xiandai yiyao weisheng* 现代医药卫生 20 (10): 937.

Zhang Jianchuan 张建川. 2010. "Aizibing fangzhi de zhengce fenxi" 艾滋病防治的政策分析 [Analysis of policies to prevent and cure AIDS]. http://wenku.baidu.com/view/1edfedf8aef8941ea76e05df.html.

Zhang Jiebin 張介賓. 1994 [1636]. *Jing Yue quanshu* 景岳全書 [The complete works of Jing Yue (Zhang Jiebin)]. Beijing: Zhongguo Zhongyiyao chubanshe.

Zhang Jin 张瑾. 2003. *Quanli, chongtu, yu biange: 1926–1937 nian Chongqing chengshi xiandaihua yanjiu* 权力，冲突，与变革：1926–1937年重庆城市现代化研究 [Power, conflict, and reform: The modernization of Chongqing 1926–1937]. Chongqing: Chongqing chubanshe.

Zhang Mingdao 张明岛 and Shao Jieqi 邵洁奇, eds. 1998. *Shanghai weisheng zhi* 上海卫生志 [Records of hygiene in Shanghai]. Shanghai: Shanghai shehui xueyuan chubanshe.

Zhang Taishan 张泰山. 2008. *Minguo shiqi de chuanranbing yu shehui—Yi chuanranbing fangzhi yu gonggong weisheng wei zhongxin* 民国时期的传染病与社会—以传染病防治与公共卫生为中心 [Infectious diseases and society during the Republican era—Placing infectious disease control and public health at the center]. Beijing: Shehui kexue wenxian chubanshe.

Zhang Taiyan 章太炎. 1936. "Shanghan lun yan jiang ci" 傷寒論演講詞 [Treatise on cold damage]. *Guoyi wenxian* 1 (1): 90–93.

Zhang Yuwen 张玉文. 2004. "Jiaoyu weisheng bu men lian shou gaige huli jiaoyu, jia kuai peiyang xun bu fa" 教育卫生部门联手改革护理教育,加快培养培训步伐 [The Education and Health Administrations are cooperating to reform nursing education and speed up the pace of training]. *Zhongguo jiaoyu bao* 中国教育报, January 16.

Zhang Zaitong 张在同 and Xian Rijin 咸日金, eds. 1990. *Minguo yiyao weisheng fagui xuanbian (1912–1948)* 民国医药卫生法规选编 (1912–1948) [Selected laws and regulations on medicine, drugs, and hygiene during the Republican era (1912–1948)]. Jinan: Shandong daxue chubanshe.

Zhang Zhongmin 张仲民. 2009b. *Wan Qing de weisheng shuji yanjiu: Chuban yu wenhua zhengzhi* 晚清的卫生书籍研究：出版与文化政治 [Literary research on hygiene at the end of the Qing: Publications and cultural administration]. Shanghai: Shanghai shudian chubanshe.

Zhao Hongjun 赵洪钧. 2006. *Huimou yu fansi: Zhong xi yi jiehe ershi jiang* 回眸与反思：中西医结合二十讲 [Looking back and reviewing: Twenty discussions of the union of Chinese and Western medicine]. Hefei: Anhui kexue jizhu chubanshe.

Zhejiang kexue jishu puji xiehui 浙江科学技术普及协会, and Zhejiang weisheng shiyanyuan 浙江卫生实验院. 1956. *Xiaomie xuexichongbing tujie* 消灭血吸虫病图解 [Charts on eliminating schistosomiasis]. Beijing: Renmin weisheng chuban she.

Zhen, Cheng 甄橙. 2008. *Yixue yu huli xue fazhan lishi* 医学与护理学发展历史 [A history of medicine and nursing]. Beijing: Beijing daxue yixue chubanshe.

Zheng Jie'an 郑介安. 1944. "Yiliao baojian xitong yu gongyi zhi bijiao yanjiu" 医疗保健系与公医制比较研究 [Comparative research on health care systems and public health service]. *Shehui Yixue* 社会医学 1 (2): 4.

"Zhiyou Sulian cai you kexue" 只有苏联才有科学 [Only the Soviets still have science]. *Kexue tongxun* 科学通讯, no. 6: 1

Zhong Huilan 鐘惠蘭. 1931. "Lun Zhongguo jiyi fazhan gonggong weisheng" 論中國急宜發展公共衛生 [Discussion of the impatient and appropriate development of public health in China]. *Zhongguo weisheng zazhi* 中國衛生雜誌, no. 22: 24–27.

Zhong Zubiao on behalf of Jiangxi sheng jiachu xuexichongbing fangzhi zhan 钟祖标, 江西省家畜血吸虫病防治站. 1998. *Jiangxi sheng jiachu xuefang zhi: 1956–1996* 江西省家畜血防志: 1956–1996 [Jiangxi gazetteer of schistosomiasis prevention of domestic animals: 1956–1996]. Nanchang: Jiangxi sheng jiachu xuefang zhi zhan.

Zhonggong zhongyang nanfang shisan sheng, shi, qu xuefang lingdao xiaozu bangongshi 中共中央南方十三省, 市, 区血防领导小组办公室, ed. 1978. *Song wenshen: Huace* 送瘟神: 画册 [Farewell to the God of Plague: Pictorial work]. Beijing: Zhonggong zhongyang nanfang shisan sheng, shi, qu xuefang lingdao xiaozu bangongshi.

"Zhongguo de yixue jiaoyu" 中國的醫學教育 [Medical education in China]. 1933. *Zhonghua yixue zazhi* 中華醫學雜誌 19 (2): 205.

Zhongguo fanglao xiehui 中國防癆協會. 1954. "Shanghai shi yi jiu wu san nian tui xing ka jie miao gongzuo zongjie baogao" 上海市一九五三年推行卡介苗工作總結報告 [Shanghai 1953 BCG work summary report]. *Fanglao tongxun* 防癆通訊 7 (4): 17–19.

———. 1980. "Wu Shaoqing jiaoshou shishi" 吴绍青教授逝世 [Professor Wu Shaoqing has died]. *Zhongguo fanglao tongxun* 中国防癆通讯, no. 2.

Zhongguo kexue jishu xiehui 中国科学技术协会, ed. 1991. *Zhongguo kexue jishu zhuanjia zhuanlve, yixue bian, zhongyixue juan 1* 中国科学技术专家传略: 医学编: 中医学卷一 [Biographical sketches of scientific and technological experts in China: Medicine; first volume on Chinese medicine]. Beijing: Renmin weisheng chubanshe.

Zhongguo weisheng nianjian bianji weiyuanhui 中国卫生年鉴编辑委员会. 2000. *Zhongguo weisheng nianjian* [Yearbook of hygiene in China]. Beijing: Renmin weisheng chubanshe.

"Zhongguo xiyi gaodeng yuanxiao shexiao nianbiao tongji" 中国西医高等院校设校年表统计 [Annual statistics for higher education institutes of Western medicine established in China]. 1987. In *Zhongguo yixue baike quanshu: Yixueshi* 中国医学百科全书: 医学史 [Encyclopedia of medicine in China: History of medicine], edited by Li Jingwei 李经纬 and Cheng Zhifan 程之范, 410–411. Shanghai: Shanghai kexue jishu chubanshe.

Zhongguo yiyao gongsi 中国医药公司, ed. 1990. *Zhongguo yiyao shangye shigao* 中国医药商业史搞 [The history of pharmaceutical commerce in China]. Shanghai: Shanghai shehui kexueyuan chubanshe.

"Zhonghua jiaoyujie" 中華教育界 [The world of Chinese education]. 1913. *Faming* 法命, June: 80–82.

Zhonghua quanguo minzhu funü lianhe hui, ertong fuli bu 中華全國民主婦女聯合會, 兒童福利部. 1953. "Xuanchuan puji xinfa jiesheng he you'er zhishi" 宣傳普及新法接生和幼兒智識 [Universal outreach on new knowledge about childbirth methods and child care]. *Xin Zhongguo funü* 新中國婦女, June: 6.

Zhonghua renmin gongheguo weishengbu 中华人民共和国卫生部. 2010. *2010 Zhonguo weisheng tongji nianjian* 2010中国卫生统计年鉴 [China health statistics yearbook 2010]. Beijing: Zhongguo xiehe yike daxue chubanshe.

"Zhongyang renmin zhengfu weisheng bu guanyu zuzhi tuixing 'zuzhi liaofa' de zhishi" 中央人民政府卫生部关于组织推行'组织疗法'的指示 [The Central People's Government Department of Public Health directive to organize the implementation of histotherapy]. 1951. *Zhonghua xinyi xuebao* 中华新医学报 2 (3): 165.

Zhou Enlai 周恩来. 1984 [1950]. "Wei gonggu he fazhan renmin de shengli er fendou" 为巩固和发展人民的生理而奋斗 [The struggle to consolidate and develop the people's physiology]. In *Zhou Enlai xuanji* 周恩来选集 [Selected works of Zhou Enlai], Vol. 2, edited by Zhonggong zhongyang wenxian bianji weiyuanhui 中共中央文献编辑委员会, 48. Beijing: Renmin chubanshe.

Zhou Fengwu 周风悟, Zhang Qiwen 张启文, and Cong Lin 丛林, eds. 1981–1985. *Ming laozhongyi zhi lu* 名老中医之路 [The paths of famous and venerable Chinese doctors]. 3 vols. Jinan: Shandong kexue jishu chubanshe.

Zhou Yutong 周予同. 1934. *Zhongguo xiandai jiaoyu shi* 中國現代教育史 [A history of education in modern China]. Shanghai: Shanghai liangyou tushu yinshua gongsi.

Zhu Binsheng 朱滨生. 1947. *Nigulayefu: Fenmianwutong fa zhong zhi shengli qushi* 尼古拉葉夫: 分娩無痛法中之生理學趨勢 [The physiological dynamics in Nikolaiev's painless method of delivery]. *Sulian Yixue* 苏联医学 3 (5): 7–9.

Zhu Chao 朱潮, ed. 1988. *Zhongwai yixue jiaoyushi* 中外医学教育史 [History of Chinese and foreign medical education]. Shanghai: Shanghai yike daxue.

Zhu Chao 朱潮 and Zhang Weifeng 张慰丰. 1990. *Xin zhongguo yixue jiaoyu shi* 新中国医学教育史 [A history of medical education in the new China]. Beijing: Beijing yike daxue and Zhongguo xiehe yike daxue.

Zhu Dan 朱炎. 1949. "Zenyang ban jiesheng xunlianban" 怎樣辦接生訓練班 [How to manage midwife training]. *Xin Zhongguo funu* 新中國婦女, November: 9.

Zhu Hengbi 朱恆壁. 1932. "Shiba niandu Zhongguo yixue jiaoyu zhi yi pie" 十八年度中國醫學教育之一瞥 [A quick glance at medical education in China in the year 18 (1929)]. *Yiyao pinglun* 醫藥評論, no. 25: 30.

Zhu Huiying 朱慧颖. 2009. "Minguo shiqi de weisheng yundong chutan—Yi Tianjin wei li" 民国时期的卫生运动初探—以天津为例 [A first exploration of hygiene movements in the Republican era: Using Tianjin as an example]. In *Qing yilai de jibing, yiliao he weisheng: Yi shehui wenhua shi wei shijiao de tansuo* 清以来的疾病、医疗和卫生—以社会文化史为视角的探索 [Disease, healing, and hygiene since the Qing: An exploration from the angle of social and cultural history], edited by Xinzhong Yu 余新忠, 357–370. Beijing: Sanlian shudian.

Zhu Kangjiu 王康久, ed. 1996. Beijing weisheng da shi ji, di yi juan 北京卫生大事记 (第一卷) [Record of major events in public health in Beijing. Vol 1]. Beijing: Beijing kexue jishu chubanshe.

Zhu Liangchun 朱良春, ed. 2000. *Zhang Cigong yi shu jingyan ji* 章次公医术经验集 [Collection of Zhang Cigong's experiences in the medical arts]. Changsha: Hunan kexue jishu chubanshe.

Zhu Youxian 朱有獻. 1932. "Riben xuezhi" 日本學制 [Japan's educational system]. *Zhongguohua jiaoyujie* 中國華教育界, no. 1: 23.

——. 1987. *Zhongguo jindai xuezhi shiliao* 中国近代学制史料 [Historical materials on the history of educational systems in modern China]. 2nd ed. Vol. 1. Shanghai: Huadong shifan daxue chubanshe.

"Zi waijiaobu wei pin qing Laximan deng san xi yuan wei ben bu guwen qing cha zhao wen" 咨外交部為聘請拉西曼等三西員為本部顧問請查照文 [Consulting the Foreign Ministry on inviting Rajchman and three Western personnel to serve as advisors to this department: Please note and act accordingly]. 1929. *Weisheng gongbao* 衛生公報 1 (3): 62.

ZRGGW (Zhonghua renmin gongheguo guojia weisheng he jihua shengyu weiyuanhui) 中华人民共和国国家卫生和计划生育委员会. 2009. "2015 nian 80% yi shang nong cun yun chan fu jiang zhuyuan fenmian" 2015年80%以上农村孕产妇将住院分娩 [By the year 2015, at least 80 percent of pregnant rural women will give birth in a hospital]. February 2. http://www.moh.gov.cn/fys/s3581/200902/85f85253631d47049d368500775 8d583.shtml.

Zutangshan jiaoyang yuan 组堂山教养院. 1958. "Zutangshan jiaoyang yuan dui jingshen bing ren shi zen yang jinxing guanli gongzuo de?" 祖堂山教养院对精神病人是怎样进行管理工作的 [How does the Zutangshan Care and Education Home manage mental patients?]. *Zhonghua shenjing jingshen ke zazhi* 中华神经精神科杂志 4: 259–262.

ZYHJF (Zhonghua yixue hui jiehebingxue fenhui) 中华医学会结核病学分会. 1997. *Zhongguo jiehebing xue ke fazhan shi* 中国结核病学科发展史 [History of the development of the scientific study of tuberculosis]. Beijing: Dangdai Zhongguo chubanshe.

Archives

Note on archival citations: This volume uses in-text parenthetical citations following the *Chicago Manual of Style*. To conform with this style while also accommodating the particular demands of citing a variety of English- and Chinese-language archives, the in-text citations for archival materials give an acronym representing the name of the archive, followed by the date of the particular document. To aid the reader in locating more information about these primary sources, each document is cited below. The materials are organized by archive and listed in chronological order by year.

ABCFM (American Board of Commissioners for Foreign Missions archives), 1810–1961, Houghton Library, Harvard University, Cambridge, MA

Shaowu Documents. 1930–1939. Vol. 2. Item 41, Reports.

ABMAC (American Bureau for Medical Aid to China records), 1937–1949, Rare Book and Manuscript Library, Columbia University, New York, NY

"National Health Administration, May 1941." 1941. Box 21, folder "National Health Administration 1940–41."

Chu, C. K. (Zhu Zhanggeng). 1942a. "National Institute of Health in 1942: An Annual Report." Box 42, folder "National Health Administration 1942."

King, P. Z (Jin Baoshan). 1942b. Letter to Lauchlin Currie. May 2. Box 21, folder "National Health Administration, King, P. Z., 1942–43."

"National Health Administration of the ROC, November 1942, (A Brief Review of the Work)." 1942c. Box 21, folder "National Health Administration 1942."

Yao, K. F. (Yao Kefang). 1942d. "A Brief Account of Kweichou Health Work." Received November 12. Box 21, folder "National Health Administration 1942."

"Report of the Kweichu Hsien Health Station, 1943." 1943. Box 20, folder "National Health Administration General."

King, P. Z. 1944a. Letter to Van Slyke. September 8. Box 21, folder "National Health Administration, King, P.Z."

King, P. Z. 1944b. Letter to G. P. Waung. September 23. Box 21, folder "National Health Administration, King, P.Z."

"Conference on the Present Medical Situation in China." 1946. Box 18, folder "Medical Conference June 1946."

Chu, C. K. (Zhu Zhanggeng). n.d.a. "Training of Public Health Personnel in 1939–40." Box 21, folder "National Health Administration 1940–41."

"Health Program of the National Health Administration." n.d.b. Box 21, folder "National Health Administration 1940–41."

King, P. Z. n.d.c. "The Chinese NHA . . ." Box 21, folder "National Health Administration 1940–41."

——. n.d.d. "The Chinese NHA During the Sino-Japanese Hostilities." Box 21, folder "National Health Administration 1940–41."

"Public Health during 1940–1942, by P. Z. King." n.d.e. Box 21, folder "King, P. Z., 1942–43."

AFSCA (American Friends Service Committee Archives), American Friends Service Committee, Philadelphia, PA

American Friends Service Committee. 1949. "Inventory of Drugs Now in Medical Storeroom." September 25. Box "Foreign Service 1951," folder "Country, China, Projects, Chungmou Hospital 1950."

Friends Service Unit (China). 1950. "Summary Report of the F.S.U. (China)." September 15. Box "Foreign Service 1950," folder "Country, China, F.S.U. 1950."

American Friends Service Committee. n.d. "Work of the Friends Unit (China): Short Statement by the Chungking Section." Box "Foreign Service, 1950," folder "Project, Clinic (South Bank) Chungking, 1950."

AH (Guoshiguan 國史館 [Academia Historica]), Taipei, Taiwan, Republic of China

Chongqing shi weisheng ju gongzuo baogao 重慶市衛生局工作報告 [Chongqing Bureau of Public Health work report]. 1946. October. File 090-183, 12b.

CMA (Chongqing shi dang'an ju 重庆市档案局 [Chongqing Municipal Archives]), Chongqing, People's Republic of China

"Chongqing shi weisheng ju gongzuo baogao" 重慶市衛生局工作報告 [Chongqing Bureau of Public Health work report]. 1938a. December 5–10. File 66-1-2.

"Yan Fuqing zhi Jiang shizhang zhi cheng" 顏福慶至蔣市長之呈 [F. C. Yen to Mayor Jiang]. 1938b. November 18. File 53-1-386.

"Yan Fuqing zhi Chongqing shizhengfu zhi cheng, han" 顏福慶至重慶市政府之呈, 函 [F. C. Yen letters to Chongqing municipal government]. 1938c. June 30–July 16. File 66-1-6, 32–44.

"Chongqing shi weisheng ju 28 nian xialing fang huoluan jihua" 重慶市衛生局28年夏令防霍亂計劃 [Chongqing Bureau of Public Health 1939 summertime cholera prevention plan]. 1939a. File 162-1-20, 45–46.

"Gong sili yiyuan diaocha biao" 公私立醫院調查表 [Survey of public and private hospitals]. 1939b. May. File 66-1-1.

"Gong sili yiyuan diaocha biao" 公私立醫院調查表 [Survey of public and private hospitals]. 1939c. November 20. File 66-1-1, 41.

"Gong sili yiyuan qingkuang zhi dianbao" 公私立醫院情況之電報 [Telegram transmitting the current conditions of public and private hospitals]. 1939d. November 20. File 66-1-1, 41.

"Chongqingshi jiaowai gong sili yiyuan zhensuo yilanbiao" 重慶市郊外公私立醫院診所一覽表 [A table of public and private hospitals and clinics in the outskirts of Chongqing]. 1940a. August. File 66-1-3, 182–183.

"Chongqing shi weisheng ju gongzuo baogao" 重慶市衛生局工作報告 [Chongqing Bureau of Public Health work report]. 1940b. File 66-1-3, 167, 223.

"Chongqing shi weisheng ju gongzuo baogao" 重慶市衛生局工作報告 [Chongqing Bureau of Public Health work report]. 1940c. January–June. File 66-1-3, 171.

"Chongqing shi weisheng ju gongzuo baogao" 重慶市衛生局工作報告 [Chongqing Bureau of Public Health work report]. 1940d. March–August. File 66-1-3, 167–168.

"Chongqing shi weisheng ju gongzuo baogao" 重慶市衛生局工作報告 [Chongqing Bureau of Public Health work report]. 1940e. August. File 66-1-3, 101.

"Chongqing shi weisheng ju gongzuo baogao: Chongqingshi yu shijiao zhi gong sili yiyuan diaochabiao" 重慶市衛生局工作報告: 重慶市與市郊之公私立醫院調查表 [Chongqing Bureau of Public Health work report: Table of private and public hospitals in Chongqing proper and in the suburbs]. 1940f. August. File 66-1-3.

"Chongqing shi weisheng ju gongzuo baogao" 重慶市衛生局工作報告 [Chongqing Bureau of Public Health work report]. 1940–1941. September 1940–February 1941 File 66-1-3, 198.

"Shili chuanranbing yiyuan xianzai qingxing ji jianglai banli gejie" 市立傳染病醫院現在情形及將來辦理各節 [Current conditions and future plans of the Municipal Infectious Diseases Hospital]. 1942. October. File 66-1-6, 115–116.

"Chongqing shi weisheng ju gongzuo baogao" 重慶市衛生局工作報告 [Chongqing Bureau of Public Health work report]. 1943a. File 66-1-2, 203–204.

"Chongqing shi weisheng ju gongzuo baogao" 重慶市衛生局工作報告 [Chongqing Bureau of Public Health work report]. 1943b. November. File 66-1-2, 204.

"Chongqing shi weisheng ju gongzuo baogao" 重慶市衛生局工作報告 [Chongqing Bureau of Public Health work report]. 1944a. File 66-1-2.

"Chongqing shi weisheng ju gongzuo baogao" 重慶市衛生局工作報告 [Chongqing Bureau of Public Health work report]. 1944b. January–March. File 66-1-2, 16.

"Chongqing shi weisheng ju gongzuo baogao" 重慶市衛生局工作報告 [Chongqing Bureau of Public Health work report]. 1944c. July–October 11. File 66-1-2, 81, 84, 86, 87.

"Chongqing shi weisheng ju gongzuo baogao" 重慶市衛生局工作報告 [Chongqing Bureau of Public Health work report]. 1944d. November 1–14. File 66-1-2, 96, 99.

"Peidu Zhongyiyuan dang'an" 陪都中醫院檔案 [Wartime capital Chinese Medicine Hospital files]. 1944–1945. Files 163-2-19; 163-2-24.

"Zhongshang yiyuan yusuan dang'an" 重傷醫院預算檔案 [Trauma Hospital budget documents]. 1945. March–June. File 53-19–1920.

Chongqing shi weisheng ju gongzuo baogao 重慶市衛生局工作報告 [Chongqing Bureau of Public Health work report]. n.d.a. File 66-1-2, 4.

"Chongqing shi yiyuan dang'an" 重慶市醫院档案 [Chongqing Municipal Hospital files]. n.d.b. File 165-2-3.

"Chongqing shi weishengju yiyuan dang'an" 重慶市衛生局醫院档案 [Chongqing Bureau of Public Health hospital records]. n.d.c. File 66-1-6.

"Chongqing shi weishengju 33 nian gongzuo jihua" 重慶市衛生局33年工作計劃 [Chongqing Bureau of Public Health work plans for 1944]. n.d.d. File 66-1-4, 12.

CMB (China Medical Board of New York archives), Rockefeller Foundation Archives and Rockefeller Archive Center, Tarrytown, NY

Memorandum, "The Purpose of the Founding of the Chair of Hygiene." 1921. September 26. Record group IV, series 2B9, box 75, folder 525.

Grant, John B. 1923. "A Proposal for a Department of Hygiene for Peking Union Medical College." Record group IV, series 2B9, box 75, file 42, folder 531.

Houghton, Henry S. 1924. Memorandum to Roger S. Greene. December 27. Record group IV, series 2B9, box 75, folder 525.

Carter, W. S. 1925a. Letter to Russell. December 14. Record group IV, series 2B9, box 75, folder 528.

Grant, John B. 1925b. Letter to Hsueh Tu-pi. February 13. Record group IV, series 2B9, box 76, folder 532.

"Health Station—First Quarter Review." 1925c. December 24. Record group IV, series 2B9, box 66, folder 465, 1.

"Monthly Reports." 1925d. September, November. Record group IV, series 2B9, box 66, folder 465.

"Public Health in Peking." 1925e. Page 2 of attachment in J. B. Grant, "Plans for Public Health Work in China 1925." Record group IV, series 2B9, box 76, folder 532.

"Rural Public Health." 1925f. Page 1 of attachment in J. B. Grant, "Plans for Public Health Work in China 1925." Record group IV, series 2B9, box 76, folder 532.

Grant, J. B. 1925g. "Plans for Public Health Work in China 1925." Record group IV, series 2B9, box 76, folder 532.

Grant, John B. 1926. Letter to Greene. December 13. Folder 465.

Greene, Roger S. 1927a. Interoffice memo to Henry S. Houghton. March 23. Record group IV, series 2B9, box 66, folder 466.

Memo to Greene. 1927b. July 27. Record group IV, series 2B9, box 66, folder 466.

"19 August 1938 Minutes of the Peiping Union Medical College Governing Council." 1938. Box 104, folder 747, "Nurses Staff Nieh, V."

Chow Meiyu (Guiyang). 1939. Letter to Salley Jean, New York. April 23. Record group IV, series 2B9, box 100, folder 719, "Nurses Staff (Chow Mei-Yu)."

Tsur, Y. T. 1945. Letter to Dr Sao-Ke Alfred Sze. August 25. Box 104, folder 747, "Nurses Staff Nieh, V."

Yuan, I. C. 1946. Letter to Dr. Alan Greg. May 31. Box 104, folder 747, "Nurses Staff Nieh, V."

American Bureau for Medical Aid to China Inc. n.d.a. Invitation for November 2 event featuring Col. Chow Mei-Yu (China army nursing service) and Col. Florence A. Blanchfield (U.S. Army nurses corps). Record group IV, series 2B9, box 100, folder 525.

"Nurses Staff (Chow Mei-Yu)." n.d.b. Record group IV, series 2B9, box 100, folder 719.

DCM (Drexel University College of Medicine), Legacy Center, Archives and Special Collections, Philadelphia, PA

"Reifsnyder, M. Elizabeth." 1881.

HPA (Hangzhou shi dang'an ju 杭州市档案局 [Hangzhou Prefectural Archives]), Hangzhou, Jiangsu, People's Republic of China

Hangzhoushi weishengju 杭州市卫生局 [Hangzhou prefecture health bureau]. "Hangzhou diqu nongcun shengchan dadui he shengchandui weisheng zuzhi qingkuang" 杭州地区农村生产大队和生产队卫生组织情况 [Survey of health organizations in production teams and production brigades in rural areas of Hangzhou prefecture]. 1976. Vol. 87-3-307.

JSDA (Jiangsu sheng dang'an ju 江苏省档案局 [Jiangsu Provincial Archives]), Nanjing, Jiangsu, People's Republic of China

"Jiangsu sheng Songjiang zhuanyuan gongshu, weishengke, guanyu chengli zhuanqu bingchong fangzhizhan ji 1952–1956 nian xuexichongbing fangzhi gongzuo de zongjie baogao, fu: Qingpu xian meiqi huoshao mieluo qingkuang baogao" 江苏省松江专员公署,卫生科,关于成立专区病虫防治站及1952–1956年血吸虫病防治工作的总结报告,附:青浦县煤气火烧灭螺情况报告 [Summary reports of Health office of Jiangsu Songjiang Commissioner Office on establishing prefectural pest prevention and treatment station, and on prevention and treatment of schistosomiasis from 1952 to 1956, with attached report on Qingpu county eliminating oncomelania by burning with gas]. 1951–1957. March 26, 1951–April 18, 1957. File 3235, 41 (yongjiu 永久 [permanent]).

"Jiangsu sheng weishengting. Dangzu, shengwei guanyu fangzhi xuexichongbing, nvgongbing bing de zhishi ji ting dang zu guanyu nvgongbing bing de diaocha he lianhe zhensuo qianfei chuli de baogao" 江苏省卫生厅. 党组, 省委关于防治血吸虫病, 女工病病的指示及厅党组关于女工病病的调查和联合诊所千费处理的报告 [Jiangsu Provincial Department of Health, Party Unit, Party Provincial Committee's directives on prevention and treatment of schistosomiasis, female workers' diseases, and Party Unit of Provincial Health Department's reports on the study of female workers' diseases and funding for joint treatment clinics]. 1956a. March 1–December 19. File 3119, 198 (duanqi 短期 [short-term]).

"Zhonggong Jiangsu shengwei, chuwuhai aiguo weisheng yundong, lingdao xiaozu bangongshi. wo shi xuefang gongzuo jiahua, diaochabaogao, tongzhi" 中共江苏省委, 除五害爱国卫生运动, 领导小组办公室. 我室血防工作计划, 调查报告, 通知 [Proposals, study reports and announcements of the Leadership Small Group Office of Eliminating Five-Pests Patriotic Health Campaign of Jiangsu Provincial Committee of CCP on prevention of schistosomiasis]. 1956b. June 23. File 3119, 231 (changqi 长期 [long-term]).

"Jiangsu weishengting, bangongshi, bensheng xuefang, fangyi he yaozheng gongzuo zongjie ji xuefang gongzuo guihua, Hongshizihui gongzuo baogao" 江苏卫生厅, 办公室, 本省血防, 防疫和药政工作总结及血防工作规划, 红十字会工作报告 [Reports of Jiangsu Provincial Department of Health and Office on prevention of schistosomiasis, epidemic prevention and drug administration, and proposal on prevention of schistosomiasis, and Red Cross work report]. 1957. February 10–December 28. File 3119, 322 (changqi 长期 [long-term]).

JXDA (Jiangxi sheng dang'an ju 江西省档案局 [Jiangxi Provincial Archives]), Nanchang, Jiangxi, People's Republic of China

"Jiangxi sheng weishengting, Jiangxi shengwei chuhai miebing lingdao xiaozu bangongshi, 1953 nian, Pengze weisheng yuan xuexichongbing zhiliao zongjie" 江西省卫生厅, 江西省委除害灭病领导小组办公室, 1953年, 彭泽卫生院血吸虫病治疗总结 [1953 summary report of Jiangxi Provincial Department of Health and Leadership Small Group Office for Eliminating Pests and Diseases on treatment of schistosomiasis at Pengze Health Clinic]. 1953. File X111-02-057.

"Zhonggong zhongyang, shengwei, Nanchang diwei, fangzhi xuexichongbing jiuren xiaozu, wuren xiaozu he sheng aiguo weisheng yundong weiyuanhui guanyu fangzhi xuexichongbing gongzuo de baogao, zongjie, yijian" 中共中央、省委、南昌地委、防治血吸虫病九人小组、五人小组和省爱国卫生运动委员会关于防治血吸虫病工作

的报告、总结、意见 [Reports, summaries and suggestions of Central Committee of CCP, Provincial Committee, Nanchang City Committee, Schistosomiasis Prevention and Treatment Nine-Person Small Group, Five-Person Small Group and Provincial Patriotic Health Campaign Committee on prevention of schistosomiasis]. 1957. File X009-01-010.

"Weishengbu, guojia tiwei, caizheng, jiaoyubu guanyu weisheng, tiyu gongzuo de guiding, tongzhi" 卫生部、国家体委、财政、教育部关于卫生、体育工作的规定、通知 [Regulations and announcements of Ministry of Health, State Sports Commission, Ministry of Finance, Ministry of Education on health and sports]. 1966. File X035-05-539.

MCANYP (Medical Center Archives of New York-Presbyterian/Weill Cornell), New York, NY

Chow Mei-Yu. 1944. "Development of Army Nursing School in China." Master's thesis, Massachusetts Institute of Technology. Mary Beard (1876–1946) Papers. Box 1, file 3.

NLM (National Library of Medicine), Bethesda, MD

Zhongguo fanglao xiehui 中國防癆協會. 1938. "Unforgivable Mistakes." Chinese Public Health Advertisement Collection, file 133F.

Shanghai fanglao xiehui 上海防癆協會. 1953–1954. "Under the leadership of the CCP, central government and Chairman Mao, we have started the FFYP. . . ." Chinese Public Health Poster Collection, file 1005.

RAC (Rockefeller Archive Center), Tarrytown, NY

Grant, John B. 1921a. Letter to S. H. Chuan. December 9. Record group IV, Rockefeller Foundation, series 1, box 78, folder 1803.

Pearce, Richard M. 1921b. March 7. Record group IV, Rockefeller Foundation, series 1, box 78, folder 1802.

Grant, John B. 1922. Letter to Heiser. January 13. Record group IV, Rockefeller Foundation, series 1, box 78, folder 1803.

Williamson, C. C. 1923. Letter to John B. Grant. March 20. Record group IV, Rockefeller Foundation, series 1, box 78, folder 1805.

Grant, John B. 1925. Correspondence. Record group V, IHB/D, series 1.2, box 235, folder 3006, "J.B. Grant."

Gray, G. Douglas. 1927. Letter to Huang (Zifang). August 22. Record group I, Rockefeller Foundation, series 601, box 44, folder 366.

Grant, John B. 1928a. Attachment to his third annual report on the Health Station. November 2. Record group V, Rockefeller Foundation, series 3, box 219, folder 2736, 1.

Grant, John B. 1928b. Letter to Heiser. September 3. Record group I, Rockefeller Foundation, series 601, box 45, folder 368.

"Excerpts from J.B. Grant's Notes of October 1929." 1929a. Record group I, Rockefeller Foundation, series 601, box 45, folder 368.

"First Quarterly Report Ending September 30, 1929, Rural Health Demonstration, Kao-Chiao, the Municipality of Greater Shanghai, China." 1929b. Record group V, Rockefeller Foundation, series 3, box 220, folder 2742, 1–3.

"Sixth Quarterly Report Ending Dec. 31, 1930, Kao Chiao Rural Health Demonstration Station, Bureau of Public Health, City Government of Greater Shanghai." 1930a. Record group V, Rockefeller Foundation, series 3, box 220, folder 2743.

Li Ting-an. 1930b. "The Health Station of the First Health Area, Beiping." Record group I, Rockefeller Foundation, series 601, box 44, folder 366, 2–5.

Grant, John B. 1931a. Letter to Victor Heiser. March 16. Record group I, Rockefeller Foundation, series 601, box 45, folder 373.

Li Ting-an. 1931b. "The 6th Annual Report of the Health Station," submitted to John B. Grant. August 15. Record group V, Rockefeller Foundation, series 3, box 219, folder 2739, 5.

First National Midwifery School. 1932. *First National Midwifery School, Peiping.* Record group I, Rockefeller Foundation, series 601, box 45, folder 373.

"Fellowships 1934–40." 1934–1940. Record group I, Rockefeller Foundation, series 1, file 601E 42 349.

Yen, Jimmy. 1937. Letter to Mr. Fosdick. September 25. Mass Education Movement 1937–1939. Record group I, Rockefeller Foundation, series 601, box 7, folder 72.

"China Health Training of Personnel: Annual Report, 1945." 1945a. Record group V, IHB/D, series 3, box 218.

"China—Health, Training of Personnel: First Semi-Annual Report for 1945." 1945b. Record group V, IHB/D, series 3, box 218.

Tennant, Mary. 1948. Officer's Diary. August 16. Rockefeller Foundation diaries, file "12–2 Tennant 1932–1955."

"Chow Mei-Yu 1948, 1949, and 1948–49." 1948–1949. Rockefeller Foundation, file 10.1 22 601E.

"Biographical Files of John B. Grant." n.d.a. Rockefeller Foundation.

"Interoffice Correspondence from JBG." n.d.b. Subject: Interview with Miss Beard. Record group I, Rockefeller Foundation, series 1, box 37, folder 298, "Peiping College Nursing School 1929–1952."

"Resolutions on Shanghai health Units." n.d.c. Record group I, Rockefeller Foundation, series 601, box 45, folder 368.

"A Review of Government Health Services in Szechuan, China, for the period of 1939–1945." n.d.d. Record group V, IHB/D, series 3, box 218.

"Traveling Clinic of Kao-Chiao." n.d.e. Record group V, Rockefeller Foundation, series 3, box 220, folder 2742. Pictures attached.

SLRO (Suzhou shi difang zhi bangongshi 苏州市地方志办公室 *[Suzhou Local Records Office]), Suzhou, Jiangsu, People's Republic of China*

"Jinchang shi: Di shisi juan (yiyao weisheng) di er zhang (yiliao weisheng jigou)" 金阊市: 第十四卷 (医药卫生) 第二章 (医疗卫生机构) [Jinchang city: Volume 14—Medical and Health, chapter II—Institutions]. 2009a. http://www.dfzb.suzhou.gov.cn/zsbl/543327 .htm.

"Suzhou zhuanye zhi: Di yi pian yiliao" 苏州专业志: 第一篇 医疗 [Souzhou local history: Chapter 1—The Medical System]. 2009b. http://www.dfzb.suzhou.gov.cn/zsbl/349427 .htm.

"Suzhou zhuanye zhi: Di er pian (yiliao) di er zhang (Zhongyi)" 苏州专业志: 第二篇 (医疗) 第二章 (中医) [Suzhou local history: Chapter 2—TCM]. 2009c. http://www.dfzb .suzhou.gov.cn/zsbl/1639927.htm.

"Suzhou zhuanye zhi: Di er pian (yiliao) di er zhang (Xi yi)" 苏州专业志: 第二篇 (医疗) 第二章 (西医) [Suzhou local history: Chapter 2—Western medicine]. 2009d. http:// www.dfzb.suzhou.gov.cn/zsbl/1640027.htm.

SMA (Shanghai shi dang'an guan 上海市档案馆 *[Shanghai Municipal Archives]), Shanghai, People's Republic of China*

"Shanghai gonggong zujie gongbu ju weisheng chu you guan jiehebing liaoyang yuan (Hongqiao) de lishi yange yu fazhan wenxian" 上海公共租界工部局卫生处有关结核病疗养院 (虹桥) 的历史沿革与发展文件 [Shanghai public concessions' Municipal Council Health Office, on history and development documents from the Hongqiao Sanatorium]. 1913–1941. File U1-16-656.

"Shanghai gonggong zujie gong bu ju weisheng chu youguan wairen geli yiyuan feijiehe bingren ruyuan deng shixiang de wenjian" 上海公共租界工部局卫生处有关外人隔离医院肺结核病人入院等事项的文件 [Shanghai public concessions' Municipal Council Health Office, on admission documents and other matters for foreigners in the isolation hospital]. 1913–1944. File U1-16-617.

"Shanghai gonggong zujie gongbu ju weisheng chu guanyu jiehebing liaoyang yuan ruyuan guizhang ji shoufei de guiding wenxian" 上海公共租界工部局卫生处关于结核病疗养院入院规章及收费的规定文件 [Shanghai public concessions' Municipal Council Health Office, on the tuberculosis sanatorium: Regulations of admission and charges]. 1929–1942. File U1-16-655.

"Shanghai gonggong zujie gongbu ju weisheng chu guanyu jiehebing Liaoyang suo zhi shuidian, huoshi ji zhusu deng zongwu wenjian" 上海公共租界工部局卫生处关于结核病疗养所之水电、伙食及住宿等总务文件 [Shanghai public concessions' Municipal Council Health Office, on water and electricity at the tuberculosis sanatorium]. 1930–1940. File U1-16-654.

"Shanghai gonggong zujie gongbu ju weisheng chu guanyu 'Zhongguo fanglao xiehui' zuzhi ji qi huodong qingkuang wenjian" 上海公共租界工部局卫生处关于"中国防痨协会"组织及其活动情况文件 [Shanghai public concessions' Municipal Council Health Office, on the "China Anti-Tuberculosis Association" organization and activities]. 1935–1939. File U1-16-2659.

"Shanghai gonggong zujie gongbu ju weisheng chu guanyu 'Shanghai fanglao xiehui' ge weiyuanhui huiyi jilu" 上海公共租界工部局卫生处关于"上海防痨协会"各委员会会议记录 [Shanghai public concessions' Municipal Council Health Office: Records from "Shanghai Anti-Tuberculosis Association" representative meetings]. 1938–1940. File U1-16-2661.

"Shanghai fa zujie gong dong ju guanyu Shanghai Zhongguo fanglao xiehui de wenjian (yi)" 上海法租界公董局关于上海中国防痨协会的文件 (一) [Shanghai French Concession Public Health Office director, on documents from Shanghai's China Anti-Tuberculosis Association]. 1938–1942a. File U38-1-191.

"Shanghai fa zujie gong dong ju weisheng chu guanyu fanglao xiehui Shanghai yiyuan shenqing jianmian fang juan ji gai yuan shenqing diaohuan fuze renshi" 上海法租界公董局卫生处关于防痨协会上海医院申请减免房捐及该院申请调换负责人事 [Shanghai French Concession Public Health Office director, on Anti-Tuberculosis Association's Shanghai Hospital applications for waivers and hospital personnel responsible for exchange]. 1938–1942b. File U38-5-1625.

"Shanghai gonggong zujie gongbu ju weisheng chu guanyu 'Shanghai fanglao xiehui' chang wu weiyuanhui huiyi jilv" 上海公共租界工部局卫生处关于"上海防痨协会"常务委员会会议记录 [Shanghai public concessions' Municipal Council Health Office, on records from the "Shanghai Anti-Tuberculosis Association" Standing Committee meetings]. 1938–1944a. File U1-16-2664.

"Shanghai gonggong zujie gongbu ju weisheng chu guanyu 'Zhongguo fanglao xiehui' zuzhi ji qi huodong qingkuang wenjian" 上海公共租界工部局卫生处关于"中国防痨协会"组织及其活动情况文件 [Shanghai public concessions' Municipal Council Health Office, on the "China Anti-Tuberculosis Association" organization and activities]. 1938–1944b. File U1-16-2660.

"Shanghai gonggong zujie gongbu ju weisheng chu guanyu 'Shanghai fanglao xiehui' gong-zuo baogao ji xingzheng wenjian" 上海公共租界工部局卫生处关于"上海防痨协会"工作报告及行政文件 [Shanghai public concessions' Municipal Council Health Office, on "Shanghai Anti-Tuberculosis Association" work reports and administrative documents]. 1938–1945. File U1-16-2663.

"Shanghai fa zu jie gong dong ju weisheng chu guanyu dong hua yaofang shenqing yingye zhi zhao shi" 上海法租界公董局卫生处关于东华药房申请营业执照事 [Shanghai French Concession public health office director on matters of the East China Pharmacy business license application]. 1942–1943. File U38-5-1654.

"Shanghai fa zujie gong dong ju guanyu Shanghai Zhongguo fanglao xiehui de wenjian (er)" 上海法租界公董局关于上海中国防痨协会的文件 (二) [Shanghai French Concession Public Health Office director, on documents from Shanghai's China Anti-Tuberculosis Association]. 1943. File U38-1-192.

"Shanghai shi weisheng ju guanyu Shanghai fanglao xiehui juan" 上海市卫生局关于上海防痨协会卷 [Shanghai Municipal Health Bureau on the Shanghai Anti-Tuberculosis Association]. 1947. File Q400-1-4053.

"Tongde yixueyuan yu xiaxiang jiefangjun zhi xuexichongbing yanjiu tiaoji yingyang tongxue, jiaoyuan laiwang wenjian ji Shanghai jiaoqu Riben xuexichongbing fangzhi weiyuanhui de jianbao" 同德医学院与下乡解放军治血吸虫病研究调剂营养同学, 教员来往文件及上海郊区日本血吸虫病防治委员会的简报 [Correspondences between Tongde Medical School and nutritionist students and instructors of the People's Liberation Army in the countryside on study of treatment of schistosomiasis and report on Japanese schistosomiasis prevention and Treatment Committee in Shanghai rural areas]. 1949–1950. December 24, 1949–April 11, 1950. File Q249-1-137.

"1949–1950 nian Shanghai shi yiwu gongzuozhe gonghui chuanda rendaihui huibao, lvxing jiuhu gongzuo zongjie, zhigong canjia jiaoqu zhujun xuefang gongzuo gongchen shiji cailiao, weiwenxin deng" 1949–1950 年上海市医务工作者工会传达人代会汇报、游行救护工作总结、职工参加郊区驻军血防工作功臣事迹材料、慰问信等 [1949–1950 Shanghai medical workers reporting People's Congress, summaries of medical emergency work, reports of good deeds of staff attending schistosomiasis prevention work in rural areas and letters of encouragement, etc.]. 1950a. February. File C3-1-11.

"Weishengbu, Shanghai shi renmin zhengfu deng guanyu Zhongguo hongshizi hui zonghui qianjing, gaizu ji zuzhi tong ce" 卫生部、上海市人民政府等关于中国红十字会总会迁京、改组及组织通则 [Ministry of Health, Shanghai Municipal People's Government on the Chinese Red Cross move to Beijing, restructuring and reorganization]. 1950b. July–December. File B242-1-194.

"Zhengdan daxue guanyu yixueyuan zhiliao xuexichongbing juan" 震旦大学关于医学院治疗血吸虫病卷 [Aurora University's report on medical school's treatment of schistosomiasis]. 1952. January–July. File Q244-1-290.

"Shanghai shi aiguo weisheng yundong weiyuanhui guanyu Shanghai shi aiguo weisheng yundong 6 yue zhi 11 yue fen gongzuo zongjie" 上海市爱国卫生运动委员会关于上海市爱国卫生运动6月至11月份工作总结 [Shanghai Patriotic Hygiene Campaign Committee on the work summary of the patriotic hygiene campaign from June to November]. 1953a. File B242-1-535-60.

"Shanghai shi si nian lai fanglao gongzuo zongjie" 上海市四年来防痨工作总结 [Shanghai city: Summary of four years of anti-TB work]. 1953b. File B242-1-530.

"Weishengbu guanyu zhaokai quanguo fangzhi xuexichongbing huiyi jianbao ji zongjie baogao, wangjuzhang fayangao" 卫生部关于召开全国防治血吸虫病会议简报及总结报告、王局长发言稿 [Ministry of Health's news bulletin on holding a national conference on prevention and treatment of schistosomiasis and final report, and speech of Director Wang]. 1955a. November. File B242-1-815.

"Zhonggong zhongyang guanyu xiaomie xuexichong binghai zhishi ji Shanghai sanniannei xiaomie gaibing de fangzhi jihua, jiaoqu fangzhi gongzuo baogao he jianbao" 中共中央关于消灭血吸虫病害指示及上海三年内消灭该病的防治计划、郊区防治工作报告和简报 [Central Committee of CCP's directives on eliminating schistosomiasis and prevention and treatment proposals of eliminating this disease in Shanghai within three years, work report and news bulletins of prevention and treatment work in the rural areas]. 1955b. November. File B242-1-816.

"Shanghai shi youju baokan lingshou dai song yuan fuli hui. Shi gui guo huaqiao lianhe hui zhongguo fang lao xiehui shanghai shi fenhui shenqing chengli he gaizao bei'an juan" 上海市邮局报刊零售代送员福利会. 市归国华侨联合会中国防痨协会上海市分会申请成立和改造备案卷 [Shanghai Municipal Post Office, on behalf of member press and retail benefits association: Application for the establishment and improvement of the Municipal Federation of Returned Overseas Shanghai branch of the Chinese Anti-Tuberculosis Association]. 1956. File B168-1-818.

"Shanghai shi weisheng ju guanyu fei jiehebing fen qi huanzhe xia gong de yijian" 上海市卫生局关于肺结核病分期患者复工的意见 [Shanghai Municipal Ministry of Health suggestions on TB patients returning to work]. 1963. January–September. File B242-1-1510.

"Weishengbu, Shanghai shi weishengju guanyu jiaqiang Shanghai shi xuefang gongzuo de zhishi ji Shanghai shi xuefang suo genggai suoming, jianli xianchang shiyan jidi de qingshi baogao" 卫生部、上海市卫生局关于加强上海市血防工作的指示及上海市血防所更改所名、建立现场实验基地的请示报告 [Ministry of Health and Shanghai Health Bureau's directives on strengthening the work of schistosomiasis prevention in Shanghai and proposals of changing the name of Shanghai Schistosomiasis Prevention Agency and establishing laboratory and experimental base]. 1963–1964. May 1963–December 1964. File B242-1-1624.

"Shanghai shi weishengju guanyu si ge yixue yanjiusuo lingdao tizhigaige yu chengli tiaozheng keyan xiezuozu ji jiyan suobu zai chengdan hunanan, yunnan yiliaodui renwu de baogao, tongzhi" 上海市卫生局关于四个医学研究所领导体制改革与成立调整科研协作组及寄研所部再承担湖南、云南医疗队任务的报告、通知 [Report and announcements of the Shanghai Health Bureau on reforming four medical research institutes' leadership systems, and on establishing and adjusting a scientific research cooperation group and a parasitic research institute to again undertake the task of a Hunan and Yunnan medical team]. 1972a. April–November. File B242-2-206.

"Shanghai shi weishengju guanyu xuefangsuo dang an xiaohui baogao ji zhiding wenjian, dang an guanli, huiyi, jingfei baoxiao guiding yijian, yongjun gongyue" 上海市卫生局关于血防所档案销毁报告及制订文件、档案管理、会议、经费报销规定意见、拥军公约 [Shanghai Health Bureau's reports on destroyed archives of Schistosomiasis Prevention Agency and proposals on creating files, archival management, conferences and reimbursement, and pledge of supporting the army]. 1972b. January–August. File B242-3-283.

SPA (*Sichuan sheng dang'an ju* 四川省档案局 [*Sichuan Provincial Archives*]), *Chengdu, Sichuan, People's Republic of China*

"Chongqing shi weisheng ju 28 nian xialing fang huoluan jihua" 重慶市衛生局28年夏令防霍亂計劃 [Chongqing Bureau of Public Health 1939 summertime cholera prevention plan]. 1939a. File 113-1-639.

"Chongqing shi yishi, yaoshi, zhuchanshi, yaojisheng diaochabiao" 重慶市醫師, 藥師, 助產士, 藥劑生調查表 [Survey of physicians, pharmacists, and midwives in Chongqing city]. 1939b. February. File 113-1-637, 1–35.

SQDA (Shanghai shi Qingpu qu dang'an ju 上海市青浦区档案局 [Shanghai City Qingpu Area archive]), Qingpu, Shanghai, Jiangsu, People's Republic of China

"Qingpu xian, xuexichongbing fangzhizhan, benzhan xuefang gongzuo zongjie" 青浦县, 血吸虫病防治站, 本站血防工作总结 [Report on the work of the schistosomiasis prevention station, by Qingpu county Schistosomiasis Prevention and Treatment Station]. 1951. March. File 95-1-1.

"Qingpu xian renmin zhengfu, xuexichongbing fangzhi zhan, benzhan xuefang gongzuo qingkuang baogao" 青浦县人民政府, 血吸虫病防治站, 本站血防工作情况报告 [Report on the work of the schistosomiasis prevention station, by Schistosomiasis Prevention and Treatment Station of Qingpu county government]. 1952. January–October. File 95-1-2.

"Qingpu xian, xuexichongbing fangzhizhan, benzhan xuefang gongzuo jihua, zongjie" 青浦县, 血吸虫病防治站, 本站血防工作计划, 总结 [Proposal and summary of the station on schistosomiasis prevention, by Qingpu county Schistosomiasis Prevention and Treatment Station]. 1954. File 95-1-6.

"Qingpu xian renmin zhengfu, qingpu xianwei xuexichongbing fangzhi zhan, zhonggong qingpu xianwei xuefang bangongshi, guanyu fangzhi gongzuo qingkuang baogao" 青浦县人民政府, 青浦县委血吸虫病防治站, 中共青浦县委血防办公室, 关于防治工作情况报告 [Report of Qingpu county government, County Schistosomiasis Prevention and Treatment Station, Schistosomiasis Prevention and Treatment Office of Qingpu county Party Committee on the prevention and treatment of schistosomiasis]. 1956. January–December. File 95-1-11.

"Qingpu xian, xuexichongbing fangzhizhan, benzhan xuefang gongzuo jihua qingkuang baogao zongjie" 青浦县, 血吸虫病防治站, 本站血防工作计划情况报告总结 [Proposal and summary of the station on schistosomiasis prevention, by Qingpu county Schistosomiasis Prevention and Treatment Station]. 1957. File 95-1-15.

SWSMM (Songwenshen Memorial Museum 送瘟神纪念馆), Yujiang, Yingtan, Jiangxi, People's Republic of China

"Xian xuefang wuren xiaozu: Guanyu xuefang diaocha yunyong nongji fangzhi deng jihua gongzuo anpai" 县血防五人小组: 关于血防调查运用农技防治等计划工作安排 [County Schistosomiasis Prevention Five-Person Small Group, on the proposal of studying schistosomiasis prevention with agricultural techniques]. 1956. April–December. No. 1.

"Xianwei, xian renwei, xianwei xuefangban: guanyu mie luo huiyi, mie luo shiyan de tongzhi baogao" 县委, 县人委, 县委血防办: 关于灭螺会议, 灭螺试验的通知报告 [County Party Committee, County People's Committee, Schistosomiasis Prevention Office of County Party Committee: Announcement on snail elimination conference and snail elimination test]. 1957. January–December. No. 2.

"Xian xuefang lingdao xiaozu xianjin shiji, chenlieguan wenzi dagang, xuefang huibao tigang gaojian" 县血防领导小组先进事迹, 陈列馆文字大纲, 血防汇报提纲稿件 [Outstanding deeds of County Schistosomiasis Prevention Leadership Small Group, outline for description of exhibition hall and report outline of schistosomiasis prevention]. 1971. January–December. No. 1.

"Zhonggong Yujiang xianwei: Guanyu xuefang gonggu gongzuo huiyi de tongzhi, baogao, zongjie, jilu" 中共余江县委: 关于血防巩固工作会议的通知, 报告, 总结, 记录 [Yujiang County Committee of CCP: Announcements, reports, summaries and records on the conferences of strengthening the work of schistosomiasis prevention]. 1973. January–December. No. 1.

Yu Laixi, zhonggong Yujiang xianwei xuefang lingdao xiaozu bangongshi 余来喜, 中共余江县委血防领导小组办公室. n.d. *Jiangxi sheng Yujiang xian xuefang zhi: 1953–1980* 江西省余江县血防志: 1953–1980 [Yujiang county, Jiangxi schistosomiasis srevention gazetteer: 1953–1980]. Handwritten copy.

UCC (United Church of Canada archives), Toronto, Ontario, Canada

Brown, Margaret. n.d. *History of the Honan (North China) Mission of the United Church of Canada, Originally a Mission of the Presbyterian Church in Canada.* Vol. 99: 2.

ZGDE (Zhongguo di er lishi dang'an guan guancang dang'an 中国第二历史档案馆馆藏档案 [No. 2 Historical Archives]), Nanjing, Jiangsu, People's Republic of China

"Weisheng bu tongji shi weisheng tongji tubiao" 卫生部统计室卫生统计图表 [Department of Hygiene Office of Statistics: Charts of hygiene statistics]. n.d.a. Record group 327, file 93:23.

"Zhe weishengchu Hainan tequ gongshu qing bao fangzhi xuexichongbing jingfei redaibing yaopin de jihua kou youguan jiguan laiwang wenshu" 浙卫生处海南特区公署请报防治血吸虫病经费热带病药品的计划扣有关机关来往文书 [Official correspondences between Zhejiang Health Agency, Hainan Special Administrative Government Office, and related departments on the proposal of applying for funding to prevent schistosomiasis and purchasing tropical diseases medicines]. n.d.b. File 372, 176.

ZGDY (Zhongguo di yi lishi dang'an guan 中国第一历史档案馆 [No. 1 Historical Archives]), Beijing, People's Republic of China

"Weipai zhongyi jiandu" 委派中医监督 [Supervision of delegate for Chinese medicine]. n.d. Guancang xunjing bu dang'an 馆藏巡警部档案, file 150-68.

ZSDA (Zhejiang sheng dang'an ju 浙江省档案局 [Zhejiang Provincial Archives]), Hangzhou, Zhejiang, People's Republic of China

Zhejiangsheng renmin zhengfu weishengting 浙江省人民政府卫生厅 [Health Bureau of the Zhejiang Province People's Government]. 1954. "Guanyu xunlian guoying nongchang nongyeshengchan hezuoshe baojianyuan gongzuo de zhishi" 关于训练国营农场农业生产合作社保健院工作的指示 [Instructions on training health care workers for the state-owned agricultural cooperatives]. December. File J165-4-100.

Contributors

BRIDIE ANDREWS is Associate Professor of History at Bentley University and also teaches medical history at the New England School of Acupuncture. She is the author of *The Making of Modern Chinese Medicine, 1850–1960* (2014) and co-editor of *Western Medicine as Contested Knowledge* (with A. R. Cunningham, 1997) and *Medicine and Colonial Identity* (with Mary P. Sutphen, 2003).

NICOLE ELIZABETH BARNES is Assistant Professor of History at Duke University. She earned her PhD in 2012 at the University of California, Irvine, and is currently writing a book entitled *Protecting the National Body: Gender and Public Health in Wartime Sichuan, 1937–1945.*

CAROL BENEDICT is Professor of History at the Edmund Walsh School of Foreign Service and the Department of History, Georgetown University, where she teaches modern Chinese history. Her research focuses on the social and cultural history of nineteenth- and twentieth-century China with a particular focus on the social history of medicine and disease, women and gender history, and the history of Chinese material and consumer culture. Benedict's publications include *Bubonic Plague in Nineteenth-Century China* (1996) and *Golden-Silk Smoke: A History of Tobacco in China, 1550–2010* (2011).

LIPING BU is Professor of History at Alma College. She has published broadly on international educational and cultural relations and public health in journals including *American Studies,* the *American Journal of Public Health,* and *Social History of Medicine.* She is the author of *Making the World Like Us: Education, Cultural Expansion, and the American Century* (2003) and co-editor of *Science, Public Health and the State in Modern Asia* (2012) and *Public Health in Post-War Asia: International Influences, Local Transformations* (2014). She is currently writing a book on public health and modernization in twentieth-century China.

MARY BROWN BULLOCK is Executive Vice Chancellor of Duke Kunshan University and Chair of the China Medical Board. Her publications include *An American Transplant: The Rockefeller Foundation and Peking Union Medical College* (1980) and *The Oil Prince's Legacy: Rockefeller Philanthropy in China* (2011). She is the former president of Agnes Scott College and Visiting Distinguished Professor of Chinese history at Emory University.

LINCOLN CHEN is President of the China Medical Board (CMB). Celebrating its one hundredth anniversary in 2014, CMB was endowed by John D. Rockefeller as an independent American foundation that aims to advance health in China and neighboring countries of Southeast Asia in an interdependent world. CMB works by strategic philanthropy to spark innovation and strengthen partnerships in building university capacity in health policy sciences and health professional education. In earlier decades, Dr. Chen was the Taro Takemi Professor of International Health at the Harvard School of Public Health, the Executive Vice President of the Rockefeller Foundation, and representative of the Ford Foundation in India and Bangladesh.

LING CHEN worked at the China Medical Board as a Research Fellow from 2011 to June 2012 and conducted research in health philanthropy and medical history in China. Chen received her master's degree in public health at Harvard University and also holds a master's degree in dental medicine from West China University of Medical Science in China. She is currently working as a Senior Project Manager at China Resources Holdings in Hong Kong.

RACHEL CORE earned her PhD in sociology at the Johns Hopkins University, where she twice held Dean's Teaching Fellowships to teach a class called "Health and Society in Contemporary China." Fieldwork for her dissertation, "The Fall and Rise of Tuberculosis: A Study of How Institutional Change Affected Health Outcomes in Shanghai, 1928–2013," was supported by a Fulbright Fellowship. She is currently a Post-Doctoral Fellow in Medical Humanities at the Wee Kim Wee School of Communications and Information of the Nanyang Technological University in Singapore, where she is working on a book manuscript based on her dissertation.

KAWAI FAN is Associate Professor at the Chinese Civilisation Center, City University of Hong Kong. Fan earned his PhD in history from the Chinese University of Hong Kong in 1997. His research interests include the history of medicine in medieval China and the history of the anti-schistosomiasis campaign in Maoist China. He is the author of *A Guide to Chinese Medicine on the Internet* (2008), *Physicians and Patients in Medieval China* (2010, in Chinese), and *A Study of Medicine in China: Its Legacies, Inheritance and Integration during the Medieval Period* (2004, in Chinese).

XIAOPING FANG is an Assistant Professor of Modern Chinese History in the Division of Chinese at the Nanyang Technological University, Singapore. His research interests focus on the history of medicine and health in twentieth-century China. He is the author of *Barefoot Doctors and Western Medicine in China* (2012).

XI GAO is Professor of History and Medical History in the History Department of Fudan University, China. Her research interests include medical missionaries, Chinese medical modernity, and the history of medical cultural exchange between West and East. Her most recent book is *John Dudgeon: A British Missionary and Chinese Medical Modernization in the Late Qing* (2009, in Chinese).

MIRIAM GROSS is Assistant Professor of History and International and Area Studies at the University of Oklahoma, Norman. Gross received her PhD in modern Chinese history from the University of California, San Diego, in 2010. Her research focuses on the popularization and politicization of science and medicine in the countryside in modern China. Her work has been supported by the Fulbright Program, the Social Science Research Council, and the University of California Pacific Rim Research Program. She is currently working on a book about China's schistosomiasis campaign that examines the imposition of state control through science and health care and the many ways rural people fought back.

SONYA GRYPMA is Dean and Professor of Nursing and Adjunct Professor of History at Trinity Western University in Langley, BC, Canada. She is the author of *Healing Henan: Canadian Nurses at the North China Mission, 1888–1947* (2008) and *China Interrupted: Japanese Internment and the Reshaping of a Canadian Missionary Community* (2012). Sonya is also co-editor (with Ellen Fleischmann, Michael Marten, and Inger Marie Okkenhaug) of *Transnational and Historical Perspectives on Global Health, Welfare and Humanitarianism* (2013).

TINA PHILLIPS JOHNSON is Associate Professor of History and Director of Chinese Studies at Saint Vincent College in Latrobe, Pennsylvania, and Research Associate at the University of Pittsburgh Asian Studies Center. She is the author of a book on reproduction in early twentieth-century China entitled *Childbirth in Republican China: Delivering Modernity* (2011). Tina is currently working on applied public health programs in nutrition and maternal and child health in China and Southeast Asia.

SEAN HSIANG-LIN LEI is Associate Research Fellow at the Institute of Modern History, Academia Sinica, Taiwan, and Associate Professor at the Institute for Science, Technology and Society, Yangming University. His ongoing research focuses on the transformation of the Chinese body, selfhood, and moral community through the history of two competing diseases, tuberculosis and wasting disorders (*laobing*). A related recent publication is "Habituating Individuality: Framing Tuberculosis and Its Material Solutions in Republican China." His book, *Neither Donkey nor Horse: Medicine and the Struggle over China's Modernity*, will be published in 2014.

VERONICA PEARSON was a Professor in the Department of Social Work and Social Administration at the University of Hong Kong until her retirement. She has published widely in the area of mental health in China, including *Mental Health Care in China: State Policies, Professional Services and Family Responsibilities* (1995) and, with Michael Phillips and Ruiwen Wang, *Models for Change in a Changing Society: Psychiatric Rehabilitation in China* (1994). She has held a number of advisory positions with government bureaus in China related to the welfare of psychiatric patients and their families and helped to establish several model training projects in the area of psychiatric rehabilitation in China.

MICHELLE RENSHAW is a Visiting Research Fellow in Public Health within the Faculty of Health Sciences at Adelaide University, South Australia. After teaching secondary-school mathematics and science, and between a bachelor's degree in politics and postgraduate training in accounting and finance, Michelle worked as a policy writer and manager in the South Australian Public Service and lectured in Aboriginal administration at the University of South Australia. A PhD in public health and Chinese studies led to the publication of her book, *Accommodating the Chinese: The American Hospital in China, 1880–1920* (2005, 2013).

VOLKER SCHEID is Professor of East Asian Medicines and Director of the EAST*medicine* Research Centre at the Faculty of Science and Technology, University of Westminster, London. He is the author of *Chinese Medicine in Contemporary China: Plurality and Synthesis* (2002) and *Currents of Tradition in Chinese Medicine, 1626–2006* (2007). He holds a Wellcome Trust Senior Research Fellowship in the Medical Humanities, and his current research focuses on a *longue duree* history of East Asian medicines from the Song to the present, combining transregional perspectives with methodological approaches borrowed from epistemic historiography and the cultural studies of science, technology, and medicine.

JOHN R. WATT is Vice President of the ABMAC Foundation and has recently published *Saving Lives in Wartime China: How Medical Reformers Built Modern Healthcare Systems amid War and Epidemics, 1928–1945* (2014).

YI-LI WU is a historian of Chinese medicine and the author of *Reproducing Women: Medicine, Metaphor, and Childbirth in Late Imperial China* (2010), which was awarded the Margaret W. Rossiter Book Prize by the History of Science Society. She holds a PhD from Yale University and was for many years a faculty member in the Albion College history department. She is currently a Research Fellow at the EAST*medicine* Research Centre, University of Westminster, where she is writing a book on the history of trauma medicine in China.

XINZHONG YU is Professor at the College of History and Vice Director of the Key Research Institute for Social History in China, Nankai University. He completed a PhD in history at Nankai University in 2000, and was a postdoctoral fellow at Kyoto University from 2003 to 2005. He is the author of the award-wining books *Epidemics and Society in Jiangnan during the Qing Dynasty: A Study on the Social History of Medicine* (2003, in Chinese) and *Family History in the Ming and Qing Dynasties*, Vol. IV of *A General History of Chinese Family* (2007, in Chinese). He is also the editor of *Disease, Medical Treatment and Hygiene since the Qing Dynasty from the Perspective of Social and Cultural History* (2009, in Chinese).

DAQING ZHANG is Professor of History of Medicine and Director of the Institute of Medical Humanities at the Center for the History of Medicine, Peking University. He is also the Director of the Commission for the History of Medicine, Chinese Society for the History of Science & Technology. His research interests include the cultural and social history of medicine in nineteenth- and twentieth-century China, comparative history, and medical cultures since the late nineteenth century. His recent books include *A Social History of Diseases in Modern China* (2006), *A History of Medicine* (2007), and *An Introduction to the Medical Humanities* (2013), all in Chinese.

CHENG ZHEN is Professor at the Center for the History of Medicine at Peking University, where she is Dean of the Department of Medical Humanities. She is one of the associate editors of the *Chinese Journal of Medical History*. Her work focuses on the history of medical disciplines, the history of nursing, and the comparative history of Western and Traditional Chinese Medicine. She is the author of *Go into Medicine* (2005) and *Confrontation between Disease and Pattern: Comparative Study in the Eighteenth Century* (2007, in Chinese). She has also translated *A Flourishing Yin*, by Charlotte Furth (2006) and co-translated *A History of Medicine*, by Arturo Castiglioni (2013). Currently she is co-editing *The Road to True Beauty and Glory: Ti-sheng Chang's Long, Legendary Tale* (2014, in Chinese).

Index

China Disabled Persons' Federation, 147, 166
China Medical Board (CMB)
  CMB/Rockefeller Foundation fellowships, 287–291; career success of fellows, 287; fellows as graduate students, 287; institutional capacity building as goal for, 287–288, 296n2; Johns Hopkins and Harvard as dominant host institutions for public health fellows, 290–291; medical fellows, home institutions, 288–289, 288t, 296n3; medical fellows, host institutions, 289, 289t, 296n4; post-fellowship careers, 293–294; public health fellows, 289–291; significance of program, 293–296
  establishment of, 1–2
  expulsion from Maoist PRC (1951), 68n2
  goals in early 20th-century China, 54
  Grant's proposal to establish PUMC Department of Hygiene and Public Health, 214–215
  Nationalist era and, 55–59
China Medical Commission, 213, 225n2
China Medical Missionary Association, 173, 177
China–Soviet Friendship Association, 198
Chinese Academy of Preventive Medicine, 82
Chinese Anti-Tuberculosis Association (CATA): public health activities of, 95, 128–129, 145n2; TB treatment facilities founded by, 129–130
Chinese Association on Tobacco Control, 82–83
Chinese Civil War (1945–1949): Guomindang removal to Taiwan, 133; as health catastrophe, 21; hospitals during, 324–325; nursing leadership in China and, 303; TB control in Shanghai during, 132–133
Chinese Communist Party (CCP): acknowledging failure of Cultural Revolution, 258; collaboration with Soviet medicine, 197; commitment to Western-style health care system, 244, 249; glorification of women's work, 61; guiding principles for health care system, 249; health program integration with mass movements, 249; institutionalization of Chinese medicine (*see* Chinese medicine, traditional); Mao Zedong as figurehead for, 248–249; midwifery training and childbirth reforms, 59–60; officials' credibility as socialist leaders, 201; preventive medicine priority over curative program, 249; reorganization of plural medical systems, 269–270; reproductive health programs, 63;

rural health care system goals, 272; rural health movement of, 60; schistosomiasis control, 119, 121; support for Chinese tobacco industry, 77–78, 85–86; tuberculosis prevention priorities, 135; unification of Chinese and Western medicine, 249. *See also* People's Republic of China (PRC)
Chinese Intellectuals and the West, 1982–1949 (Wang), 287
Chinese Journal of Neurology and Psychiatry, 153
Chinese Journal of Nursing, 311
Chinese Journal of Practical Nursing, 311
Chinese Leprosy Association, 95
Chinese Medical Association, 95
Chinese Medical Missionary Association, 95
Chinese medicine, traditional
  Communist party and institutionalization of, 248–252, 340–341; abolition of private practice by Chinese medicine physicians, 252, 270; Academy of Chinese Medicine and, 253; acceptance into national health scheme, 245–248; admission of Chinese medicine physicians to Western medicine hospitals and clinics, 254, 332; barefoot doctors using, 272–274; foundation of Chinese Medicine colleges, 255; licensing requirements for Chinese physicians, 250–251; midwifery training and childbirth reforms, 59–60; as nation building and socialist modernization, 255–256; proposal for Chinese medical research centers, 250; recruitment of Chinese physicians into official health care system, 249; reeducation of practicing Chinese medicine physicians in Western medicine, 251–252; reeducation of Western physicians in Chinese medicine, 253–254; reintroduction of apprenticeship system, 255; subordination of Western medicine as test of political loyalty, 253–254; unification with Western medicine as guiding principle, 244, 249, 251, 254–255, 259–260
  contemporary period and, 260–263; criticism of modernization of, 262; drug research and development, 261; globalization and popularity of, 260, 262–263, 264–266, 341; neoliberal economy in, 260; plural health care system integrating, 245, 258–260, 274; rediscovery by state for rural health care delivery, 262; as resource for economics and social policy,

medical factions, 187–195; allegiances of health department leaders, 192–193, 193t; Anglo-American, structure and influence of, 189–190, 189t, 192; fluid lines of demarcation between, 191; French and Belgian, 190–191; German-Japanese, 188–189, 188t, 192; pluralism of, 192; politics and disputes among, 191–192; Qing government preference for German model, 178–179 during Republican era, 173–196

Soviet (*see* Soviet medicine and medical education)

Western models approved for use in socialist China, 194

"four horsemen of the apocalypse": health catastrophes as, 17, 20–22

"Four Principles of Health Work," 270

Framework Convention on Tobacco Control (FCTC), 83–84, 85

Fryer, John, 73

Fu Lianzhang, 200, 205, 207–208

Fujinami, Akira, 110

Gage, Nina, 302

Gamble, S. D., 37

Gan Jiehou, 286

Gao, Xi, 3, 8

Gaoqiao health station, 218–219, 225n9

gender segregation: nursing and, 298–299

General Medical Department of the Worker-Peasant Red Army, 325

General Nursing (textbook), 310

German Medical School (Qingdao), 185

Germany: influence on Japanese medical system, 178–179

Global Health Initiative, Emory University, 85

globalization of Chinese medicine, 260, 262–263, 264–266, 341

Goldstein, Joshua, 61

Gong Naiquan, 197–198

Goodrich, Sarah Boardman Clapp, 74

Grant, John B.: changing attitude toward rural public health projects, 218, 343; on China's immediate health needs, 221, 226n15; departure from Johns Hopkins model of public health education, 215; efforts to build a central Ministry of Health in China, 220–221, 222, 225nn10–12; establishment of Public Health Experimental Station, Metropolitan Police Department of Beijing, 216–217, 225n7; founding of First Health Office of Peiping, 311–312; influence on Chinese public health

administration, 184; legacy to public health profession in China, 223–224; maternal and child health efforts, 57; medical education and influences on career of, 214; mission in China, 213–214; as professor at PUMC, 213; public health in China and, 9; PUMC Department of Hygiene and Public Health and, 214–217, 225nn3–5; recruitment of personnel for public health work, 219–220; relationship with Chinese medical leaders, 215; as representative of Rockefeller Foundation International Health Board in China, 213, 225n2; service on International Board of Finance, Central Epidemic Prevention Bureau, 216; on socioeconomic development and public health, 213–214; as spirit of public health in China, 212; state medicine and disease prevention in PRC as legacy of, 223–224; support for Chiang Kai-shek, 191; support for state medicine in China, 214, 221–223, 228, 339

Gray, G. Douglas, 220–221

Great Leap Forward: famine during, 21; nursing education and, 308; schistosomiasis prevention, 107, 113; scientific research following, 115

Gross, Miriam, 2, 3, 6, 106–125, 338

Grypma, Sonya, 3, 12, 287, 297–316

Gu Yunyu, 196

Guangdong National Zhongshan University Medical College, 191

guardianship networks, 165, 167, 169

Guizhou province: Provincial Health Committee, 242; public health care during wartime, 241–242, 243n11

Guo Moruo, 199

Guomindang government (GMD). *See* Nationalist government

Hall, G. A. M, 46

Halpern, Fanny, 152

Han dynasty: schistosomiasis infections during, 108, 110

He Cheng, 114, 250, 253, 325

Health Bureau of Greater Shanghai, 217

health care: culture of, 47–48, 269; as hybrid system, 1; state responsibility for, 1, 269; *weisheng*, as system of knowledge, 174. *See also* delivery of health care; foreign models of medical care

Health Care of the Soviet Union (Zhu Binsheng), 197

water treatment: schistosomiasis prevention and, 116

Watt, John, 9, 227–243, 323, 343

WCTU (Women's Christian Temperance Union), 72–73

Wei Wenbo, 115

weisheng (healthcare): as symbol of modernization, 48

Welch, William Henry, 215, 225nn4–5, 292

Weng Naiqun, 101–102

Weng Xinzhi, 78, 82, 87n1

Wenyon, Seymour, 149–150

West China University of Medical Sciences (Chengdu): "community beds" scheme for mental health care, 165; PUMC nursing program during Sino-Japanese War, 305

Western medicine: Chinese influences on, 285; Chinese medicine compared with, 53; criticism of traditional culture, 48; introduction by medical missionaries, 174–175; limited influence on maternal and infant health prior to 1910, 54–55; medical models approved for use in socialist China, 194; Qing government and, 53–55. *See also under specific topics*

WHO. *See* World Health Organization (WHO)

Wilms, Sabine, 173

women: anti-cigarette associations in China, 74; Communist glorification of women's work, 61; hospitals for, 299, 322; insistence on right to contraception, 342; as medical missionaries, 53–54; "medicine for women" (*fuke*), 52; missionary education of, 54; mortality from secondhand smoke, 81; responsibility for health of next generation, 340; stigmatization of women who smoke, 76–77, 79

Women's Christian Temperance Union (WCTU), 72–73

Women's Union Medical College, 57. *See also* Peking Union Medical College (PUMC)

Woods, Andrew, 151–152

Work Program for Disabled Persons: in Eighth Five-Year Plan, 166–167

work units (*danwei*): creation by PRC, 133–134; dismantling of system, 141–142; health care controlled by, 62, 68n3; TB control and, 134–135

Workers' Health Care in the Soviet Union (Zhu Binsheng), 197

World Bank: funding of schistosomiasis project, 123

World Conference on Tobacco or Health, Tenth (Beijing, 1997), 82

World Health Organization (WHO): Collaborating Centre for Global Tobacco Surveillance, 85; Collaborating Centre for Tobacco or Health, 83–84; Directly Observed Therapy, Short-Course (DOTS) tuberculosis control program, 7, 47, 142–143, 145; PRC as member of, 309; on three-tier Chinese health care system, 268–269; tobacco control initiatives, 83–84

World Women's Christian Temperance Union (WWCTU), 74

Wu, Yi-Lin, 3, 5, 51–68, 342

Wu Cheng-i, 153–154

Wu Jianyun, 312

Wu Jibo, 48–49

Wu Jieping, 82, 87n2

Wu Lien-teh, 103, 128, 183, 186, 221, 321

Wu Rulun, 175

Wu Shaoqing, 132, 135, 137

Wu Tingfang, 74

Wu Yinkai, 83–84, 87n3

Wu Zheying (Lillian Wu), 302

Wu Zhongdao, 111

Wufeng Garden (hospital), 322

Wusong health station, 217–218, 225n8

Xi Gao, 173–211, 222, 326, 340

Xia Zhenyi, 151, 152

Xiao jing yiyuan (Little Well Hospital), 325

Xu Aizhu, 306

Xu Songming, 186

Xuhui District Prevention and Treatment Clinic, 135, *139*

Yan Fuqing (F. C. Yen): as Minister of Health, 221, 232, 243nn2–3; national medical education and, 186, 187; proposal for separate Health Department, 183; tuberculosis control and, 128; Wusong health station and, 185–186, 217, 225n8

Yan Yangchu (Yen, James Y. C.), 218, 306, 307

Yang, Marion (Yang Chongrui): on Grant, 212; on maternal and infant mortality, 40; midwifery reforms of, 57–58, 343; political purge for support of Ma Yinchu, 62

Yang Gonghuan, 83

Yangzi River: flooding and schistosomiasis infections, 123

Yao Kefang, 241

Ye Gongshao, 82, 87n1